DENTAL HEALTH EDUCATION
THEORY AND PRACTICE

DENTAL HEALTH EDUCATION THEORY AND PRACTICE

Christina B. DeBiase, B.S.D.H., M.A., Ed.D.
Professor and Coordinator
Degree Completion and Master of Science
Programs in Dental Hygiene
West Virginia University
School of Dentistry
Morgantown, West Virginia

LEA & FEBIGER • PHILADELPHIA • LONDON
1991

Lea & Febiger
200 Chester Field Parkway
Malvern, Pennsylvania 19355
U.S.A.
(215) 251-2230
1-800-444-1785

Library of Congress Cataloging-in-Publication Data

DeBiase, Christina B.
    Dental health education : theory and practice / by Christina B.
DeBiase.
        p. cm.
    Includes index.
    ISBN 0-8121-1366-7
    1. Dental health education. 2. Dental public health. I. Title.
    [DNLM: 1. Comprehensive Dental Care. 2. Health Education, Dental.
3. Preventive Dentistry.   WU 113 D286d]
RK60.8.D43   1991
617.6'01—dc20
DNLM/DLC
for Library of Congress   90-13344
                                                               CIP

Reprints of chapters may be purchased from Lea & Febiger in quantities of 100 or more.

PRINTED IN THE UNITED STATES OF AMERICA

Print number: 5   4   3   2   1

This book is dedicated to my loving husband, whose faith in me and encouragement have been a constant source of strength in all my endeavors, near and far; to my wonderful parents, whose love and support sustain me each day of my life; to my colleague, Catherine, for her sincere interest in my accomplishments; and to my students of the past, present, and future, who teach me the real joys of health education.

PREFACE

The field of health education is growing by leaps and bounds in response to several factors: the vast number of health concerns of modern society, consumers' demand for a voice in decisions concerning their health care, a movement toward the concepts of prevention and wellness by a growing segment of the population, and government involvement in preventing health problems to reduce health care costs.

The basic function of a health educator is to act as an educator and resource person for the general public and community agencies regarding personal and community health matters. This definition can also be applied to the dental health educator. As the scope of dentistry increases, the role of the dental health educator becomes more comprehensive. The intent of this book is to expose the licensed or student dental health educator to many of the critical health care issues that affect our society, the impact they have on dental health, and the educational techniques that can be employed to assist individuals or groups in making informed decisions on matters affecting their own health and the health of their significant others.

Dentists and dental hygienists are both referred to as the dental health educator or "he" in this text. Both are members of a team, ethically responsible for providing their patients with the necessary information to draw conclusions and make decisions that might alter their behavior. This information must be accurate, reliable, and individualized. To be an effective teacher, the dental health educator must be knowledgeable, keep abreast of current research, and be familiar with the psychology of human behavior. The health concerns and priorities of adolescents are often different from those of the elderly, for example. Therefore each chapter has been designed to focus on a stage in the life cycle of an individual. The life cycle theme serves as a basis for categorizing health care issues and patient instruction into time periods in a person's life when each issue is most relevant.

Limiting the dental health education experience to the occasional brushing and flossing spiel in the dental office and to classroom demonstrations to third graders short-changes both the general public and the dental health professional. Dental health education of the 1990s is no longer synonymous with office or school dental health alone. The purpose of this text is to broaden the professional's view of dental health to a repertoire of diverse topic areas including teething, child abuse, smokeless tobacco use, pregnancy, AIDS, and Alzheimer disease. More topics could and perhaps should have been addressed, but the list is endless. As the thirteenth century scholar Tai T'ung (*The Six Scrips: Principals of Chinese Writing*) once said, "Were I to await perfection my book would never be finished." A true dental health educator will astutely modify topics in this text as needed and supplement the list with additional subjects he finds interesting.

The last two chapters of the textbook address program development, implementation, and evaluation; and the legal and ethical concerns surrounding dental health education. A variety of appendices at the end of the text include resource persons and materials to assist the educator with patient education.

All patients have a right to dental health education, and we as professionals have a responsibility to provide that often intangible yet always invaluable service.

Morgantown, West Virginia

CHRISTINA B. DeBIASE

ACKNOWLEDGMENTS

I wish to thank several members of my family who unselfishly contributed their time and energy to this book: Daniel F. DeBiase, J.D., for the final chapter on legal implications; Henry J. Bianco, Jr., D.D.S., M.S., for his vast dental expertise, photographs, and illustrations; and Charlotte R. Bianco, A.S., for her outstanding preparation of the text.

I would also like to express my appreciation to Carol A. Spear, BSDH., M.S., for her photographs and contribution of the table clinic discussion in Chapter 11; Dennis Overman, Ph.D., for his original illustration; Jack A. Roth, D.D.S., M.A., for his assistance with the implant section; Patricia Wilbur, Gordon McGregor, and Bonny Starkey for their photographs and illustrative assistance; and all those individuals who permitted me to use their information or photographs in various applications and theories throughout the text. Special thanks to Ray Kersey and David Amundson of Lea & Febiger for their continued support and expert editorial contributions.

I am especially grateful to Frances A. Stoll, R.D.H., Ed.D., Professor Emeritus at Columbia University and author of *Dental Health Education* (five editions), who explored the field of dental health education during its infancy. Dr. Stoll's works have been an inspiration to me as a student, as an academician, and as an author.

CHRISTINA B. DEBIASE

CONTENTS

Chapter 1

GENERAL PRINCIPLES OF HEALTH EDUCATION

Look toward your health;
and if you have it praise it,
praise God and value it
next to a good conscience;
for health is the second blessing
that we mortals are capable of—
a blessing that money cannot buy.
Izaak Walton
The Compleat Angler

WHAT IS HEALTH?

Although health is universally desired, it does not have a universally shared definition. There are a variety of uses for the word health. A person can join a health club, eat healthful food, live in a health-conscious society, be a health educator, or possess a state of mental health. It is clear that health is a complex, multidimensional concept. Health can be applied to any aspect of human life depending on the individual's background and values.[1]

Models of Health

Historically health has been associated with the absence of disease or infirmity. The traditional medical model referred to health as a state of biologic normality. This microscopic view of health became the ultimate goal of medicine.[2] In the case of illness, the physician intervened to restore normal functioning. Researchers of the twentieth cen-

tury, however, explored new dimensions of health. Health came to be viewed as a process, surpassing the mere lack of disease. In 1959 H.L. Dunn described health as an integrated method of functioning oriented toward maximizing an individual's potential. His philosophy of health encompassed the following criteria:[3]

1. It involves a direction and progress toward an even higher potential of functioning rather than the achievement of an optimal level of wellness.
2. It involves the total individual, including his environment and in all of his uniqueness, rather than just the proper functioning of his eyes, heart, brain or other parts of his body, important though these may be; the ability to live, at a higher potential.
3. It is concerned with how the individual functions within the particular environment in which he lives, no matter how favorable or unfavorable it may be, and irrespective of his ability to alter it for his needs and satisfactions.

1

Newer models conceptualize man's health potential on a continuum, with optimum health at one end and death (the complete absence of health) on the other end (Fig. 1-1).[4] Degrees of health are evident at various points with "high-level wellness" or optimum health requiring a state of complete physical, mental, and social well-being. True to this definition, an individual can be rendered paraplegic as a result of a car accident. Although the person is in good physical health, he might believe he is no longer a functioning member of society. The mental confusion he experiences, related to his worth and ability to resume a normal lifestyle, places him in a temporary state of "subhealth."

Today's literature portrays health as a five-dimensional picture. These dimensions are physical, mental, social, emotional, and spiritual. A model published in 1984 also included the vocational dimension of health.[2] The sum of these dimensions fully represents human health. The complex integration of these dimensions reveals how man functions within his environment. The components of each dimension can be found in Table 1-1.[5]

Prevention

Currently modern medicine is searching for cures for diseases such as cancer, muscular dystrophy, and arthritis. Ways are being designed to boost the body's immune system to fight AIDS, and accept organ transplantation. Genetic engineering is becoming useful in mapping out certain genes for specific behavioral disorders and emotional determinants. A new orally adminis-

tered insulin and an abortion pill are being tested for use. In behavioral medicine, biofeedback and electronic monitoring have been found to exert control over blood pressure, migraine headaches, nausea, and pain.

Despite these biomedical advances, it is more beneficial to mankind to prevent disease than to treat it. Educating the public about healthful living is primary. Sophisticated health care is costly; prevention is inexpensive, and the effects are long-term. Major strides in medical and surgical techniques should continue, but an equal emphasis needs to be placed on prevention. Prevention is the sparkling dimension of health education that endows mankind with the tools and the know-how to lead a long and productive life.[6]

WHAT IS HEALTH EDUCATION?

The 1972–1973 Joint Committee on Health Education Terminology defined health education as "a process with the intellectual, psychological, and social dimensions relating to activities which increase the abilities of people to make informed decisions affecting their personal, family, and community well-being."[7] Green and his colleagues define health education as "any combination of learning experiences designed to facilitate voluntary adaptations of behavior conducive to health."[8] Health education is not incidental; it is planned. Although numerous health education messages are enhanced by marketing strategies, health education involves a great deal more

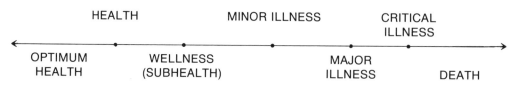

Figure 1-1. Health potential continuum. Health status scale modified from Rogers, E. S.: Human Ecology and Health, New York, Macmillan, 1960.

Table 1-1. Selected Subelements that Constitute the Major Dimensions of Human Health*

Health	Selected Subelements	Health	Selected Subelements
Physical	Functional ability of each body system	Spiritual	Life force (inspiration)
	Fitness level		Survival instincts
	Metabolism		Enthusiasm/pleasure-seeking
	Blood chemistry		Acceptance of self-limitations (death)
	Presence or absence of disease(s)		Creativity
	Presence or absence of disease-predisposing factors		Ethics/integrity/moral code
			Ability to love and be loved
	Exposure to alcohol, stress, radiation		Trust
	Flexibility		Feelings of selflessness
	Muscle tone	Vocational	Gaining new perspectives to problem solving
Emotional	Ability to relate to personal values		Impact on the quality of life of others
	Self-knowledge		
	Love of self and feelings of self-importance		Job satisfaction
			Financial "success"
	Self-perception		Advancement
	Ability to express feelings appropriately		Recognition for contributions
			Sharing of experience with co-workers
	Honesty		
	Empathy		Service to humankind
	Sexuality		Fulfillment of goals related to the "greater good"
Mental	Intelligence		
	Sexuality		Meeting new nonrecreational challenges
	Perceptions of others		
	Adaptability		Expanding professional horizons
	Decision-making ability		
	Ability to cope		
	Ability to relax		
	Tolerance		
	Judgment		

Adapted from Sorochan, Walter, D.: Self-Actualization Inventory, by Eberst, R.: Defining health: A multidimensional model. J. Sch. Health, 54:100, 1984. Reprinted with permission.

than publicity, gimmicks, or a media blitz used to sell a health program. Health education is essentially a way of working with an individual's existing knowledge, attitudes, and values that are problematic to positive health practices. For instance, when a child enters school he has numerous health attitudes and practices that have been acquired from home. Some might not be appropriate or scientifically sound and need modification; others might be adequate and require reinforcement. Providing the individual with integrated and meaningful solutions to his problematic viewpoints, through planned learning experiences, effects desirable changes in attitudes and behaviors related to health.

The methodology of health education is based largely on the scientific principles of psychology and sociology that facilitate learning and behavioral change in the individual. The key focus of health education is on the process, the individual, and active involvement. Learning is enhanced by the individual's active participation in the decision-making process and by the behavior itself.[9,10]

According to the Health Belief Model,[11] in order for an individual to display a "readiness" to take action to avoid a disease or act in a preventive manner, he would need to believe that (1) he was personally *susceptible* or *vulnerable* to a particular health condition; (2) contracting the condition would have *serious consequences;* (3) compliance with recommended behaviors would be *beneficial* by reducing the threat of contracting the condition; and (4) by attaching a certain *salience* or importance to the prevention of a particular condition he is leading himself on a path toward good health.[11,12] For example, a patient smokes three packs of cigarettes per day. The dental health educator points out the areas of cell dysplasia in the patient's mouth (seriousness). The patient's father was diagnosed with an oral carcinoma 5 years previously (susceptibility). The patient realizes the (importance) of ceasing his smoking habit and the (benefit) it will have for his overall health.

Health education not only functions by facilitating learning in the present, but endeavors to help the individual utilize this learning when challenged by similar situations in the future. This is known as the "transfer of learning."[10]

Basic Aims of Health Education

The sole responsibility for health education should not lie with the physician, the professional health educator, the public health department, the school system, the media, or the individual. The responsibility must be a shared one, each sector playing an integrated and mutually supportive part in facilitating change toward a desired behavior.

The basic aims of health education are to

1. Develop desirable health attitudes and habits
2. Create and develop a proper health consciousness that can be applied to new learning situations
3. Develop an understanding of what is necessary for maintaining a healthy body and mind
4. Teach discrimination between reliable and unreliable health information
5. Teach wise and judicious use of available health services
6. Influence health attitudes and habits of future generations

Health Education Legislation

The decade of the 1970s witnessed the emergence of health education as a significant factor in the health policy of the United States. In 1968, the Joint Commission of the National School Boards Association and the American Association of School Administrators recommended a comprehensive program of health education for students in kindergarten through grade 12. This program was designed to meet the health needs and interests of this student population and prepare these children for their roles as future citizens.[6] Most programs related to health are located within the Department of Health and Human Services (known previously as the Department of Health, Education and Welfare until May 1980, at which time a separate federal Department of Education was established). Through the Health Care Financing Administration, which governs Medicare and Medicaid programs, Health and Human Services pays hospital and medical bills for the elderly, disabled, and other beneficiaries eligible under state welfare programs. Through the Public Health Service, the Department conducts and supports activities, e.g., biomedical research; disease control, health care, and mental health programs; food and drug regulation; and health manpower, facilities, and resource planning.[13]

In 1974 the Bureau of Health Education was established in the Centers for Disease Control, one of five principal agencies of the Public Health Service. The Bureau served as the impetus for federal legislation mandating greater attention to the educational aspects of health. In 1975 the 93rd Congress passed Public Law 93-641, which identified health education as one of the major priorities of a new health planning system affecting the use of federal health resources across the country. In 1976 the National Center for Health Education was created. The 94th Congress enacted Public Law 94-317, which organized a group of authorities on health education and promotion and charged them with the task of coordinating health education activities and funding. The 95th Congress in 1978 enacted Public Law

95-626, which placed greater emphasis on prevention activities and built them more solidly into the health service system.[13,14,15]

Public Health Service activities related to dental care originate from three of five operating agencies: (1) Centers for Disease Control, Center for Prevention Services, and Center for Health Promotion and Education; (2) Health Resources and Services Administration, Bureau of Health Professions, Division of Associated and Dental Health Professions; and (3) National Institutes of Health, National Institute of Dental Research (NIDR). State and local health agencies also provide preventive dental services across the country.[16]

Categories of Health Education

As an extension of the lifestyle, health promotion, and health service goals of the 1974 Surgeon General's Report on Health Promotion and Disease Prevention, 15 major subareas of health were defined. Health education is the primary instrument for accomplishing these goals. Essentially all health education issues can be placed into one or more of the following categories:

1. Personal health care
2. Nutrition and growth
3. Body structure and function
4. Sex and family living
5. Safety and first aid
6. Prevention and control of disease
   a. Communicable
   b. Chronic
7. Community health
8. Drug abuse and alcoholism
9. Smoking education
10. Mental health
11. Environmental health
12. Consumer health
13. Dental health
14. Occupational health/health careers
15. Death education

These categories are not in order of importance, nor are they considered as separate or unrelated areas of study; rather they are interdependent and interrelated to one another. The remainder of this textbook focuses on dental health and its relationship to many of the other major health education categories.

REFERENCES

1. Seedhouse, D.: Health: The Foundations for Achievement. Chichester, U.K., Wiley, 1986.
2. Eberst, R.: Defining health: A multi-dimensional model. J. Sch. Health, 54:99–104, 1984.
3. Dunn, H. L.: What high-level wellness means. Health Values.: Achiev. High Lev. Wel., Jan/Feb, 1977.
4. Rogers, E. S.: Human Ecology and Health. New York, Macmillan, 1960.
5. Sorochan, W.: Personal Health Appraisal. New York, Wiley, 1976.
6. Willgoose, C. E.: Health Teaching in Secondary Schools. 3rd Ed. Philadelphia, Saunders, 1982.
7. 1972–73 Joint Committee on Health Education Terminology: New definitions. Health Ed. Monogr. 33:63–9, 1969.
8. Green, L. W.: Health Education Planning: A Diagnostic Approach. Palo Alto, CA, Mayfield, 1980.
9. Stoll, F. A.: Dental Health Education. 5th Ed. Philadelphia, Lea & Febiger, 1977.
10. Dewey, J.: The School and Society. Chicago, University of Chicago Press, 1900.
11. Becker, M. H.: The Health Belief Model and Personal Health Behavior. Thorofare, NJ, Charles B. Slack, 1974.
12. Kegles, S. S.: Why people seek dental care. Am. J. Public Health, 51:1306–1311, 1961.
13. Ogden, H. J.: Health education as an element of U.S. policy. Int. J. Health Educ., 23:150–155, 1980.
14. United States Code: Health Information and Health Promotion. Subsection 300u, Title 42, 1976.
15. U.S. Dept. of Health, Education and Welfare. Focal Pts., November, 1976.
16. Jong, A. W.: Community Dental Health. 2nd Ed. St. Louis, C. V. Mosby, 1988.

Chapter 2

LEARNING PROCESS AS APPLIED TO DENTAL HEALTH EDUCATION

*Learning hath his infancy,
when it is but beginning and
almost childish; then his youth,
when it is luxuriant and juvenile;
then his strength of years, when it
is solid and reduced; and lastly his
old age, when it is waxeth dry and
exhaust.*

Francis Bacon
Essays: "Of Vicissitude of Things"

THE LEARNING PROCESS

Webster's Dictionary defines learning as "a process of acquiring knowledge or skills through study, instruction or experience." If dental health education refers to those activities that attempt to impart knowledge and influence attitudes and behavior in individuals, for the purpose of improving oral health, then "those activities" must be solidly based in learning theory to be effective as change agents.[1] The learning process involves reasoning, imagination, and problem-solving. Learning so conceived is an active process, not merely a passive absorption of facts to be memorized and repeated. How individuals learn certain behaviors, e.g., oral hygiene practices or oral self-examination techniques, varies from one individual to another.

According to Coleman, four factors influence the learning process:[2] the learner, the task, the procedure, and the learning situation. Learning is expanded or limited by (1) the individual's prior knowledge, (2) the individual's basic motivations for learning, (3) the individual's needs and goals, (4) the individual's communicative relationship with the educator, and (5) the type of task to be learned and the conditions and procedures under which the learning takes place.

DENTAL HEALTH KNOWLEDGE

The prior knowledge base of the individual supplies him with the facts and procedures to know how to react in a given situation. Yacovone states that it is important not to ignore the fact "that the person is already 'behaving' when we encounter him—

maybe not as we would like him to, but 'behaving.'"[3] A person entering a dental office for the first time might have a limited knowledge base derived solely from others, e.g., peers or family who have related their dental experiences to him. Another individual's dental knowledge might have been acquired from a dental health unit in school, and still another might have had direct experience such as previously receiving an oral prophylaxis or an amalgam restoration.

Two major errors can result in a dental health learning activity if too little or too much emphasis is placed on knowledge. For example, dental health educators who fail to assess the existing knowledge and experiences of the learner before the educational encounter and treat the individual as if he were void of any dental health knowledge or experiences at all are advised to quit while they are ahead.[4] Ignoring what a patient brings to be situation will defeat the learning process. The individual will view the educator as one-sided, possessing notions that are incompatible with his lifestyle. Conversely, dental health educators who assume that increasing a patient's dental health knowledge will produce desirable dental health behaviors are operating on a misconception. Knowledge alone does not determine behavior. Knowledge does not guarantee desired behavior unless it is founded on a meaningful learning experience for the individual.

DENTAL HEALTH ATTITUDES AND VALUES

Often blocks or barriers in the environment or within a person's inner structure, e.g., his attitudes, beliefs, or values, interfere with the translation of knowledge into action. Health attitudes and values are the intermediate pieces of the puzzle; they are the reactions of the individual to the learning he has acquired. When an individual absorbs a great deal of correct information or knowledge on a health issue, he has a greater chance of developing supporting values and beliefs.

But suppose an individual has been given conflicting information. At school he is told to visit the dentist regularly, practice good oral hygiene, and avoid sweets. At home finances are low, the family's diet is high in fermentable carbohydrates, and dental care only becomes salient when pain occurs. Although poverty is an environmental roadblock to preventive dental health behavior, the more commonly faced roadblock in dental health education is the internal barrier in this example. Because the individual's value system does not allow him to perceive dental disease as a serious health condition, prevention of dental disease is of minimal importance to him. Common barriers to health education are listed in Table 2-1. Many or all of these barriers can affect compliance with dental health education. (Fear as a barrier to seeking dental care is discussed in Chapter 7.)

Can these values ever be changed? Yes, but the dental professional must be patient and never impose his values on the individual. Resistance from the individual is normal, and permanent changes in behavior are not always easy to achieve. "The characteristic stubbornness of man in reacting to unwanted pressures, together with the infinite variability of his response patterns, poses problems that require the effective educator to be artful or professional in his approach, constantly adapting his techniques to the unique requirements of the situation."[5] The educator must respect the fact that people present with many different viewpoints. These views are linked to a whole set of values, often very different from his own. To attain behavior change the educator must assess and understand the internal and external conditions that affect the way an individual thinks or acts. He must "jump into the individual's skin," so to speak, and reconstruct the chain of events that led him to his existing knowledge, attitudes, and values on dental health. "Educational efforts must be initiated at an elemental level that matches the status of the patient."[6] Assessment can be accomplished through careful

Table 2-1. Barriers Operating in Health Education Programs

Ethnic and cultural conflicts

Differences in meaning assigned to scientific terms by the layman and the professional

Negative aspects of the medical setting (physical features, status, relationships, negative connotations of treatment)

Personal and group values (e.g., low level of importance placed on preventive dental care)

Group memberships and attitudes (e.g., religious, political)

Form and content of messages improperly designed for speed and simplicity of understanding and for fitting easily into present habits of thought of the recipient

Illiteracy: This limits all conceivable directions of original messages as well as feedback

Poverty (cost of medical care)

Technical unsophistication—scientific vs. unscientific treatment

Habit

Availability of services: physical location, policies, and attitudes toward special groups

Lack of faith in treatment

Denial of existence of illness

Belief in personal invulnerability to disease

Differing opinions

Safety of suggested procedures

Transportation problems

Convenience (e.g., availability of baby-sitters)

Attitudes toward body

Fear, anxiety levels

Education levels

Generalized educational approach; lacking individual assessment of patient needs

Insincerity of educator or patient

observation of the patient's behavior and active listening.

DENTAL HEALTH SKILLS

Higher level learning involves the application of information gained through instruction to the performance of certain activities. A patient might be able to describe an approved method for brushing his teeth, but if he cannot demonstrate brushing his teeth by this technique and plaque is not thoroughly removed from the teeth, then the skill has not been learned.[7] Frequently, the dental health educator will find deficiencies in a patient's skill level when observing the patient's oral hygiene practices. Watching the patient carefully as he performs his oral hygiene and offering him clear, explicit solutions to correct these deficiencies is essential. Hands-on prompting in conjunction with verbal instructions enhances learning because the patient sees as well as hears what is necessary to perfect his skills.[8] The educator should observe the patient's technique again to ensure that he has understood the suggestions given and possesses the dexterity to accomplish them.

Skills are progressive and ongoing; they become fine-tuned over time with repetition and reinforcement. Once a basic skill has been mastered, more advanced techniques can be learned. When teaching a skill it is particularly important that the educator communicate appropriate directions to the patient that are realistic to his level of understanding and dexterity, and avoid instruction overload or teaching the patient too many skills too quickly.

Stages of Learning

The "learning ladder" depicts man's progression from knowledge absorption to value adoption (Fig. 2-1).[9] The length of time a patient remains at a particular stage varies. *Unawareness*, the first step in the learning process, occurs when the patient has incomplete or inaccurate dental health information, e.g., fluoride causes cancer or soft teeth are inherited. *Awareness* arises when correct information is obtained but it lacks personal meaning for the patient. A patient enters the *self-interest* stage when he realizes the information is personally meaningful. The dental health educator can enhance this realization by the effective use of value clarification. Value clarification exercises allow the patient to reflect on the level of importance oral health has to him personally and how it fits into his lifestyle[10] (Fig. 2-2).[11] If a patient recognizes that his dental health values are not consistent with

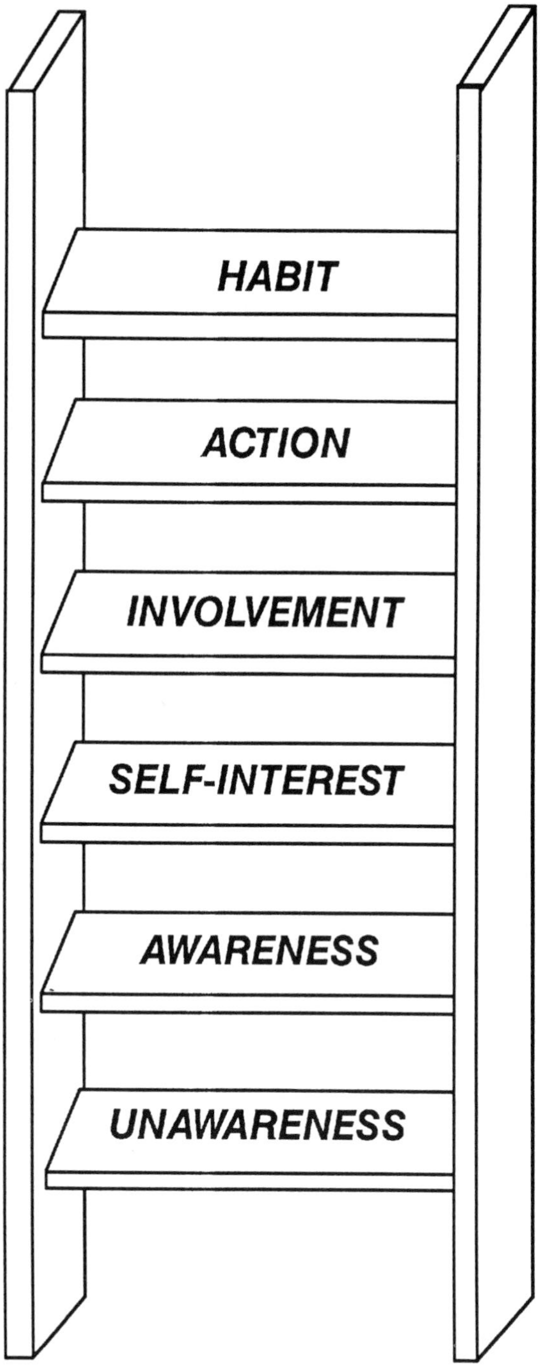

Figure 2-1. The learning ladder. From Harris, N. O., and Christen, A. G.: Primary Preventive Dentistry. 2nd Ed. Norwalk, CT, Appleton and Lange, 1987, p. 391.

I. My teeth are important to me for the following reasons:
  1. _____
  2. _____
  3. _____
  4. _____
  5. _____

II. Please rate on a scale of 1–10 (1 = lowest value 10 = highest value) the value you place on the following:
  1. A color television _____
  2. A clean and bright smile _____
  3. A dependable car _____
  4. The ability to chew food _____
  5. Relaxing home environment _____
  6. The ability to taste and appreciate food _____
  7. A stereo or music system _____
  8. Oral health _____
  9. Freedom from pain _____
  10. An occasional vacation _____
  11. General health _____

III. In the space provided below, please write a short paragraph describing how you feel about the way your teeth look, what condition you think they are in, and how long you expect to keep them.

_____
_____
_____
_____

Figure 2-2. Oral health values clarification exercise. From Horowitz, L. G., Dillenberg, J., and Rattray, J.: Self-care motivation: A model for primary preventive oral health behavior change. J. Sch. Health, 57:116, 1987. Reprinted with permission.

his behavior, he experiences cognitive dissonance. Old ideas are discarded for new ones, tension is felt, and the inclination to act results. This is referred to as the *involvement* stage. Quickly the patient hastens to act. The *action* stage is the level at which the patient tests new concepts and practices suggested by the educator. For example, after 5 days of keeping a diet diary, the patient begins to notice the extensive amount of sweets he consumes. Each day he tries new snack substitutions that do not contain sucrose. He begins experiencing self-satisfaction and gratification in his accomplishments and is now motivated to eliminate the imbalance of values and practice in his life by making permanent cognitive and behavioral adjustments that produce a long-term habit.[12] Once a habit has been formed a new value has been established.

MOTIVATION

In addition to assessing the patient's prior dental health knowledge and determining where dental health fits into his value system, it is important to explore what motivates the patient. When a high value is placed on dental health, motivation increases the chance that the individual will not only improve his dental health practices but will be committed to them over a long period of time, despite any external barriers that may exist, e.g., lack of finances or transportation. Motivation is defined as the internal and external driving forces that prompt an individual to act. It is the drive that pushes an individual to satisfy a need. These driving forces take many forms and influence the way an individual thinks, feels, and responds.

The process of motivation involves four basic factors: (1) the driving force, (2) action by the individual, (3) the need or goal to be achieved, and (4) some form of satisfaction of an individual's needs.[7] For example, a patient begins to experience bleeding gums, halitosis, and a bad taste in his mouth. He is not uncomfortable, but he has the desire to have the unpleasant odor eliminated (*drive*). He calls his dentist's office for an appointment (*action*). The dental hygienist gives the patient an oral prophylaxis and a fluoride treatment (*goal*). The patient is content with the outcome of fresh breath (*satisfaction*). When attempting to interact with a patient on the importance of routine oral prophylaxis and home care, the dental health educator should identify the sources of motivation that are likely to spark the patient's interest in good oral health even if his interests are not dentally related.[6] The motivating force for the individual in the previous example was the unpleasant odor and taste in his mouth and the importance of not appearing offensive, rather than the

elimination of gum disease and concern over eventual tooth loss. Although many patients know that halitosis can be a symptom of periodontal disease, they are still motivated by the alleviation of short-term symptoms rather than the long-term prevention of disease. The educator should use halitosis as a salient point for initiating discussion on the effects of periodontal disease and the role of toothbrushing and flossing in preventing the odor and subsequently the disease. The resultant desired oral hygiene behavior is accomplished by using the patient's own source of motivation.

Types of Motivation

Two types of motivation exist. Intrinsic motivation is self-generated; it is innate and originates from strong drives within the individual such as hunger, thirst, and anxiety. Motivation derived from the satisfaction of these internal forces is more likely to induce long-term changes in attitudes and behaviors. The relief of anxiety or the contentment within that a patient feels after receiving a good dental checkup might be motivation enough for the patient to continue proper oral hygiene practices.

Extrinsic motivators or incentives reside outside of the patient, within his environment. External incentives can be used by the dental health educator to motivate an individual to perform a desired task or stop an undesirable one. Persuasive techniques can take the form of material rewards, praise or encouragement, punishment or removal of rewards, and fear appeals or threats from another source.[9] For example, fear appeal might persuade a patient to cease a smokeless tobacco habit. His chewing behavior has produced all of the typical clinical signs, e.g., keratosis, gingival recession, and stain. The dental health educator emphasizes the patient's vulnerability to oral cancer and illustrates the many undesirable consequences of this disease through hideous photographs.

Only after the patient and the dental health educator have found a common perceptual ground on the concepts of suscep-

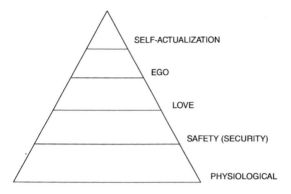

Figure 2-3. Maslow's hierarchy of needs. The hierarchy is arranged in pyramid form to represent the levels one must attain before full potential has been reached; general needs exist at the base of the structure. From Harris, N. O., and Christen, A. G.: Primary Preventive Dentistry. 2nd Ed. Norwalk, CT. Appleton & Lange, 1987, p. 31.

tibility, severity of oral disease, and the benefits and salience of proper dental health practices can they proceed to meet the needs of the patient.[6]

NEEDS

Satisfaction of a need is the goal of a behavior. Maslow's theory of self-actualization is based on the hierarchic relationship of five basic needs: physiologic, safety, belongingness and love, esteem, and self-actualization.[13] These levels can be arranged in the form of a pyramid (Fig. 2-3).[9] *Physiologic* needs consist of life-sustaining elements such as food, water, oxygen, and sleep. *Safety* needs emerge during childhood when the individual begins to have control over his own physiologic functioning; safety includes protection from physical threat or harm. After physiologic and safety needs have been fairly well gratified, *identity* needs surface; they include a sense of belonging, the giving and receiving of affection, a desire for identity and social recognition, and the expression of love. When an individual desires to be successful, self-confident, and respected, *esteem* needs arise.

Finally, if one is fortunate enough to fully develop his potential—to be all that he is capable of—then he has reached *self-actualization;* complete maturation has been achieved. "Unlike the disease-orientation process which encourages the practicing of healthful behaviors in order to prevent disease, self-actualization encourages healthful living behaviors by enabling people to utilize their own capacities more fully."[14] Proper assessment of a patient's level of need will guide the educator in designing motivational strategies and assure that realistic goals are established relative to dental health. The dental health educator's role is to bring each patient as close to "ideal" as he is capable of being.

Need vs. Demand

Historically, dentistry in the United States has responded to dental care demands to a greater extent than it has the dental needs of society. Individuals with higher incomes and educational levels have classically demanded or sought dental care at a higher rate than their lower socioeconomic status counterparts. But times are changing. In 1969, statistics showed that only 37% of the population visited the dentist at least once yearly. In 1987, American Dental Association statistics revealed this figure had increased to 77%.[15] Nonetheless, dental needs still exist for the impoverished, elderly, medically compromised, and disabled. For those individuals who have demanded care routinely in the past, the focus of their dental needs has changed from repair to prevention and wellness. In dentistry specifically, this value of wellness relates to esthetics and self-esteem.[15,16]

GOALS

Higher level needs do not emerge until lower level needs are satisfied. Therefore, when the educator and the patient are formulating a dental health plan with goals or outcomes for desired behavior, they must tailor the program to meet the individual's present needs. Goals must provide a realistic solution to the health problems of an individual. When needs change, new goals might be indicated. Goals must be attainable.[6] If they are set at an unrealistic level for the patient, the educator is setting the patient up for failure, frustration, and abandonment of the effort. For example, an adult patient routinely misses work because of pain associated with caries. A goal consisting of a caries-free checkup within 6 months of the initial treatment appointment is established. If the patient is successful at the recall visit the original goal might be modified. Similarly, a periodontal patient continues to experience inflammation and an increase in pocket depth levels. The goal for this patient might be stated as "periodontal maintenance characterized by a reduction in inflammation and a stabilization of pocket depths within 3 months of the initial treatment appointment."

OBJECTIVES

Objectives or specific activities designed to reach goals should be meaningful and appealing to the patient.[6] The approach used to develop these activities should be directed by the individual's values, motives, and needs, coupled with sincerity and sensitivity to these needs by the educator.[17] Consider the previous patient with extensive dental caries. The tasks or general objectives that would enable this patient to meet his goal of caries control might include a gradual modification in diet that would reduce the intake of sucrose, meticulous oral hygiene practices, and multiple fluoride therapy. In order for a patient to understand what is clearly expected of him, each general objective must be subdivided into specific successive approximations of the desired behavior. For example, a patient can reach the general objective of reducing foods containing sucrose from his diet by (1) reading labels and identifying sucrose and other available forms of sugar in various foods, (2) preparing snacks that are not cariogenic, and (3) limiting the intake of sweets, if consumed at all, to mealtime. Eliminating sugars entirely from the diet would require major lifestyle changes and might be an unrealistic expectation of the patient.

In the periodontal patient example, the general objective for attaining the goal of periodontal maintenance involves an office and home care oral hygiene regimen. It is suggested by the dental health educator that the patient accomplish his home care regimen by specific objectives that outline the use of a rotary toothbrush and irrigating device. The individual's finances are low and he feels he cannot meet his objectives. Instruction in the use of more affordable manual products is necessary so that the objectives are attainable for the patient.

Although objectives are activities designed for the patient, they must also be measurable for the dental health educator so that he can determine if the objectives have been reached. Additionally, objectives should be explained at an appropriate level of understanding for the patient. An individual's personal and intellectual maturity and adjustment affect his attention span, his level of comprehension, his objectivity, and his ability to concentrate. Instruction based on clearly defined, realistic, attainable, and meaningful goals and objectives, at a language level understandable to the patient, enhances the communication process and facilitates learning.

COMMUNICATION

Communication is an essential and important component of all education. Communication is an ongoing, continuously changing process. Each participant is simultaneously affected by the other through an interaction of content and relationship.[18] Interpersonal or informal two-way communication between patient and dental health educator must exist if the patient is to be actively motivated to change his attitudes and behavior.

During interpersonal communication the following chain of events occurs:[19]

1. The sender has a message to communicate.
2. He encodes or transforms his mental information into a series of written or verbal and nonverbal symbols that he hopes the receiver will understand.
3. The message is sent.
4. The receiver reads or listens to and observes the message and decodes it by attaching personal meaning to the information.
5. The receiver now responds by providing feedback relevant to how he interpreted the message.
6. The original speaker receives and interprets the feedback and the cycle begins again (Fig. 2-4).[20]

Verbal vs. Nonverbal Communication

There are two major encoding systems available to humans. The first of these is verbal or written language. Language is a complex system of shared symbols that provides humans with a medium for expressing their thoughts and feelings to others. Nonverbal communication is the second system available to humans. During a normal conversation, it is believed that approximately two-thirds of the actual meaning is indirectly communicated through nonverbal messages.[21] These messages involve a more visual or auditory exchange such as gestures, eye contact, facial expressions and voice cues, e.g., changes in tone or rhythm. The nonverbal system is a more primitive form of conveying information about emotions, attitudes, and preferences. It is the universal mechanism for communication when individuals do not possess command of a language.

Informal/Interpersonal Communication

Studies suggest that 30 to 70% of dental patients do not comply with home care and diet recommendations because they are dissatisfied with the interpersonal communication skills of the dental health educator. Patient cooperation can be affected by an educator's ability to communicate sensitivity and caring.[22] Hornsby and his colleagues comment: "If a dentist has established rapport or has formed a positive relationship with patients, then he is more likely to positively change their oral hygiene procedures. . . . More than the giving of information is needed. A strong positive relationship is necessary for the patient to act upon the information."[23] The dental health educator must take the initiative to assist the patient in revealing his values, needs, and possible concerns. This can be accomplished by displaying a genuine concern for the patient's problems through tactful questioning, intent listening, supportive nonverbal expressions, and nonjudgmental feedback. Despite how the educator feels about the patient's ideas, he should not criticize or reject them. Criticism or rejection only blocks communication; the patient becomes defensive and ceases to express his opinion.[6]

Accurate interpersonal communication is paramount in health education. The degree of accuracy can be enhanced by several factors: (1) the educator's ability to adjust the complexity of the message based on the patient's frame of reference, (2) the educator's ability to anticipate possible objections the patient might have to his message, (3) both parties reducing the rate and length of time of message transmission, (4) both parties asking questions when information is unclear or overwhelming, and (5) most important, the ability of one individual to actively listen while the other actively communicates and vice-versa. Imagine the 7-year-old patient who asks why he must brush his teeth so often and is given a detailed description of the pathophysiology of caries and periodontal disease. Too much infor-

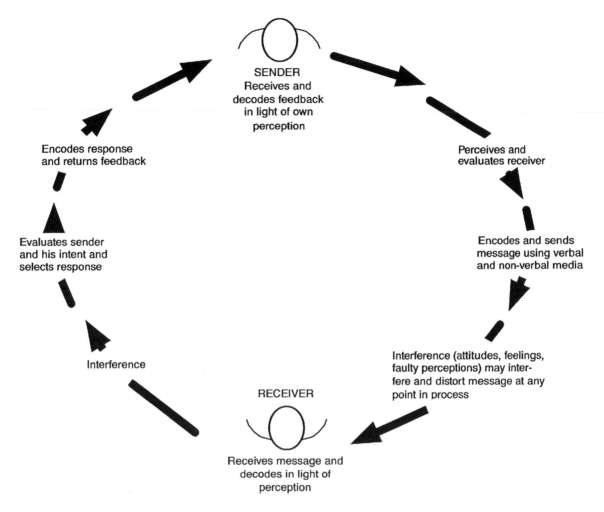

Figure 2-4. One-to-one communication. From Brill, N.: Working with People: The Helping Process. 2nd Ed. Philadelphia, Harper & Row, 1978, p. 35.

mation has been presented, above the cognitive level of the child, and consequently little or nothing has been learned. It is similarly detrimental to speak below the patient's intellectual level of understanding.

Listening

Research shows that people listen at only about 25% efficiency.[24] Poor listeners miss significant information, experience more misunderstandings than good listeners, and often find that people have difficulty feeling close to them.[25] A good listener is attentive, doesn't interrupt or give unsolicited advice, establishes and maintains good eye contact, and acknowledges the speaker by head nodding and leaning forward.[9]

The technique of active listening includes paraphrasing, verifying consequences, and preparing to listen.[26] Paraphrasing requires that the educator repeat in his own words what the patient has said to verify that communication was accurately understood, e.g., "Do you mean that you are concerned about the anesthesia or about the actual extraction of your wisdom teeth?" Verifying consequences confirms requests, e.g., "That's correct, you will be placed on our recall program and will be called when you are due for your next dental cleaning." Preparation improves listening if the educator is able to think through what a patient is likely to say before he says it, e.g., "Let's talk about your recent diagnosis of diabetes after I finish taking your blood pressure."[27]

Formal Communication

Although most dental health education is interpersonal, conducted informally at the office setting, frequently dental health educators have the opportunity to speak publicly in a formal setting, e.g., PTA or health department. After analyzing the target group (Chapter 11) and the topic, the health educator can prepare the speech. A speech or lecture should be well organized, clearly focused, and brief. A key to effective public speaking is the use of relevant verbal or visual examples to emphasize a point. The use of slides or transparencies is an ideal way to get the audience's attention.[28]

Carefully chosen audiovisual aids can enhance the educational process, but it is important to remember that they are just that—aids. To be effective they must be accurate, relevant, and personalized. Audiovisual aids cannot take the place of personal influence in changing peoples's attitudes and behavior;[29] they are an adjunct. Trying to get patients to read printed material is more difficult than getting them to watch a slide show because it requires more patient compliance and people read at varying rates of comprehension—and some do not read at all. Pamphlets are most effective when given to the patient by the dental health educator and reinforced with verbal instruction.[30] The use of media in program development is discussed in Chapter 11.

THE LEARNING SITUATION

"The type task to be learned, its size, complexity, and clarity, and the conditions and procedures under which learning is to take place—in short, the learning situation itself—must also be factored into the equa-

tion."[14] The particular task to be learned (cognitive-knowledge, affective-emotional, or psychomotor skill or action) influences the patient's rate of learning and the educator's approach to the subject matter. For example, a patient might master the verbal description of how to floss in one session, whereas it might take several appointments and practice at home for him to become proficient in the actual technique of flossing his own teeth. Learning is obviously less difficult when the learning task is clearly defined and the educator presents small amounts of material at one time, letting the patient set his own pace. Sequential learning involves instruction in a stepwise fashion with review and reinforcement of each step prior to moving ahead. The educator must be cognizant of how fast and how much a patient can learn at one time. What might be a small step to one individual can be an unrealistic one to another.[31]

Learning is also enhanced by establishing a fixed time and place for health educator–patient interaction. The reliability or stability of the environment signifies the importance of the task to be learned. It is equally significant to maintain the continuity of care; the educator should remain the same if possible throughout the patient's instruction to supervise the patient's practices. Once a good rapport has been established with the patient and the patient recognizes the educator's interest in him and his ability to perform a desired task, desirable changes will more readily take place.

Remember that the educator's control over the patient's ability to change his behavior is merely one of planning, organizing, and administering learning experiences congruent with the patient's background, motivations, and needs. The patient's active involvement in the educational process ultimately determines its success or failure.[32] Helping patients assume responsibility for their own dental health status is the primary function of a dental health educator.[33] A patient's commitment to a set of dental health goals and objectives is directly proportional to the level of participation he is willing to

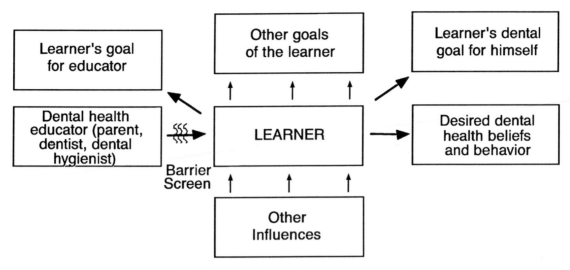

Figure 2-5. Young's model of the dental health education process. From Young, M. A. C.: Dental health education: An overview of selected concepts and principles relevant to programme planning. Int. J. Health Educ., *13*:2, 1970.

accept in developing them.[9] Active involvement in one's own objectives and goals makes them more meaningful and eases the transfer of behavior into one's real life experiences.

During the learning process, the educator must continually provide feedback to the patient related to his progress. A minimal amount of time should elapse between a behavior and a report of the results of a behavior if learning is to remain uninterrupted. The longer feedback is delayed, the more a patient forgets what was done and what changes were made. Feedback in the form of positive reinforcement increases the probability that a behavior will be repeated.[34] If a patient is having difficulty with a behavior, the educator should point out the problem areas, give solutions to correct the difficulties, and praise him for the skills he is performing correctly.

By using these patient education principles as guidelines, the educator can assess his teaching techniques and make improvements as needed. Effective patient education assists patients in becoming responsible for the improvement of their oral health.

DENTAL HEALTH EDUCATION MODEL: A SUMMARY

An individual's knowledge, attitudes, values, motives, needs, goals, and communication skills plus the influence of peers, family, educators, and the mass media all play a role in shaping his actions or behavior.[35]

Socioeconomic factors such as education and income have been shown to greatly affect the demand for dental care. The interaction of all of these factors must be considered when designing and implementing an individualized dental health education program. Young has done just that in a model he created in 1970 (Fig. 2-5).[36]

REFERENCES

1. Burt, B. A.: The prevention connection: Linking dental health education and prevention. Int. Dent. J., 33:188–95, 1983.
2. Coleman, J. D.: Psychology and Effective Behavior. Palo Alto, CA, Foresman, 1969.

3. Yacovone, J. A.: Translating research in the social and behavioral sciences for more effective use in community dentistry. J. Public Health Dent., *36*:155, 1971.

4. Jong, A. W. (ed.): Community Dental Health. 2nd Ed. St. Louis, C. V. Mosby, 1988.

5. Knutson, A. L.: The Individual, Society, and Health Behavior. New York, Russell Sage, 1965.

6. Young, W. O. (Ed.): Motivating patients to accept preventive services. Dent. Clin. North Am., July 1965, pp. 525–533.

7. Stoll, F. A.: Dental Health Education. 5th Ed. Philadelphia, Lea & Febiger, 1977.

8. Weinstein, P., Getz, T., and Milgrom, P.: Oral Self Care. Reston, VA, Reston Publishing, 1985.

9. Harris, N. O., and Christen, A. G.: Primary Preventive Dentistry. 2nd Ed. Norwalk, CT, Appleton & Lange, 1987.

10. Read, D. A., Simon, S., and Goodman, J.: Health Education: The Search for Values. Englewood Cliffs, NJ, Prentice-Hall, 1977.

11. Horowitz, L. G., Dillenberg, J., and Rattray, J.: Self-care motivation: A model for primary preventive oral health behavior change. J. Sch. Health, *57*:114–118, 1987.

12. Badura, A.: Self-efficacy: Toward a unifying theory of behavioral change. Psychol. Rev., *84*:191–202, 1977.

13. Maslow, A. H.: Toward a Psychology of Being. 2nd Ed. New York, D. Van Nostrand, 1968.

14. Ross, H. S., and Mico, P. R.: Theory and Practice in Health Education. Palo Alto, CA, Mayfield Publishing, 1980.

15. Press, B. H.: United States: Old needs, new expectations. J. Public Health Dent., *48*:103–105, 1988.

16. Strom, T. (Ed.): Dentistry in the '80s: A changing mix of services. J. Am. Dent. Assoc., *116*:617–624, 1988.

17. Moss, S. J. (Ed.): Contemporary Dentistry: Persuasive Prevention. Cincinnati, Crest Professional Services, Proctor and Gamble Co.; Medcom, Inc., 1975.

18. Geboy, M. J.: Communication and Behavior Management in Dentistry. Baltimore, Williams & Wilkins, 1985.

19. Haney, W. V.: Communication: Patterns and Incidents. Homewood, IL, Richard D. Irwin, 1960.

20. Brill, N.: Working with People: The Helping Process. 2nd Ed. Philadelphia, Harper & Row, 1978.

21. Knapp, M. L.: Essentials of Nonverbal Communication. New York, Holt, Rinehart & Winston, 1980.

22. Sackett, D. L.: The magnitude of compliance and non-compliance. *In* Compliance with Therapeutic Regimens. Edited by D. L. Sackett and R. B. Haynes. Baltimore, John Hopkins Press, 1976.

23. Hornsby, J. L., Denneen, L. J., and Heid, D. W.: Interpersonal communication skills development: A model for dentistry. J. Dent. Educ., *39*:728–732, 1975.

24. Nichols, R. G.: Listening is a 10-part skill. Nation's Business, *45*:26–29, 1957.

25. Lassen, M. K.: Listening can be the key to communication. R.D.H., *3*:21–26, 1983.

26. Nichols, R. G.: Do we know how to listen? Practical help in a modern age. Speech Teacher, *10*:120, 1961.

27. Chambers, D. W., and Abrams, R. G.: Dental Communication. Norwalk, CT, Appleton-Century-Crofts, 1986.

28. Breckon, D. J., Harvey, J. R., and Lancaster, R. B.: Community Health Education. Rockville, MD, Aspen, 1985.

29. Oskamp, S.: Attitudes and Opinions. New York, Prentice-Hall, 1977.

30. Bourne, T.: How to improve your patient's dental IQ. Dent. Mgmt., *23*:38–40, 1983.

31. Huntley, D. E.: Five principles of patient education. Dent. Hyg., *53*:420–423, 1979.

32. Shou, L.: Active-involvement principle in dental health education. Comm. Dent. Oral Epidemiol., *13*:128–132, 1985.

33. Alderman, M. K.: Self-responsibility in health care/promotion: motivational factors. J. Sch. Health, *50*:22–25, 1980.

34. Skinner, B. F.: Contingencies of Reinforcement. New York, Appleton-Century-Crofts, 1969.

35. Lewin, K.: Field Theory in Social Science. New York, Harper and Brothers, 1951.

36. Young, M. A. C.: Dental health education: An overview of selected concepts and principles relevant to programme planning. Int. J. Health Educ., *13*:2, 1970.

Chapter 3

DENTAL DISEASE AND SOCIETY

*We believe that the conditions of perfect
health, either public or personal, are seldom or
never attained, though attainable; that the
average length of human life may be very much
extended, and its physical power greatly
augmented; that in every year thousands of lives
are lost which might have been saved—and
that measures for prevention will affect infinitely
more than remedies for the cure of disease.*

Lemuel Shattuck
1850

DENTAL CARIES

The World Health organization defines dental caries as a "localized, post-eruptive, pathological process of external origin involving softening of the hard tooth tissue and proceeding to the formation of a cavity."[1] According to Wilkins, "dental caries is a disease of the dental calcified structures (enamel, dentin, and cementum) which is characterized by decalcification of the mineral components and dissolution of the organic matrix."[2]

Dental caries has afflicted mankind to some degree since hunting and gathering were replaced by agriculture as the primary source of food.[3] Early in history, attrition and root surface caries seemed to predominate. There is historic evidence of the prominence of root surface decay in the Egyptians dating back at least 6000 years.[4] Frequently the crowns of teeth were found to be free of caries, but root surface involvement was present. The prevalence was also found to increase proportionally with the age of the individual. It was not until the

seventeenth century that the prevalence of enamel caries actually increased. Refinement of the diet and the increased consumption of sugar are chiefly responsible for the pattern of caries as it has been known up through the 1970s.[3,5]

Causes

Dental caries is produced by the interrelationship of four factors: the susceptible tooth surface (host), specific microorganisms (bacteria), fermentable carbohydrates predominantly in the form of sucrose (substrate), and (time) (Fig. 3-1).[6]

Dental plaque is composed of a variety of acidogenic microorganisms. Streptococcus mutans is the specific causative microorganism implicated in dental caries. These microorganisms have the potential to synthesize carbohydrates into extracellular polysaccharides (dextrans, levans, and other glucans and fructans) and intracellular polysaccharides, which are stored. Extracellular polysaccharides assist in the formation

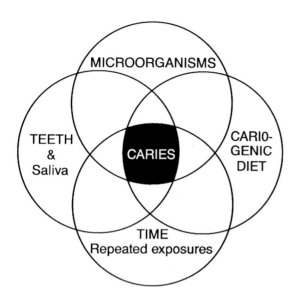

Figure 3-1. Dental caries process. The four circles illustrate the factors involved in the development of dental decay; the area of overlap indicates caries. Adapted from Newbrun, E.: Cariology. 2nd Ed. Baltimore, Williams & Wilkins, 1983, and Wilkins, E. M.: Clinical Practice of the Dental Hygienist. 6th Ed. Philadelphia, Lea & Febiger, 1989, p. 383.

and adherence of plaque to the tooth. Streptococcus mutans, Streptococcus sanguis, and Streptococcus mitis are involved in enamel caries, whereas Actinomyces viscosus and Actinomyces naeslundii are involved in root caries.[1]

When a fermentable carbohydrate is eaten, enzymes in the bacterial plaque break down the foodstuff and form an acid. The acid demineralizes the tooth surface, and eventually, with repeated exposures to fermentable carbohydrates, particularly sucrose, a carious lesion results. In the absence of cariogenic foods, stored intracellular polysaccharides can convert to an acid. The formation of acid begins immediately when the sucrose from food becomes incorporated into the bacterial plaque. The pH drops to an average level of 5.0 and remains at that acidity for approximately 20 minutes for each cariogenic exposure. It takes 1 to 2 years from the initial attack of organic acids on the tooth surface to form a clinically detectable carious lesion.[7]

A diminished salivary flow can also con-

tribute to caries by interfering with the proper oral clearance of cariogenic foodstuffs. The natural buffering capacity of the saliva, which functions to neutralize acids formed during carbohydrate fermentation, is impaired when salivary volume decreases. Flow rate is less in females, when in darkness, when lying down, and diminishes with age or during warmer weather.[8] (Further discussion of xerostomia is included in Chapter 9).

Epidemiology

One of the unique features of dental caries is its ability to remain a lifelong disease in so many individuals by the succession of lesions throughout the dentition.[8] Who is most susceptible to decay? The host factors of location of caries, race, age, sex, heredity, and emotional disturbances are significant variables in the search for the answer to this question. Environmental variables such as geographic location, nutrition, fluoride, and oral hygiene are also responsible in determining an individual's or a group's susceptibility to caries.

HOST FACTORS

Location of Caries. The significance of the location of caries requires observation of the tooth surface attacked, the frequency with which different teeth are attacked in the mouth, and the presence of bilateral symmetry.[8] There are four main types of caries attack by surfaces:

1. *Pit-and-fissure caries* (occlusal) is the easiest to detect and the first to appear.
2. *Proximal or smooth-surface caries* is seen later in the life-span of deciduous teeth and during ages 15 to 35 years in permanent teeth.
3. *Cervical caries* occurs uniformly throughout life and borders the free margin of the gingiva, making it highly susceptible to plaque accumulation.
4. *Root caries* occurs in more advanced years.

The mandibular incisors are usually the last teeth in the dentition to experience decay. Although these teeth appear to be protected by the action of the submandibular and sublingual salivary glands, the maxillary first molars have not been afforded the same resistance by the parotid gland. These variations have not been explained. Bilateral symmetry is extremely helpful in tracing the route(s) caries will take in an individual. Evidence that the concept of bilateral attack actually exists makes it a useful indicator for also determining when and what type of preventive measure should be used to stop the spread of caries.[8]

Race. Recent studies of the adult working population continue to indicate that blacks have a lower caries rate than the corresponding white population (Table 3-1).[9] Because of tooth loss, estimates of caries prevalence become erratic beyond age 35. When employed blacks were asked to give the main reason for their last dental visit, 26% replied "to have a tooth pulled"; of the employed whites, 9.4% cited extraction as their main reason for seeking dental care.[9] This lack of preventive orientation toward dentistry among the black population can be attributed to low socioeconomic status and educational level. In general, dental care seeking behavior is directly proportional to income and educational level. Cultural differences also relate to diet and availability of and demand for dental care.[10] Whites in the United States generally seek dental care more frequently than do blacks (Table 3-2).[9]

Age. The idea that caries was essentially a disease of childhood is now known to be fiction. By the close of the 1970s it became evident that the prevalence of caries, particularly among America's youth, was declining sharply. Today, half of United States children ages 5 to 17 years are clinically caries-free in their permanent dentition (Table 3-3).[11] Only 4% of the adult working population ages 18 to 64 can make that same claim (Table 3-4).[9]

The 1979–1980 National Caries Prevalence (NCP) survey of U.S. school children aged 5 to 17 revealed that, on the average, a school child had at least one permanent tooth surface affected by caries by age 8, 4 surfaces by age 12, and 11 by age 17.[12] In comparison, the NIH study of 1986–1987 indicates less than one (0.71) carious surface in the 8-year-old, fewer than three (2.66) surfaces in the 12-year-old, and 8 in the average 17-year-old. Among children between 5 and 17 years of age, the mean number of decayed, missing, and filled tooth surfaces (the DMFS rate) has declined by 1.7 in 7 years (Table 3-5).[11]

In 1985 the mean DFS (decayed and filled surfaces) for the age group 18 to 19 years was 12, increasing to a mean DFS of 29 for the oldest employed persons. The average for

Table 3-1. Mean Decayed and Filled Surfaces (DFS) for Employed Persons by Race and Age, U.S. 1985

Age Group	Whites	Blacks
18–19	12.038	10.404
20–24	14.510	12.192
25–29	18.083	15.125
30–34	22.499	13.486
35–39	27.315	14.240
40–44	32.053	19.230
45–49	33.346	15.006
50–54	32.412	15.938
55–59	31.534	11.548
60 and over	30.341	10.212
All ages	24.513	14.306

U.S. Public Health Service, National Institute of Dental Research: Oral Health of United States Adults and Seniors: 1985–86. National Institutes of Health. Publication #(PHS) 87-2868, U.S. Dept. of Health and Human Services, 1987.

Table 3-2. Percentage Distribution of Employed Persons by Time of Last Visit for Dental Care and Race, U.S. 1985

Time of Last Visit	Whites	Blacks
Within past 12 mo	60.9	42.9
1 to 2 years	20.6	26.4
3 to 5 years	9.9	16.3
Over 5 years	7.9	12.7
Never received care	0.7	1.4
Unknown	0.1	0.35

U.S. Public Health Service, National Institute of Dental Research: Oral Health of United States Adults and Seniors: 1985–86. National Institutes of Health. Publication #(PHS)87-2868, U.S. Dept. of Health and Human Services, 1987.

Table 3-3. Percentages of Children Who Were Caries-Free in Two National Surveys

Age	1979–80	1986–87
5	95.4	97.3
6	89.7	94.4
7	76.5	84.2
8	58.6	75.0
9	50.6	65.5
10	37.9	55.7
11	33.7	45.0
12	26.9	41.7
13	21.1	34.0
14	19.6	27.7
15	14.9	21.8
16	11.8	20.0
17	10.7	15.6
All ages	36.6	49.9

U.S. Public Health Service, National Institute of Dental Research: Caries Prevalence in U.S. Schoolchildren 1986–1987. National Institutes of Health, Publication #(PHS)89-2247, U.S. Dept. of Health and Human Services, 1989.

Table 3-5. Age-Specific Prevalence of Caries in Permanent Teeth, 1979–80 and 1986–87

Age	Mean DMFS	
	1979–80	1986–87
5	0.11	0.07
6	0.20	0.13
7	0.58	0.41
8	1.25	0.71
9	1.90	1.14
10	2.60	1.69
11	3.00	2.33
12	4.18	2.66
13	5.41	3.76
14	6.53	4.68
15	8.07	5.71
16	9.58	6.68
17	11.04	8.04
All ages	4.77	3.07

U.S. Public Health Service, National Institute of Dental Research: Caries Prevalence in U.S. Schoolchildren 1986–1987. National Institutes of Health. Publication #(PHS)89-2247, U.S. Dept. of Health and Human Services, 1989.

all ages was 23 decayed and filled surfaces. The adult population surveyed appeared to have achieved a very high level of restorative care for coronal caries, over 92% of carious surfaces having been restored.[9]

The prevalance of root surface carious lesions increases with age. Caries are more likely to occur when gingival recession exposes root surfaces, making them vulnerable

Table 3-4. Percentages of Dentate Employed Persons with No Decayed or Filled Teeth (DFT) by Age, U.S. 1985

Age Group	Males	Females	Total
18–19	7.89	6.65	7.28
20–24	8.23	4.20	6.28
25–29	6.75	3.68	5.37
30–34	3.00	3.29	3.12
35–39	3.33	1.46	2.51
40–44	2.82	2.41	2.63
45–49	5.26	2.70	4.17
50–54	2.27	4.79	3.32
55–59	4.08	1.78	3.11
60 and over	3.28	1.10	2.39
All ages	4.70	3.14	4.00

U.S. Public Health Service, National Institute of Dental Research: Oral Health of United States Adults and Seniors: 1985–86. National Institutes of Health. Publication #(PHS)87-2868, U.S. Dept. of Health and Human Services, 1987.

to bacterial plaque. Twenty-one percent of the working population and 67% of the senior citizen population had some evidence of root surface caries (Table 3-6).[9] (Root caries is discussed in further detail in Chapters 7 and 10.)

Sex. Regardless of age, females generally have a slightly higher DFS than males (Fig. 3-2).[9,11] The difference is minimal enough to be explained by the earlier eruption of teeth in females, making the oral cavity at risk for a longer period of time.[13] Females also tend to value their oral hygiene more than males[14,15] and visit the dentist more frequently (Table 3-7).[9]

Interestingly, males show a substantially higher rate of root surface caries than females (Table 3-6), a reversal of the trend found in coronal decay.

Heredity. It is widely accepted that dental caries varies from family to family[8,15,16] and that inheritance of specific tooth structures conducive to decay, e.g., malformed teeth and deep grooves, can occur. What is unknown is whether these tendencies are actually genetic or only represent the passage of dietary or behavioral traits through family indoctrination. Mansbridge found caries ex-

Table 3-6. Percentages of Dentate Employed Persons and Seniors with at Least One Decayed or Filled Root Surface by Age Group and Sex, U.S. 1985

Age Group	Males	Females	Total
18–19	5.53	7.78	6.64
20–24	7.25	5.29	6.30
25–29	10.55	8.00	9.41
30–34	15.76	11.01	13.67
35–39	19.86	16.33	18.30
40–44	29.49	20.08	25.26
45–49	36.66	28.92	33.36
50–54	44.41	38.93	42.14
55–59	44.43	40.63	42.83
60–64	59.00	47.82	54.42
65–69	70.13	60.01	63.79
70–74	66.05	63.91	64.59
75–79	70.72	70.91	70.86
80 and over	67.21	60.69	62.88

U.S. Public Health Service, National Institute of Dental Research: Oral Health of United States Adults and Seniors: 1985–86. National Institutes of Health Publication #(PHS)87-2868, U.S. Dept. of Health and Human Services, 1987.

Table 3-7. Percentage Distribution of Employed Persons by Time of Last Visit for Dental Care and Sex, U.S. 1985

Time of Last Visit	Males	Females
Within past 12 mo	55.0	63.0
1–2 years	21.5	20.6
3–5 years	11.8	9.2
>5 years	9.7	6.6
Never received care	1.4	0.4
Unknown	0.7	0.3

U.S. Public Health Service, National Institute of Dental Research: Oral Health of United States Adults and Seniors: 1985–86. National Institutes of Health. Publication #(PHS)87-2868, U.S. Dept. of Health and Human Services, 1987.

perience between identical twins to be more similar than that of fraternal twins and that unrelated pairs of children displayed less resemblance than either type of twin.[17] He concluded that although caries experience might be influenced by genetic factors, environmental variables had a stronger effect on the causation of caries.

Emotional Disturbances. Anxiety has been considered by some to affect caries rate. One study showed sharp peaks in the caries incidence of those experiencing acute stress, with a return to their previous caries rate during periods of more normal mental health.[18] Another study indicated that stress increased caries experience by affecting salivary flow and pH.[19] A third study demonstrated a higher dental caries experience in hospitalized manic-depressive patients than in the hospital population at large.[20]

ENVIRONMENTAL FACTORS

Geographic Location. Countries that are more developed economically and whose people have a higher socioeconomic status generally have a higher prevalence of dental caries, particularly in urban areas. Poorer countries such as those in central Africa and India experience less dental caries because the people still consume foodstuffs obtained from hunting and subsistence farming, both of which produce diets high in protein and fiber and low in fermentable carbohydrates.[21]

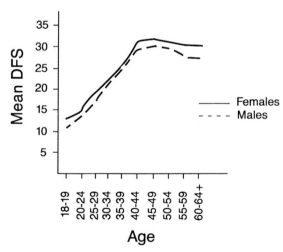

Figure 3-2. Mean decayed and filled surfaces (DFS) for employed persons by age and sex, U.S. 1985. U.S. Public Health Service, National Institute of Dental Research: Oral Health of United States Adults and Seniors: 1985–86. National Institutes of Health. Publication #(PHS)87-2868, U.S. Dept. of Health and Human Services, 1987.

Even though the United States is a highly developed country, there are still variations in caries experience from region to region. This phenomenon can be explained by the presence or absence of fluoride in the drinking water, the level of fluoride available, and climate differences, which alter the amount of water consumed. In the United States, approximately 9 million people live in 1,909 communities where natural fluoride occurs in the water supply at a level of 0.7 ppm or above. Other areas of the country require that fluoride be added to the water supply. Currently 7,700 communities in the United States provide fluoridated water to over 121 million Americans. This translates to approximately 61% of the nation's population receiving fluoride benefits.[22,23] Standards for acceptable fluoride in the drinking water are set at one part per million fluoride. For warmer or colder climates, the fluoride concentration can be adjusted from 0.6 to 1.2 ppm F, based on the amount of water consumed; the warmer the climate, the lower the concentration of fluoride because more water is ingested (Table 3-8).[24]

Nutrition. Caries prevalence is directly related to the frequency of between-meal snacking. It is not the amount of sugar one ingests, but the frequency of between-meal exposures that accounts for dental caries susceptibility. When a cariogenic food is eaten with a meal, its decay-producing potential is reduced because of the presence of proteins and fats in the other foods consumed. Proteins and fats such as peanuts and cheese create a plaque pH of 6 or higher and exert a strong buffering action by neutralizing plaque acids.[7]

The physical form of sugars is also important in the development of caries. More retentive sugars place the oral environment at a greater risk. If sugar-containing solutions such as soft drinks are consumed frequently, however, they also produce caries.

Fluoride. Until this past decade, dental caries was considered to be a pandemic health issue. Fluoride has been cited as one of the major reasons for the recent decline in caries across the country.[25] Fluoride functions to inhibit dental caries through four basic mechanisms:

1. Fluoride reduces the enamel's solubility by converting hydroxyapatite in enamel to stable fluorapatite, which resists demineralization when exposed to acids.[26]
2. Fluoride is antibacterial; in high concentrations it might inhibit the acid production of Streptococcus mutans.
3. Systemic fluoride traveling through the bloodstream bathes the outermost layer of enamel of developing teeth, making them resistant to acid attack once they have erupted and have been exposed to plaque and dietary sugars.[26] Continuous exposure to fluoride after eruption sustains the fluoride-rich outer layer and accelerates the maturation of the tooth enamel.[27]
4. Fluoride remineralizes a subsurface lesion by forming larger, well-formed, insoluble crystals that are more resistant to acid attack and by enhancing the incorporation of minerals (calcium and phosphorus) into the lesion. When the remineralization process surmounts the damage incurred by demineralization, caries can be arrested and the lesion repaired.[28]

Oral Hygiene. Plaque control is an extremely important factor to be considered in the prevention and control of caries. One cannot rationalize that oral hygiene practices alone will lower the incidence of caries, in light of the multifactorial causes of

Table 3-8. Fluoride Levels Recommended for Cool and Warm Climates

Annual Average of Maximum Daily Air Temperatures (degrees Fahrenheit)	Recommended Control Limits (F concentration ppm)		
	Lower	Optimum	Upper
50.0–53.7	0.9	1.2	1.7
53.8–58.3	0.8	1.1	1.5
58.4–63.8	0.8	1.0	1.3
63.9–70.6	0.7	0.9	1.2
70.7–79.2	0.7	0.8	1.0
79.3–90.5	0.6	0.7	0.8

U.S. Public Health Service: Public Health Service Drinking Water Standards 1962. Publication #(PHS)956. Washington, DC, Government Printing Office, 1962.

caries already mentioned in this chapter. The problem with oral hygiene procedures is that individuals are not consistent in their plaque control efforts, are often poorly motivated, and many use poor brushing and flossing technique.[29,30] Poor technique often results from lack of knowledge, disinterest, or the presence of malaligned teeth or other orodental anomalies that make home care difficult. When oral hygiene is performed optimally, as in the studies conducted by Lindhe and Axelsson,[31-34] caries in children can be nearly eradicated. In this research, meticulous plaque control was carried out on children by trained dental auxiliaries at set intervals.

PERIODONTAL DISEASE

Periodontal disease refers to a group of diseases[35] that involve pathologic destruction of the periodontium or the supporting structures of the teeth, e.g., gingiva, cementum, periodontal ligament, and alveolar bone.

Periodontal disease, like caries, was also found in ancient skulls. Studies show that severe bone loss was present in individuals at a rather early age, indicating that periodontal problems affected ancient people more seriously than dental caries.[3,36]

Causes

The causes of periodontal disease are multifaceted; they consist of a complex set of local factors (irritants) and systemic factors (the body's response to the irritants).[37] Like caries, the major local agent responsible for this disease is bacterial dental plaque.

Approximately 200 different bacterial species have been isolated from plaque[37] (Table 3-9). The pathogenicity of plaque (as in the case of juvenile periodontitis) is proportional to the quality of the plaque rather than its quantity. A new diagnostic tool, the DNA probe,* has a paper point. It is inserted subgingivally for 10 seconds and sent to the laboratory to determine the type of bacteria in the sulcus. Once the organism is identified the patient can be treated more efficiently.

Periodontal disease can be inflammatory as in gingivitis or periodontitis or noninflammatory as in occlusal trauma. After 1 to 4 days of plaque accumulation, initial subclinical changes occur such as vasodilation, leukocytic infiltration (predominantly polymorphonucleated leukocytes or PMNs, and macrophages), slight collagen loss, and production of exudate.[38-40]

After 1 to 2 weeks of plaque accumulation, early gingivitis becomes apparent. In addition to accentuation of the initial features, an influx of T lymphocytes, rete peg formation, and damage to the fibroblasts results. Edema and bleeding on probing become evident. Soft plaque deposits usually transform into mineralized calculus during this period. Calculus provides a larger surface area of roughness, which enhances the collection of additional plaque on the teeth.

Beyond 14 days, chronic gingivitis is established. It is characterized by further involvement of the previous manifestations plus a thin, ulcerated crevicular epithelium that deepens as a result of subgingival plaque deposition. Mature plasma cells enter the cellular infiltrate and become the dominant defense cells. To this point, only gingival tissue has been implicated; no bone loss has occurred.

Inflammatory destruction, caused by some forms of gingivitis, eventually spreads laterally and apically, adversely affecting periodontal ligament and bone. Bone loss and pocket formation define this condition as periodontitis.[37-43]

Epidemiology

The epidemiology of periodontal disease has become one of the major challenges of the dental profession today. Estimating the

---

* Bio Technia Diagnostics: DMD$_x$ test for periodontitis. Diagnostic kit. Cambridge, MA.

Table 3-9. Predominant Bacterial Flora and Conditions Associated with Different Periodontal Disease States

Periodontal Classifications	Bacterial Flora and Conditions
Early gingivitis	Actinomyces sp., Streptococcus sp.
Established gingivitis	Treponema sp., Veillonella sp., Fusobacteria sp., Bacteroides sp.
Adult periodontitis	Actinomyces sp., Streptococcus sp., Treponema sp., Bacteroides gingivalis, Bacteroides intermedius, Fusobacteria nucleatum, Eikenella corrodens, Wollinella recta
Early-onset periodontitis	
Prepubertal periodontitis	Actinobacillus actinomycetemcomitans, Selenomonas sputigena, Bacteroides intermedius, Eikenella corrodens
Juvenile periodontitis	Actinobacillus actinomycetemcomitans, Capnocytophaga sp.
Rapidly progressive periodontitis	Bacteroides sp., Capnocytophaga sp., Actinobacillus actinomycetemcomitans
Necrotizing ulcerative gingivitis	Treponema sp., Fusobacteria sp., Bacteroides intermedius

Periodontics associated with systemic disease	Conditions:
	     Down syndrome
	     Type I diabetes
	     Papillon-Lefevre syndrome
	     HIV infection

"Refractory" periodontitis (does not respond to therapy)	Actinobacillus actinomycetemcomitans, Bacteroides gingivalis, Bacteroides intermedius.

Adapted from American Academy of Periodontology: Proceedings of the World Workshop in Clinical Periodontics. Princeton, NJ, July 23–27, 1989, pp. I 23–24; American Academy of Periodontology: Perspectives on Oral Antimicrobial Therapeutics. Littleton, MA, PSG Publishing, 1987, p. 9; and Allen, D. L., McFall, W. T., and Jenzano, J.: Periodontics for the Dental Hygienist. 4th Ed. Philadelphia, Lea & Febiger, 1987, p. 39.

prevalence of periodontal disease is difficult. Signs of the disease are much more subjective than those of caries, and because the disease undergoes periods of exacerbation and remission, determining the status of the disease process at a given time is tedious. Also, measures to detect the disease, e.g., radiographs, crevicular fluid, and probing depths, are not standardized, making studies of larger populations arduous.[44]

In 1980, the need for effective preventive programs for periodontal disease became a national health issue.[45] A shared emphasis in dental caries and periodontal disease had emerged.

Examination of a number of host factors such as race, age, sex, systemic disease, emotional disturbances, and intraoral distribution assists in developing an understanding of who is more susceptible to periodontal disease. Environmental variables such as geographic location, nutrition, fluoride, and oral hygiene are important.

HOST FACTORS

Race. In the United States, periodontal disease is of greater prevalence and is more severe among blacks than whites.[46–48] Orientals and individuals from India immigrating to the United States have also shown greater levels of periodontal involvement.[49,50] These differences might be due to religious beliefs, education and socioeconomic status more than race (see discussion of environmental factors).

Age. Periodontal disease has always been defined as the most common cause of tooth loss over the age of 35. Although it remains true that periodontal disease does increase with age, the full scope of the varying degrees of this condition must be reviewed.

The 1979–1980 NCP survey of United States schoolchildren (ages 5 to 17 years) reported that 92% had moderate gingival treatment needs, 3% had severe needs, and 5% had no gingival treatment needs.[12]

Sixty percent of the adult population is afflicted with some form of periodontal disease. Forty-four percent of the employed group (18 to 64) in the 1985–1986 NIH study had at least one gingival site that bled on gentle probing, and nearly 47% of the senior group (65 and over) showed gingival bleeding on probing. Seventy-seven percent of the employed sample and 95% of the seniors had some evidence of attachment loss (Table 3-10).[9] A longitudinal study conducted by Loe and his colleagues illustrated that even in cases of excellent oral hygiene, some loss of attachment occurs with age. Nevertheless, loss of attachment progresses much more rapidly in conditions of poor oral hygiene.[51–53]

Americans who grew up prior to World War II did not gain the benefit of preventive

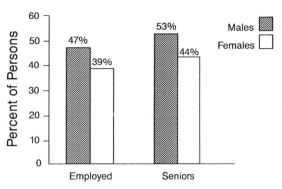

Figure 3-3. Prevalence of gingival bleeding, U.S. 1985. U.S. Public Health Service, National Institute of Dental Research: Oral Health of United States Adults and Seniors: 1985–86. National Institutes of Health. Publication #(PHS)87-2868, U.S. Dept. of Health and Human Services, 1987.

dental programs. Consequently, the 1985–1986 adult survey found many older Americans to be suffering from oral health problems. Forty-two percent of those 65 years and older were edentulous.[9,54]

Sex. Males tend to have a higher rate of periodontal disease at all levels than do females. In the 1985–1986 NIH study, 47% of employed males had bleeding in at least one site, compared to 39% of employed females. Similar differences were found in the senior group (Fig. 3-3).[9]

Only 13% of employed males and 20% of the employed females surveyed were calculus-free. On the average 39% of the employed males and 62% of the male seniors had calculus (either supragingival, subgingival, or both), compared to 29% of employed females and 50% of the female seniors examined (Fig. 3-4).[9]

Eighty percent of the employed males and 98% of male seniors compared to 73% of employed females and 94% of female seniors had at least one site where the loss of attachment was 2 mm or greater. Approximately 8% of the employed group and 34% of the seniors had at least one site with attachment loss of 6 or more millimeters (Fig. 3-5).[9] A mean attachment loss of 2.04 mm was found in the employed male group, with a 1.8-mm loss for females of the same group. The employed population experienced ap-

Table 3-10. Percentages of Employed Persons and Seniors with Attachment Loss* by Age Group and Sex, U.S. 1985

Age Group	Males	Females	Total
18–19	52.71	50.30	51.53
20–24	64.55	55.07	59.97
25–29	70.89	62.54	67.14
30–34	77.22	74.32	75.95
35–39	83.85	76.59	80.67
40–44	82.92	80.89	82.02
45–49	89.34	83.69	86.94
50–54	96.58	88.51	93.24
55–59	97.36	86.41	92.74
60–64	95.67	89.11	92.94
65–69	98.13	94.10	95.47
70–74	98.63	93.23	95.24
75–79	97.19	93.81	94.89
80 and over	96.56	93.48	94.32

* ≥2 mm.

U.S. Public Health Service, National Institute of Dental Research: Oral Health of United States Adults and Seniors: 1985–86. National Institutes of Health. Publication #(PHS)87-2868, U.S. Dept. of Health and Human Services, 1987.

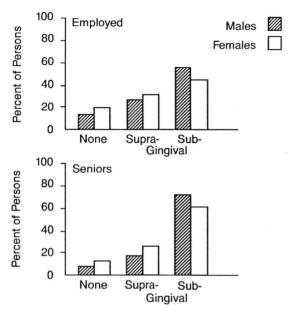

Figure 3-4. Percentage of persons with calculus: U.S. adult population 1985. U.S. Public Health Service, National Institute of Dental Research: Oral Health of United States Adults and Seniors: 1985–86. National Institutes of Health Publication #(PHS)87-2868, U.S. Dept. of Health and Human Services, 1987.

proximately six affected sites per person. The mean loss of attachment increased to 3.54 mm for males and 2.99 mm for females. On the average, seniors sustained nine affected sites per person.[9]

Systemic Disease. The systemic disorders that predispose an individual to periodontal disease are malnutrition, vitamin deficiencies, endocrine changes (e.g., puberty, pregnancy), and debilitating diseases (e.g., diabetes, tuberculosis, kidney disease, leukemia, viral infections, allergies, and heavy-metal poisonings).[8,55,56] These maladies rarely initiate periodontal disease, but they accentuate the effects of an already existing periodontal condition. For instance, an acute form of leukemia can produce oral mucosal ulcerations, gingival enlargement, and bleeding. (See Chapter 9 for further discussion of leukemia.) A patient with pernicious anemia, a deficiency of intrinsic factor necessary for the absorption of vitamin B_{12}, frequently displays gingiva that is inflamed at the margin and contrastingly pale

throughout the mucosa.[55] The diabetic patient also has an increased incidence of gingivitis and periodontal disease. This is often complicated by oral moniliasis and peripheral neuropathy (which presents orally as a burning tongue).[57]

Emotional Disturbances and Habits. A study of over 100 psychiatric patients conducted by Belting and Gupta confirmed that the incidence of periodontal disease was significantly higher among persons with emotional disturbances than the general population, regardless of age or frequency of toothbrushing.[58]

Habits, whether occupational or emotionally related, can also contribute to periodontal disease. For example, the carpenter who holds nails in his mouth, the tailor who bites thread, and the musician who plays a woodwind instrument all place undue stress on certain teeth. Nail, lip, or cheek biting, and bruxism are neurotic habits that also conduce to periodontal disease.[8] Habitual pipe smokers usually hold the pipe stem between the same teeth on one side of their mouth creating stress on these teeth. Thermal irritation of the gingiva and oral mucosa from tobacco smoking and smokeless chewing tobacco habits can produce a cellular dysplasia known as keratosis. Long-term use of tobacco, particularly in its smokable form, is implicated in both oral and lung cancer. (Smoking is discussed in greater detail in Chapters 6 and 7.) Another habit, "toothbrushing mania," also causes changes in the peridontium. This is seen in the individual who presents with cervical abrasion and gingival recession subsequent to vigorous, improper toothbrushing techniques, with a history or current use of a hard toothbrush.

Trauma from Occlusion. In addition to habits, the forces of occlusion can result in periodontal disease by placing excessive stress on the periodontium, or, conversely, by not providing sufficient stimulation to these supporting structures, inducing morphologic changes in the bone and periodontal ligament. Prematurely contacting teeth, poorly contoured restorations, missing teeth, decayed teeth, and ill-fitting appliances can exert occlusal forces destructive to alveolar bone that eventually produce

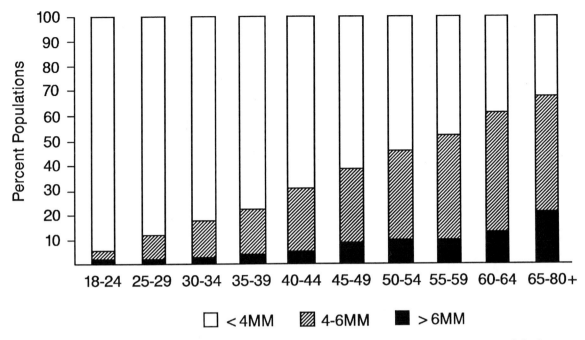

Figure 3-5. Percentages of persons by most severe loss of attachment and age group: adult dentate population, U.S. 1985. U.S. Public Health Service, National Institute of Dental Research: Oral Health of United States Adults and Seniors: 1985–86. National Institutes of Health. Publication #(PHS)87-2868, U.S. Dept. of Health and Human Services, 1987.

tooth mobility without pocket formation. The periodontal ligament adapts by becoming wider. Disuse atrophy or a lack of stimulation to the periodontal ligament of a tooth out of occlusion will result in a thinning of the ligament and bony trabeculae without gingival recession. Trauma superimposed on a site where periodontal disease exists produces more bone loss than periodontitis alone.[8,37,55]

Malocclusion can produce areas of interproximal food impaction. Chronic gingival irritation of the interdental papilla(e) results where the food continually accumulates and can eventually lead to destructive periodontal disease.[8] Occlusal trauma alone cannot initiate inflammatory periodontal disease.[37] *Intraoral Distribution.* Maxillary molars and mandibular central incisors are the teeth most frequently affected by periodontal disease; mandibular molars follow closely in vulnerability. The teeth least prone to periodontal problems are the maxillary canines and the mandibular premolars.[59]

In the 1985–1986 NIH study assessing the oral health of adults, the majority of persons with probing depths beyond 4 millimeters had them on mesial sites rather than buccal. Gingival recession was more prevalent on buccal sites.[9]

ENVIRONMENTAL FACTORS

Geographic Location. Russell's worldwide studies indicate regional differences in periodontal disease, but these differences are not clearly demarcated by countries.[60] This finding offers little evidence for a relationship between periodontal disease and race or ethnicity. Instead Russell[46] and his colleagues[61] suggest the degree of urbanization and in particular, the educational background of the people to be more important and inversely proportional to the level of periodontal disease in a given area. *Nutrition.* Retained food and a poor diet can increase an individual's chances of developing periodontal disease by enhancing microbial growth in the gingival crevice, interfering with the immune response, and inhibiting connective tissue repair following insult from plaque and calculus deposits.[7,62,63]

The breakdown and collection of food in and around the gingival crevice leads to increased microbial growth in that area. These bacteria produce enzymes that gradually destroy the periodontium.[7]

Protein is necessary for phagocytic activity. Therefore, a diet low in protein will increase the severity of a periodontal infection by impairing the body's immune response.[7,64]

Deficiencies in vitamins C, A, B complex, and folic acid and minerals iron, zinc, and calcium can also contribute to periodontal disease.[7] Aboard the old sailing ships, a deficiency of vitamin C, known as scurvy, produced acute periodontitis followed by a loss of teeth. A deficiency in niacin has been known to produce necrotizing gingivitis.[8] Vitamin deficiency oral lesions usually manifest as ulcerations, glossitis, and cheilitis.[2]

The physical consistency of the foods consumed also influences an individual's periodontal health. Although fibrous foods do not remove plaque as was once believed, they do stimulate salivary flow and consequently aid in the removal of food debris from the oral cavity. The mastication of firmer foods, as opposed to a soft diet, strengthens the periodontal ligament through exercise. In addition, a diet that emphasizes fibrous food rather than soft foods that are high in sucrose inhibits the formation of a substrate on which supragingival bacterial plaque can form.[7]

Fluoride. Fluoride, in addition to its reputation for promoting a tooth's resistance to decay, has also been heralded for its efficacy as an antiplaque and antigingivitis agent. Stannous fluoride in particular, in the form of a mouthrinse or dentifrice, has been demonstrated to be effective in reducing plaque accumulation by metabolically disrupting plaque bacteria, specifically Streptococcus mutans.[27,65–67]

Oral Hygiene. The relationship between periodontal disease and oral hygiene is well documented in the United States and other countries.[68–75] In a healthy individual, poor oral hygiene will, in most cases, lead to periodontal disease and eventual loss of teeth.[48] Conscientious oral hygiene techniques achieve oral cleansing and gingival stimulation, both of which are necessary for the maintenance of optimum oral health. Additional benefits of an active oral physiotherapy regimen include improved appearance, fresh breath, increased taste acuity, and a feeling of personal cleanliness.[37]

THE ROLE OF PREVENTION IN THE CONTROL OF DENTAL CARIES AND PERIODONTAL DISEASE

Preventive dentistry encompasses all of dentistry; it involves those practices aimed at the eradication of dental diseases. There are three basic levels of prevention. *Primary prevention* refers to the prepathogenesis stage and involves those actions that prevent the invitation of disease, e.g., daily toothbrushing and flossing. *Secondary prevention* entails those services that attempt to interrupt pathogenesis so as to stop the progression and recurrence of disease, e.g., preventive resin and early diagnosis and prompt treatment of a small atypical lesion on the lip. *Tertiary prevention* includes those rehabilitative services aimed at restoring the loss of function resultant from a disease process, e.g., implants and prostheses.[76]

The remainder of this chapter focuses on the preventive measures directed toward the bacteria, the tooth, and the substrate of the two major plaque diseases, dental caries and periodontal disease.

Preventive Measures Directed Toward the Bacteria

TOOTHBRUSHING

The fundamental home care instrument used for plaque control is the toothbrush.[77]

A soft, multitufted nylon bristle toothbrush is preferred. The bristles should be hollow to prevent the harboring of microorganisms, and the ends of the bristles should be polished and rounded to remain flexible and nonirritating to the oral tissues. Bristle height may vary depending on the manufacturer's philosophy on cleaning. The size of the toothbrush head may vary, but it should be small enough to reach crowded or narrow areas of the arch and large enough to cover several teeth during one brushing stroke.[37] Toothbrushing should be thoroughly accomplished at least once daily. Deciding on a brushing sequence in the mouth and following that pattern each time the teeth are brushed is recommended. Adequate toothbrushing should take approximately 5 minutes; the average toothbrushing time, however, is only 67 seconds.[78] The palate and the tongue should also be cleansed with a posterior-to-anterior brushing stroke.

The choice of a brushing technique must be individualized based on the patient's oral environment, manual dexterity, and degree of motivation. Information on specific toothbrushing techniques can be gained from innumerable other texts. For health education purposes, these are necessary to know, but most importantly the patient must master thoroughness and be guided by the dental health educator toward methods that meet his individual needs. A patient might find it necessary to use several methods to clean his teeth adequately.[26] Some techniques might be more difficult than others with a manual toothbrush if the individual has impaired motor coordination. (Toothbrush modifications are discussed in Chapter 8.)

Automatic toothbrushes are excellent motivators and coordination tools for children and the disabled. Studies comparing automatic toothbrushes with manual brushes have not demonstrated automatic toothbrushes to be more effective.[37] Yet, two impressive mechanical plaque removal devices were recently placed on the market that appear to be exceptions to the rule. Interplak[79] features a rotation/reverse rotation motion. A study conducted at University of Missouri–Kansas City reported a significant improvement in subgingival and interproximal plaque removal with Interplak as compared to that obtained with the manual toothbrushing method.[78] The manufacturer recommends use of a small amount of gel toothpaste only and rinsing of the toothbrush head daily to prevent clogging.

Rota-dent[80] functions like a prophy angle and has the ability to reach hard-to-clean areas such as fixed bridges and furcations. Based on the results of a recent study, the Rota-dent was found to be more effective than the conventional manual brush in decreasing gingival inflammation in the anterior region.[81] In addition, its design makes it excellent for cleaning occlusal fissures (Fig. 3-6).[78]

Regardless of the type of toothbrush used or the brushing method employed, patients should be advised to change their toothbrushes frequently, particularly after an upper respiratory illness.

DISCLOSING AGENTS

Solutions or tablets of erythrosin dye assist in the visualization of bacterial plaque. These products are ideal for chairside instruction and are often suggested for home use to help the patient evaluate his plaque control techniques in his routine surroundings. As the patient becomes more proficient in his home care, less reliance on disclosing products is necessary. Fluorescein dye, which is only visible with a special filtered light, can also be used to disclose plaque[37] (Fig. 3-7).

DENTAL FLOSS

No toothbrushing method has been found to be as good as dental floss or tape for the removal of plaque from the interproximal surfaces.[26] Studies indicate that waxed, unwaxed, and flavored products all clean effectively.[82] Recommendations for making a choice should be based on tightness of contacts, restorative quality, and patient preference.[37] Yarn, pipe cleaners, and gauze strips can also be used interproximally.

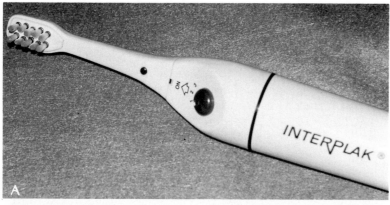

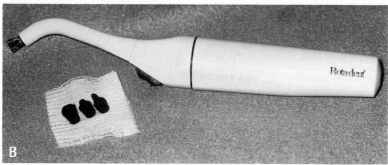

Figure 3-6. The most current electric toothbrushes recommended. A. Interplak. B. Rota-dent.

Super Floss and floss threader devices act as needles to assist in threading floss under a tight contact, orthodontic appliance, or bridge (Fig. 3-8). (See Chapter 7 for technique.) Floss carriers or holders are ideal for patients who experience difficulty manipulating dental floss, such as arthritics, and for caregivers of the disabled. (See Chapter 8.)

OTHER INTERDENTAL CLEANING DEVICES

Some patients have oral conditions that require special aids other than a toothbrush and dental floss to accomplish plaque control. Such special aids include: *Periodontal aids*—mounted toothpicks or plastic tips that are useful in adapting to irregular root surfaces, particularly in areas of recession and furcation involvement; to avoid trauma, the wooden tip should be softened before applying it to the gingival margin.

Rubber tip stimulators and wooden wedge-shaped Stimudents—primarily used to massage interdental tissues. This type of massage is ideal for molding desirable papillary form after periodontal surgery.[37]

Interproximal brushes—small brushes attached to handles, which adapt well to wide embrasures where interdental papillae have been lost. This brush is excellent for cleaning exposed proximal surfaces in these areas. Proxabrushes are also available in a travel size. (See Fig. 3-9.)[37]

Remember not to bombard the patient with too many devices too soon. This only serves to confuse the patient.

IRRIGATION DEVICES

Toothbrushes, floss, and interdental devices have only limited access to subgingival plaque. The pulsating action of the oral irrigator fitted with a special cannula, on the other hand, can disrupt the quality of the plaque that proliferates subgingivally by detoxifying it.[26] The use of these devices to deliver antimicrobial agents into the gingival crevice might make irrigation a routine part of preventive care in the future.[37,83,84]

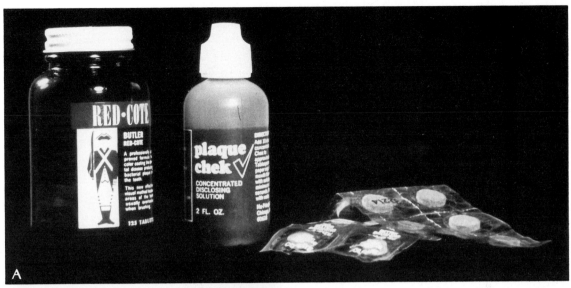

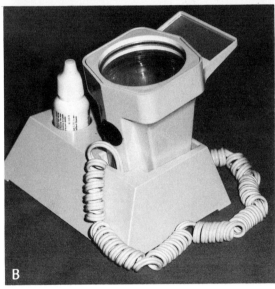

Figure 3-7. A. Disclosing solution and tablets. B. Plak-Lite for disclosure of bacterial plaque.

CHEMOTHERAPEUTIC AGENTS

Many chemical agents exert a bacteriostatic and bacteriocidal effect on dental plaque and should be used as supplements to mechanical plaque removal. The five categories of antiplaque agents include antibiotics, antiseptics, enzymes, plaque modifiers that alter the structure or activity of plaque, and agents that impede the attachment of plaque to the tooth surface.

Placement of synthetic fibers impregnated with tetracycline into a periodontal pocket has been proven effective, particu-larly in the treatment of localized juvenile periodontitis. This controlled or slow-release delivery system is more concentrated and has a longer duration than the systemic administration of an antibiotic. Metronidazole has also been shown to possess some merit as an adjunctive antibiotic.

Control of supragingival plaque and gingivitis has been accomplished by the use of chlorhexidine (Peridex) and Listerine mouthrinses, the only two mouthrinses claiming antimicrobial activity that are accepted by the American Dental Association's Council on Dental Therapeutics for

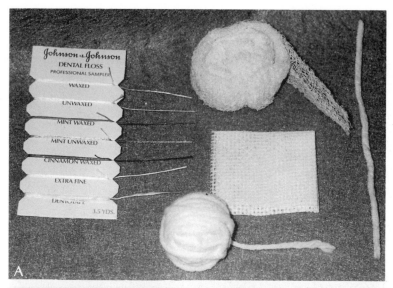

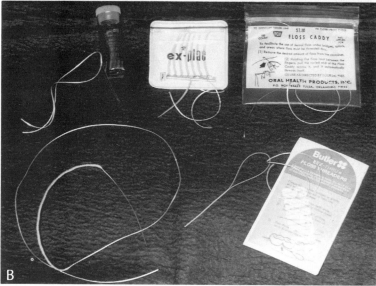

Figure 3-8. A. Types of floss and other interproximal flossing adjuncts. B. Super Floss and other floss-threading devices.

their safety and effectiveness (Fig. 3-10). Listerine, an over-the-counter preparation, contains three essential oils that inhibit microbial growth, reducing plaque and gingivitis by 25% to 35%. The prescription mouthrinse Peridex, containing 0.12% chlorhexidine gluconate, has been known to cause a reduction in plaque by 40% to 50% and gingivitis by 30% to 50%.[85] A recent study found lozenges containing 5 mg chlorhexidine dissolved orally three times daily to be highly effective when rinsing is difficult.[86]

Rinses do not permeate subgingivally, but when a liquid, e.g., water or an antimicrobial agent, is applied subgingivally through an oral irrigating syringe or device delivering the solution deep into a periodontal pocket, it has greater potential.[87,88] Brownstein et al. found irrigation with 0.06% chlorhexidine superior in reducing gingivitis, bleeding on probing, and plaque than rinsing with 0.12% chlorhexidine twice daily.[89]

Stannous fluoride (1.64%) has been shown to exert an antimicrobial effect on dental plaque. A reduction in the number of spirochetes and motile rods results from subgingival irrigation with stannous fluo-

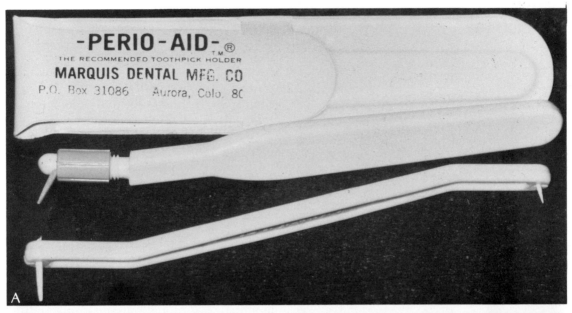

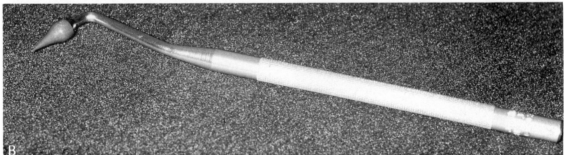

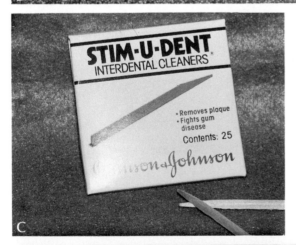

Figure 3-9. Plaque-control adjuncts. A. Perio-aid. B. Rubber-tipped stimulator. C. Wooden Stim-U-Dent. D. Proxabrush.

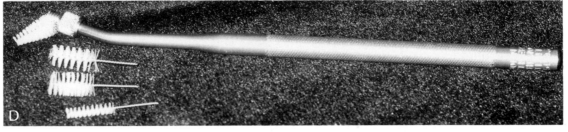

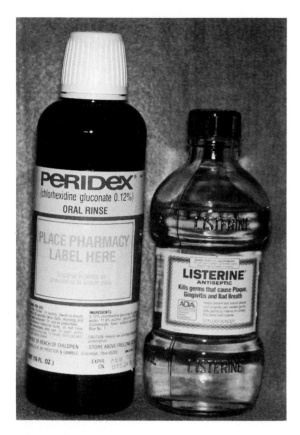

Figure 3-10. Chlorhexidine (Peridex) and Listerine: the only antimicrobial mouthrinses currently accepted by the ADA, Council on Dental Therapeutics.

ride.[37] Both chlorhexidine and stannous fluoride have the disadvantages of staining teeth and tooth-colored restorations and creating a bitter taste. Chlorhexidine also increases calculus formation. If chlorhexidine and fluoride rinses are prescribed simultaneously, the fluoride should not be used for at least 30 minutes after the Peridex rinse to avoid a drug interaction.

Sanguinarine, the antiplaque agent in Viadent, appears to remain incorporated in dental plaque up to 4 hours after rinsing. Its action might be the result of this plaque-retentive property coupled with its antimicrobial activity.[26,90,91] The efficacy of Viadent as an antiplaque agent improves when both dentifrice and mouthwash are used. Three additional antimicrobial solutions, saline, iodine, and hydrogen peroxide, have also been dispensed through subgingival delivery systems. An irrigation device must be purchased that tolerates the given solution decided on. Subgingival cannulae are included, and the device should be operated at the lowest pressure to avoid trauma. Supragingival water irrigation continues to be suitable for the removal of materia alba and other oral debris from the crowns of teeth, particularly as an adjunct to toothbrushing, for the surgical or orthodontic patient. Subgingival water irrigation is therapeutic in reducing bleeding and gingivitis, but because plaque is not soluble in water, such irrigation has no antimicrobial effect. The American Academy of Periodontology contraindicates the habitual use of hydrogen peroxide because of its potential carcinogenicity.

The manufacturer of Plax, a prebrushing mouthrinse formulation containing sodium lauryl sulfate (an anionic surfactant), attributes its effectiveness to a combination of detergent and antibacterial properties. Manufacturer claims that this product whitens teeth and the degree to which Plax enhances the physical removal of plaque over toothbrushing alone remain questionable.[92]

Tartar-control dentifrices have also gained some notoriety recently. Their active ingredients, the soluble pyrophosphates, function by interfering with the crystalline growth of calcium phosphate, therefore inhibiting the formation of supragingival calculus on a clean tooth surface. These toothpastes do not possess antiplaque properties.[90]

DENTAL PROPHYLAXIS

The state of the art in nonsurgical periodontal therapy includes plaque control and some chemotherapeutic agents as previously mentioned, plus scaling and root planing in conjunction with systemic antibiotics. Although adjunctive measures promote healthy tissue response, their duration is short and cannot replace effective scaling and root planing in cases of typical adult periodontitis.[87]

In relation to caries, an oral prophylaxis does not come without its disadvantages.

The fluoride-rich outer layer of enamel can be removed during polishing. For this reason the polishing paste used should contain fluoride, and the procedure itself should be followed routinely with a topical fluoride application.[8]

Preventive Measures Directed Toward the Tooth

FLUORIDE

Water fluoridation has been successful in reducing caries prevalence by 50% to 65% in the permanent dentition of individuals who have consumed water containing fluoride from birth.[93] The greatest protection afforded by fluoride occurs on the smooth surfaces of teeth; the occlusal pits and fissures gain the least benefit. Between 1980 and 1987, the greatest decline in caries by surface type was on the mesial-distal surfaces (54%). (Fig. 3-11.)[11]

Community water fluoridation is considered one of the most dramatic public health developments of the twentieth century because of its effectiveness, safety, ease of implementation, minimal cost, ease of public compliance, and ability to serve all people regardless of education or socioeconomic status.[76]

Fluoridation of school water supplies is often accomplished when central water provisions lack fluoride. The recommended level of fluoride for school programs is 4.5 times the optimum level prescribed for community usage.[94] School water fluoridation, like community water fluoridation, has topical effects on newly erupted teeth in addition to systemic effects on developing teeth.[76]

Dietary fluoride supplements in the form of tablets, lozenges, vitamin supplements, or drops are ideal when the community or school water supply cannot be adjusted optimally. Fluoride supplements also function both topically and systemically. The process of chewing and swishing the remains of a tablet produces a topical effect, whereas the swallowing process leads to the systemic incorporation of fluoride into the developing tooth. When a tablet cannot be chewed, drops are available that can be applied directly to the teeth or added to sugarless juice or water. Milk should not be used as a vehicle for fluoride supplements because it binds fluoride ions and slows absorption.[76,95] (Dosage recommendations for fluoride supplementation are reviewed in Chapter 4.)

Fluoride can also be applied directly to the teeth by the use of *topical solutions or gels, mouthrinses, and dentifrices.* Professionally applied topical fluoride preparations are concentrated, approved systems that are applied directly to the teeth, which have been dried, by using contoured trays that provide complete coverage of all tooth surfaces, or cotton tip applicators and cotton roll isolation. These systems do not require a prophylaxis prior to application and are normally kept in contact with the teeth for 4 minutes. Although the composition of advertised "1-minute gels" is no different from that of the approved 4-minute topical system, the time factor precludes its acceptance by the ADA as a professionally applied topical fluoride. Silverstone* advocates 1-min-

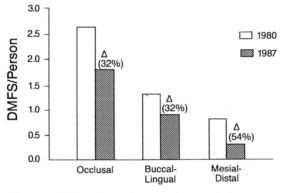

Figure 3-11. Prevalence of dental caries (DMFS) by surface type, 1980 and 1987. U.S. Public Health Service, National Institute of Dental Research: Caries Prevalence in U.S. Schoolchildren 1986–1987. National Institutes of Health. Publication #(PHS)89-2247, U.S. Dept. of Health and Human Services, 1989.

_____

* Oral B Laboratories, Focus interview with Dr. Leon Silverstone, 1989.

Table 3-11. Amounts of Fluoride in Professionally Administered Topical Fluoride Treatments

Agent	Frequency	F Concentration (%)	Volume (ml)	Total Amount of F (mg)
2% NaF	series of 4 every 3 yr	0.91	2.5	22.8
8% SnF_2	1 or 2/yr	1.95	5	97.5
10% SnF_2	1 or 2/yr	2.44	5	122
APF	1 or 2/yr	1.23	5	61.5

From Woodall, I. R. et al.: Comprehensive Dental Hygiene Care. 3rd Ed. St. Louis, C. V. Mosby, 1989, p. 554. Adapted from Heifetz, S. B., and Horowitz, H.S.: The amount of fluoride in current fluoride therapies: Safety considerations for children. ASDC J. Dent. Children, *51*:257, 1984.

ute gel applications because the majority of fluoride uptake occurs within the first minute of exposure and the shorter regimen reduces gel ingestion. Since acidulated phosphate fluoride (APF) gels must be more acidic (pH≤4.0) to be effective, a shorter exposure time would also prevent the etching of porcelain or composite resin restorations. Approved professionally applied fluorides include 2% sodium fluoride, 8% stannous fluoride, and 1.23% APF (Table 3-11). Aqueous stannous fluoride is obtained in powdered form and is mixed with distilled water immediately prior to use. Sodium fluoride is available in solution and is given in a series of appointments. APF is marketed as a solution or gel. Thixotropic gels are recommended because of their adherence to the tooth surface and excellent interproximal diffusion. Gels, usually in 0.4% stannous fluoride, 0.5 to 1% acidulated phosphate fluoride, or 1.1% to 2% neutral NaF concentration, are formulated for daily home care use when individuals need additional protection, e.g., against rampant caries. Generally home care gels are applied with a toothbrush for 1 minute, after which excess gel is expectorated.[76] Studies indicate that a 0.4% stannous fluoride gel is also effective in the reduction of pain associated with dentinal hypersensitivity when it is used twice daily for up to 4 weeks.[96]

Approximately 17% of Americans ages 5 to 17 years use fluoride mouthrinses.[97] Mouthrinsing involves a 1-minute swish with 10 ml of sodium fluoride either as a 0.05% solution daily or a 0.2% solution weekly.[76] An APF mouthrinse formulation containing 0.044% fluoride is also available. Presently, Act and Fluorigard are the two accepted over-the-counter rinses available for daily use. There appears to be no significant difference in effectiveness between the daily and weekly rinsing formats. On the basis of concerns about accidental overingestion, the American Dental Association Council on Dental Therapeutics has limited the amount of sodium fluoride per container to 264 mg. This amount is considered within the boundaries of safety for ingestion at one time.[8]

Dentifrices containing fluoride are used by approximately 89% of all dentate Americans.[97] Currently, fluoride is the single additive in dentifrices known to have a caries-preventive effect. Persons residing in fluoridated areas have been known to experience additional anticaries benefits from the use of a fluoridated dentifrice.[98-100] Toothpastes with fluoride combined with other forms of fluoride therapy have had even greater success in controlling caries.[101] Table 3-12 lists the various dentifrices carrying ADA approval or acceptance.[90,102]

Multiple fluoride therapy incorporating the various combinations of fluoride treatment forms previously discussed provides maximal caries protection. The extent of caries control is generally related to the number of times the teeth are exposed to fluoride and the length of time the fluoride is in contact with the teeth. Although various forms of fluoride have differing caries-reduction capabilities and differing concentrations of fluoride, studies indicate that lower concentrations of fluoride applied more frequently

Table 3-12. Accepted or Approved Fluoride Dentifrices

Dentifrice Name	Fluoride Source	Abrasive System	Year of Acceptance or Approval
Crest*	SnF_2	$Ca_2P_2O_7$	1964
Colgate MFP*	Na_2PO_3F	$(NaPO_3)n + CaHPO_4$	1969
Gleem	NaF	$Ca_2P_2O_7$	1973
Macleans Fluoride	Na_2PO_3F	$CaCO_3$	1976
Aquafresh	Na_2PO_3F	$CaCO_3 + SiO_2nH_2O$	1978
Aim*	SnF_2	SiO_2nH_2O	1979
Aim	Na_2PO_3F	SiO_2nH_2O	1980
Colgate MFP	Na_2PO_3F	$CaHPO_42H_2O$	1980
Crest	NaF	SiO_2nH_2O	1981

* These formulations were replaced with newer formulations with same product name during 1981.

From Harris, N. O., and Christen, A. G.: Primary Preventive Dentistry. 2nd Ed. Norwalk, CT, Appleton & Lange, 1987, p. 221.

are of greater benefit than higher concentrations spaced over longer intervals of time[27] (Table 3-13). When prescribing multiple fluoride therapy, the dental health educator must continually assess a child's exposure to avoid the possibility of dental fluorosis.[103]

A 3-year study of children in a nonfluoridated Finland community reported that xylitol gum-chewing in combination with multiple fluoride therapy reduces the risk of caries more than fluoride therapy alone.[104] In general, when brushing and flossing are not feasible, chewing gum, whether sweetened or sugar-free, for at least 20 minutes immediately after meals increases salivary flow and raises the salivary pH, therefore neutralizing caries activity.[105]

PIT AND FISSURE SEALANTS

Over half of all carious lesions in children occur in the occlusal pits and fissures, where fluorides are least effective. This is a considerable problem because the occlusal surfaces represent only 12.5% of the total number of tooth surfaces susceptible to decay. A preventive solution emerged in the late

Table 3-13. Relative Benefit, Practicality, and Cost of Different Fluoride-Preventive Measure

Preventive Measure	Expected Caries Reduction (%)	Practicality	Approximate Cost per Person per Year ($)
Water fluoridation, community*	35–50	Excellent	0.20–0.50
Fluoride supplementation	35–50		
Individual*		Poor	10.00–20.00
Group		Excellent	8.00–12.00
Topical fluoride therapy (liquid)†	20–40	Fair§	20.00
Fluoride dentifrice, approved type†	10–20	Good	15.00
Fluoride rinses† ‖	20–60	Good	2.00–5.00

* Operates preeruptively and posteruptively.

† Operates posteruptively only.

§ Requires approximately one hour professional chair time per year.

‖ Once a week at school with paid supervisors.

From Dunning, J. M.: Principles of Dental Public Health. 4th Ed. Cambridge, MA, Harvard University Press, 1986, p. 256.

1960s and early 1970s with the development of dental resins referred to as sealants.[26] The American Dental Association granted sealants full acceptance in 1976.[106]

The sealant functions by adhering firmly to the enamel surface, creating a physical barrier that isolates the occlusal pits and fissures from the oral environment.[107] The procedure for sealant application is described in Table 3-14. Maintenance of a dry field throughout the entire procedure is imperative.

Numerous sealant materials currently exist and can be classified based on the method by which they are cured or hardened and whether or not they contain fillers or coloring agents (Table 3-15). The most common chemical agents used in sealants are bisphenol A and glycidyl methacrylate (Bis-GMA).

Table 3-14. Technique for Sealant Application

1. **Select tooth** based on the (a) deep morphology of the pits and fissures and (b) degree of eruption, which must be sufficient to maintain a dry field
2. **Educate the patient** regarding (a) the tooth or teeth to be sealed, (b) the function of sealants, (c) the procedure involved, (d) the types of sealants available, and (e) the average longevity of sealants
3. **Clean tooth**
   a. Prophy (do not use a polishing paste which contains oil or fluoride)
   b. Rinse thoroughly
   c. Dry with compressed air (check air stream to ensure there is no moisture in the line)
4. **Isolate tooth**
   a. Isolate the tooth to be sealed from contamination with oral fluids by using a rubber dam, cotton rolls, or bibulous (absorbent) shields
   b. Dry tooth thoroughly for 10 seconds
5. **Apply etchant**
   a. Place etchant (35% to 50% concentration of phosphoric acid) on the tooth surface with a small plastic sponge or cotton pledget held with cotton pliers
   b. Gently daub the solution onto the tooth surface; do not rub
   c. Saturate the tooth surface for approximately 1 minute (check the manufacturer's specifications)
6. **Rinse** etched surface for at least 10 seconds; suction
7. **Reisolate** if necessary
8. **Dry tooth**
   a. Dry tooth thoroughly for at least 10 seconds
   b. Check etched enamel for a chalky, dull appearance
9. **Apply sealant**
   a. Mix universal and catalyst in a 1:1 ratio no longer than the time designated by the manufacturer (autopolymerized)
   b. Apply sealant to the etched surface within the alloted time period
   c. Allow sealant to cure completely before checking with an explorer
   or
   a. Apply sealant to the etched surface (light polymerized); no mixing is required
   b. Expose the sealant to the light source for approximately 20 seconds (check manufacturer's directions)
   c. Check sealant with an explorer to ensure that all the occlusal grooves are filled (if there are voids, additional sealant can be added without etching as long as the field remains dry)
10. **Rinse sealant**
11. **Remove rubber dam, cotton rolls, or shields**
12. **Check occlusion**
    a. Use articulating paper to check the occlusion
    b. Reduce sealant with slow-speed bur if necessary
13. **Educate the patient** by explaining (a) the need for a fluoride application after sealant placement; and (b) the need for examination of the sealant at routine recall appointments to assess retention. Allow the patient to view the sealant also so he can observe the status of the sealant on a monthly basis during home care procedures

Table 3-15. Pit and Fissure Sealant Materials

Brand Name	Manufacturer	Base Material	Filler	Type of Cure	Color
Concise White Sealant System	3M Dental Products 3M Center St. Paul, MN 55101	Bis-GMA	None	Autocure	White titanium dioxide
Delton Clear	Johnson & Johnson Dental Products 20 Lake Drive E. Windsor, NJ 08561	Bis-GMA	None	Autocure	Clear
Delton Tinted	Johnson & Johnson Dental Products 20 Lake Drive E. Windsor, NJ 08561	Bis-GMA	None	Autocure	Amber 0.07% annatto
Helio Seal	Vivadent P.O. Box 304 Tonawanda, NY 14151	Urethane dimethacry-late	2% SiO_2	Visible light	White aluminum dioxide
Nuva Cote	Caulk The L. D. Caulk Div. P.O. Box 359 Milford, DE 19963	Bis-GMA	50–64% filled lithium aluminum silicate	UV light	Tooth colored
Nuva Seal	Caulk The L. D. Caulk Div. P.O. Box 359 Milford, DE 19963	Bis-GMA	None	UV light	Clear
Oralin Clear	S. S. White Dental Products 3 Parkway Philadelphia, PA 19102	Bis-GMA	None	Autocure	Clear
Oralin Pink	S. S. White Dental Products 3 Parkway Philadelphia, PA 19102	Bis-GMA	None	Autocure	Bright pink 0.01–0.001% rhodomine B
Prisma-Shield	Caulk The L. D. Caulk Div. P.O. Box 359 Milford, DE 19963	Bis-GMA	50–64% filled lithium aluminum silicate	Visible light	Tooth colored
Visio-Seal	Espe-Premier Norristown, PA	Bis-GMA	None	Visible light	Translucent pink

Retention rate studies on sealants indicate that 85% of all chemically cured sealants are expected to be completely retained 1 year from the time of initial placement.[108] The Kalispell study showed that although this retention figure dropped to 56% after 5 years, there remained a 92% reduction in caries in these originally sealed teeth.[109] This is in all probability due to acid etching, which permits tags of sealant to penetrate enamel and be retained there long after the bulk of the sealant has been lost.[110–112] Increased retention can also be related to improved materials and meticulous application technique.

Sealants are recommended for (1) teeth with deep fissures, fossae or lingual pits; (2) teeth with intact occlusal surfaces where a contralateral tooth is carious or has been restored; and (3) teeth that have recently erupted. Studies demonstrate that incipient carious lesions that have been sealed properly will not progress and will arrest over a period of time.[107] A sealant is contraindicated when (1) a frank carious lesion is present, (2) caries exist on other surfaces of the same teeth being considered, (3) a restoration is already present, and (4) the patient's behavior prevents the use of an adequate dry field during the procedure.[27]

Although sealants have been proven effective and have been shown to be the only preventive service that provides patients with a level of long-term protection, their use by professionals and the public's awareness of sealants has been relatively low.[113] Dental health educators must educate the public regarding the value of sealants, so they will be able to make informed decisions concerning their feasibility for themselves and their children.

Preventive Measures Directed Toward the Disease Substrate: Nutritional Counseling

Human carbohydrate intake consists of approximately 47% starch and 53% sugar. The average American consumes about 2.5 pounds of caloric sweeteners per week. Over 70% of this sugar is derived from foods and beverages that are presweetened through processing. Sugar is the major food additive currently used in the United States. In addition to desserts and soft drinks, sugar in its various forms, e.g., glucose, fructose, and sucrose, can be found in salad dressings, most canned foods, cured meats, frozen TV dinners, ketchup, and breakfast cereals, to name a few.[7]

Not all patients eat an excess of sugary foods. For those individuals who do and who are highly susceptible to caries, dietary counseling can be beneficial. A simple initial screening is required to review a patient's typical dietary intake over the past 1 to 5 days, based on the educator's preference. This assessment will assist in identifying possible dietary excesses or deficiencies relevant to sugar and caries as well as numerous other disorders, e.g., sodium and hypertension, cholesterol and atherosclerosis, and vitamin C and poor wound healing. The dental health educator's role is to offer advice on food selection, alternate

snacks, and preparation of foods based on the patient's likes and dislikes. The educator is also responsible for exploring the reasoning behind why, when, and where the patient eats certain foods. Responsibility for making dietary modifications lies with the patient. After the dental health educator has succeeded in involving the patient in the planning and implementation of his own dietary program, a series of follow-up appointments are made to evaluate the patient's cooperation.

Diet counseling does not succeed with everyone. People who agree to counseling must be willing to expend a great deal of effort to alter their eating habits. They must give a high priority to preventive health care which translates in their desire to preserve their natural dentition for a lifetime.

DENTAL DISEASE AND PREVENTION: A SUMMARY

Despite strides made in dentistry over the past two decades, dental caries and periodontal disease continue to be the most dominant of dental diseases as well as two of the most common afflictions known to man. The major impact these diseases have on society warrants the implementation of nationwide preventive dental health education programs. These programs must be tailored to meet the specific dental health needs of a variety of target groups, from the unborn child to the elderly.

A significant part of prevention entails not only educating the populace about the necessity for making routine visits to the dentist and practicing good dental health habits, but also involves the maintenance of a preventive philosophy on the part of the dental health educator. A surface white spot lesion should not be penetrated with explorer and restored, but should be treated noninvasively with fluoride. A patient with light to moderate calculus and inflamed gingival tissue should not merely receive an oral prophylaxis during the appointment; equal time should be spent on oral hygiene measures that will enable him to prevent the recurrence of gingivitis in his own mouth. Thirty-minute appointments will not accomplish this goal.

The accent of the 1990s and future decades will be on prevention and aesthetics. Health education creates an aware, responsible individual, actively involved in his own personal health and fitness. It can therefore be expected that this person will also be interested in the prevention of oral diseases and the attainment of a beautiful smile.

REFERENCES

1. World Health Organization: The Etiology and Prevention of Dental Caries. WHO Technical Report Series, #494. Geneva, World Health Organization, 1972.
2. Wilkins, R. M.: Clinical Practice of the Dental Hygienist. 6th Ed. Philadelphia, Lea & Febiger, 1989.
3. Moore, W. J., and Corbett, M. E.: The distribution of dental caries in ancient British populations. I. Caries Res., 5:151–168, 1971.
4. Leigh, R. W.: Dental pathology of Indian tribes of varied environmental and food conditions. Am. J. Phys. Anthropol., 15:315–325, 1931.
5. Young, W. O., Burt, B. A., and Striffler, D. F.: The epidemiology of oral diseases. In Dentistry, Dental Practice, and the Community. 3rd Ed. Philadelphia, W. B. Saunders, 1983.
6. Newbrun, E.: Cariology. Baltimore, Williams & Wilkins, 1983.
7. Nizel, A. E., and Papas, A. S.: Nutrition in Clinical Dentistry. 3rd Ed. Philadelphia, W. B. Saunders, 1989.
8. Dunning, J. M.: Principles of Dental Public Health. 4th Ed. Cambridge, MA, Harvard University Press, 1986.
9. U.S. Public Health Service, National Institute of Dental Research: Oral Health of United States Adults and Seniors: 1985–86. National Institutes of Health. Publication #(PHS)87-2868, U.S. Dept. of Health and Human Services, 1987.
10. Martinsson, T.: Socioeconomic investigation of schoolchildren with high and low caries frequency. Odont. Rev., 23:93–113, 1972.
11. U.S. Public Health Service, National Institute of Dental Research: Caries Prevalence in U.S. Schoolchildren 1986–1987. National Institutes of Health. Publication #(PHS)89-2247, U.S. Dept. of Health and Human Services, 1989.
12. Office of Disease Prevention and Health Promotion: Disease Prevention and Health Promotion: The Facts. U.S. Public Health Service. Palo Alto, Bull Publishing, 1988.
13. Klein, H., and Palmer, C. E.: Sex differences in dental caries experience of elementary schoolchildren. Pub. Health Rep., 53:1685–90, 1938.
14. U.S. Public Health Service, National Center for Health Statistics: Oral hygiene in adults; United States, 1960–62. Kelly, J. E., Van Kirk, L. E., and Garst, C. C. Publication #(PHS)1000-Ser. 11 No. 16. Washington, DC, Government Printing Office, 1966.
15. U.S. Public Health Service, National Center for Health Statistics: Basic data on dental examination findings of persons 1-74 years: United States, 1971–1974. Kelly, J. E. and Harvey, C. R. DHEW publication #(PHS) 79-1626-Ser. 11-No. 214. Washington, DC, Government Printing Office, 1979.
16. Ringelberg, M. L., Matonski, G. M., and Kimball, A. W.: Dental caries experience in three generations of families. J. Pub. Health Dent., 34:174–180, 1974.
17. Mansbridge, J. N.: Heredity and dental caries. J. Dent. Res., 38:337–347, 1959.
18. Dunning, J. M.: Measurement of short-term changes in dental caries associated with stress: Four case reports. J. Prev. Dent., 6:291–295, 1980.
19. Burstone, M. S.: The psychosomatic aspects of dental problems. J. Am. Dent. Assoc., 33:862–871, 1946.
20. Dunning, J. M., Hyde, R. W., and Dalton, P. J.: Dental disease in psychiatric patients. J. Dent. Res., 30:806–814, 1951.
21. Moller, I. J.: Impact of oral diseases across cultures. Int. Dent. J., 28:376–380, 1978.
22. U.S. Public Health Service, Center for Disease Control: Fluoridation Census 1985. U.S. Dept. of Health and Human Services, 1988.
23. McCann, D. (Ed.): Fluoride and oral health: A story of achievements and challenges. J. Am. Dent. Assoc., 118:529–540, 1989.
24. U.S. Public Health Service: Public Health Service Drinking Water Standards 1962. Publication #(PHS)956. Washington, DC, Government Printing Office, 1962.
25. Granath, L., and McHugh, W. D.: Basic Prevention for the Individual. In Systemized Prevention of Oral Disease: Theory and Practice. Granath, L., and McHugh, W. D. Boca Raton, CRC Press, 1986.
26. Woodall, I. R., et al: Comprehensive Dental Hygiene Care. St. Louis, C.V. Mosby, 1989.
27. Harris, N. O., and Christen, A. G.: Primary Preventive Dentistry. 2nd Ed. Norwalk, CT, Appleton & Lange, 1987.
28. Silverstone, L. M.: Caries and remineralization. Dent. Hyg., 57:30–36, 1983.
29. Heifetz, S. B., et al.: Programs for the mass control of plaque; an appraisal. J. Pub. Health Dent., 33:91–95, 1973.
30. Sutcliffe, P.: A longitudinal clinical study of oral cleanliness and dental caries in schoolchildren. Arch. Oral Biol., 18:765–770, 1973.
31. Axelsson, P., and Lindhe, J.: The effect of a preventive programme on dental plaque, gingivitis, and caries in schoolchildren: Results after one and two years. J. Clin. Periodontol., 1:126–138, 1974.
32. Axelsson, P., and Lindhe, J.: Effect of fluoride on gingivitis and dental caries in a preventive program based on plaque control. Community Dent. Oral Epidemiol., 3:156–160, 1975.
33. Axelsson, P., Lindhe, J., and Waseby, J.: The effect of various plaque control measures on gingivitis and caries in schoolchildren. Community Dent. Oral Epidemiol., 4:232–239, 1976.
34. Lindhe, J., and Axelsson, P.: The effect of proper oral hygiene and topical fluoride application on caries and gingivitis in Swedish schoolchildren. Community Dent. Oral Epidemiol., 1:9–16, 1973.
35. Ranney, R. R.: Pathogenesis of periodontal disease. In International Conference on Research in the Biology of

Periodontal Disease. Chicago, University of Illinois School of Dentistry, 1977.

36. Moore, W. J., and Corbett, M. E.: The distribution of dental caries in ancient British populations. II. Caries Res., 7:139–153, 1973.

37. Allen, D. L., McFall, W. T., and Jenzano, J.: Periodontics for the Dental Hygienist. 4th Ed. Philadelphia, Lea & Febiger, 1987.

38. Listgarten, M. A.: Structure of the microbial flora associated with periodontal health and disease in man. J. Periodontol., 47:1, 1976.

39. Listgarten, M. A., and Hillden, L.: Relative distribution of bacteria at clinically healthy and periodontally diseased sites in humans. J. Clin. Periodontol., 5:115, 1978.

40. Socransky, S. S., et al.: New concepts of destructive periodontal disease. J. Clin. Periodontol., 11:21, 1984.

41. Weinmann, J. P.: Pathway of inflammation to underlying periodontal structures. J. Periodontol., 12:71, 1941.

42. Page, R. C., and Schroeder, H. E.: Pathogenesis of inflammatory periodontal disease. Lab. Invest., 33:235, 1976.

43. Page, R. C., et al.: Rapidly progressive periodontitis: A distinct clinical condition. J. Periodontol., 54:197, 1983.

44. Rambler, R. W., and Dull, H. B. (Ed.): Closing the Gap: The Burden of Unnecessary Illness. New York, Oxford University Press, 1987.

45. Periodontal disease in America: A personal and national tragedy [reprint of 1980 JPHD article]. Dent. Hyg., 58:10–18, 1984.

46. Russell, A. L.: Some epidemiological characteristics of periodontal disease in a series of urban populations. J. Periodontol., 28:286–293, 1957.

47. Douglass, C. W., et al.: National trends in the prevalence and severity of periodontal diseases. J. Am. Dent. Assoc., 107:403–412, 1983.

48. Russell, A. L.: World epidemiology and health. In Environmental Variables in Oral Disease. Edited by S. J. Kreshover and F. J. McClure. American Association for the Advancement of Science, Publication #81, Washington, DC, 1966.

49. Anderson, B. G.: Hypertrophic gingivitis among Chinese. Nat. Med. J. China, 15:453–454, 1929.

50. Mehta, F. S., et al.: Relative importance of the various causes of tooth loss. All-India Dent. Assoc. J., 30:211–221, 1958.

51. Loe, H., et al.: The natural history of periodontal disease in man: Study design and baseline data. J. Periodont. Res., 13:550–562, 1978.

52. Loe, H., et al.: The natural history of periodontal disease in man: Tooth mortality rates before 40 years of age. J. Periodont. Res., 13:563–572, 1978.

53. Loe, H., et al.: The natural history of periodontal disease in man: The rate of periodontal destruction before 40 years of age. J. Periodontol., 49:607–620, 1978.

54. Sheridan, P. (Ed.): National Institute of Dental Research: 40 years of progress. J. Am. Dent. Assoc., 116:837–844, 1988.

55. Glickman, I.: Clinical Periodontology. 3rd Ed. Philadelphia, W. B. Saunders, 1964.

56. Stoll, F. A.: Dental Health Education. 5th Ed. Philadelphia, Lea & Febiger, 1977.

57. Lynch, M. A. (Ed.): Burket's Oral Medicine: Diagnosis and Treatment. 7th Ed. Philadelphia, J. B. Lippincott, 1977.

58. Belting, C. M., and Gupta, O. P.: Incidence of periodontal disease among persons with neuropsychiatric disorders. J. Dent. Res., 39:744–745, 1960.

59. Bossert, W. A., and Marks, H. H.: Prevalence and characteristics of periodontal disease of 12,800 persons under periodic dental observation. J. Am. Dent. Assoc., 52:429–442, 1956.

60. Benjamin, C. M., Russell, A. L., and Smiley, R. D.: Periodontal disease in rural children of 25 Indiana counties. J. Periodontol., 28:294–298, 1957.

61. Newmann, M. G., and Socransky, S. S.: Predominant cultivable microbiota in periodontosis. J. Periodont. Res., 12:120, 1977.

62. Navia, J. M.: Research advances and needs in nutrition in oral health and disease. In Nutrition in Oral Health and Disease. Edited by R. L. Pollack and E. Kravitz. Philadelphia, Lea & Febiger, 1985.

63. Navia, J. M.: Nutrition in oral health and disease. In A Textbook of Preventive Dentistry. 2nd Ed. Edited by R. E. Stallard. Philadelphia, W. B. Saunders, 1982.

64. Nisengard, R. J.: The role of immunology in periodontal disease. J. Periodontol., 48:505, 1977.

65. Svanberg, M., and Rolla, G.: Streptococcus mutans in plaque and saliva after mouthrinsing with SnF_2. Scand. J. Dent. Res., 90:292–298, 1982.

66. Svanberg, M., and Westergren, G.: Effect of SnF_2 administered as a mouthrinse or topically applied on Streptococcus mutans, Streptococcus sanguis, and lactobacilli in dental plaque and saliva. Scand. J. Dent. Res., 91:123–129, 1983.

67. Tinanoff, N., and Weeks, D. B.: Current status of SnF_2 as an antiplaque agent. Pediatr. Dent., 1:199–204, 1979.

68. Lovdal, A., et al.: Incidence of clinical manifestations of periodontal disease in light of oral hygiene and calculus formation. Am. Dent. Assoc. J., 56:21–33, 1958.

69. Russell, A. L., and Ayers, P.: Periodontal disease and socioeconomic status in Birmingham, Alabama. Am. J. Pub. Health, 50:206–214, 1960.

70. Russell, A. L., et al.: Periodontal disease and nutrition in South Vietnam. J. Dent. Res., 44:775–782, 1965.

71. Schei, O., et al.: Alveolar bone loss as related to oral hygiene and age. J. Periodontol., 30:7–16, 1959.

72. Sheiham, A.: The epidemiology of chronic periodontal disease in Western Nigerian schoolchildren. J. Periodont. Res., 3:257–267, 1968.

73. Sheiham, A.: Dental cleanliness and chronic periodontal disease: Studies on populations in Britain. Brit. Dent. J., 120:413–418, 1970.

74. Todd, J. E.: Children's Dental Health in England and Wales, 1973. London, Her Majesty's Stationary Office, 1975.

75. U.S. Public Health Service, National Center for Health Statistics: Periodontal disease in adults: United States, 1960–62. Kelly, J. E., and Van Kirk, L. E. Publication #(PHS)1000-Ser. 11-No. 12, Washington, DC, Government Printing Office, 1972.

76. Jong, A. W. (Ed): Community Dental Health. 2nd Ed. St. Louis, C. V. Mosby, 1988.

77. Bass, C. C.: The optimum characteristics of toothbrushes for personal oral hygiene. Dent. Items, 70:696, 1948.

78. Toon, S.: Rubbing out the bad guys. R. D. H., 7:10–11, 15, 1987.

79. Interplak electric toothbrush, Bausch and Lomb Oral Care Division, Inc., 5243 Royal Woods Pkwy, Suite 100, Tucker, GA 30084.

80. Rota-dent electric toothbrush, Pro-Dentec Co., Batesville, AK.

81. Mueller, L. J., et al.: Rotary electric toothbrushing: Clinical effects on the presence of gingivitis and supragingival dental plaque. Dent. Hyg., 61:546–549, 1987.

82. Lobene, R., and Soparker, P.: Use of dental floss, effect on plaque and gingivitis. Clin. Prev. Dent., 4:5, 1982.

83. Lang, N. P., and Raber, K.: Use of oral irrigation as a ve-

hicle for the application of antimicrobial agents in chemical plaque control. J. Clin. Periodontol., 8:177, 1981.

84. Eakle, W. S., Ford, C., and Boyd, R. L.: Depth of penetration in periodontal pockets with oral irrigation. J. Clin. Periodontol., 13:39, 1986.

85. McCann, D. (Ed.): Periodontal research: Exploring new horizons. J. Am. Dent. Assoc., 119:481–489, 1989.

86. Kaufmann, A. Y., et al.: Reduction of dental plaque formation by chlorhexidine dihydrochloride lozenges. J. Periodont. Res., 24:59–62, 1989.

87. Strom, T. (Ed.): Nonsurgical antibacterial approaches to periodontal treatment. J. Am. Dent. Assoc., 116:22–32, 1988.

88. Vick, V., and Ciancio, S. C.: Chemical Warfare. R. D. H., 8:30–34, 1988.

89. Brownstein, C., et al.: Gingival irrigation with chlorhexidine resolves naturally occurring gingivitis. Presented at the American Academy of Periodontology meeting, San Antonio, Texas, 1987.

90. Sherrill, C. A., and Krouse, M.: A critical look at recent dentifrice claims. Dent. Hyg., 60:410–411, 1986.

91. Southard, G. L., et al.: Sanguinarine, a new antiplaque agent: Retention and plaque specificity. J. Am. Dent. Assoc., 108:338, 1984.

92. Ciancio, S. G. (Ed.): Lack of efficacy of a prebrushing rinse. Biol. Therapies in Dent., 5:1, 3–4, 1989.

93. Horowitz, H. S., et al.: School fluoridation studies in Elk Lake, Pennsylvania, and Pike County, Kentucky: Results after eight years. Am. J. Pub. Health, 58:2240, 1968.

94. Dental caries prevention in primary care projects. U.S. Dept of Health and Human Services, Public Health Service, 1985.

95. Ripa, L.: A guide to the use of fluorides for the prevention of dental caries. J. Am. Dent. Assoc., 113:502, 1986.

96. Blong, M. A., et al.: Effects of a gel containing 0.4 percent stannous fluoride on dentinal hypersensitivity. Dent. Hyg., 59:489–492, 1985.

97. Ismail, A. I., et al.: Findings from the dental care supplement of the national health interview survey, 1983. J. Am. Dent. Assoc., 114:617–621, 1987.

98. Lind, O. P., et al.: Anticaries effect of a 2% Na$_2$PO$_3$F-dentifrice in a Danish fluoride area. Community Dent. Oral Epidemiol., 4:7–14, 1976.

99. Marthaler, T. M.: Caries inhibition by an amine fluoride dentifrice: Results after 6 years in children with low caries activity. Helv. Odont. Acta, 18:35–44, 1974.

100. von de Fehr, F. R., and Moller, I. J.: Caries-preventive fluoride dentifrices. Caries Res., 12(Suppl. 1):31–37, 1978.

101. Horowitz, H. S., et al.: A program of self-administered fluorides in a rural school system. Community Dent. Oral Epidemiol., 8:177–183, 1980.

102. Council on Dental Therapeutics: Fluoride compounds. In Accepted Dental Therapeutics. 40th Ed. Chicago, American Dental Association, 1984.

103. Tobin, E. A.: Dental fluorosis in children in the 1980s: A review of the literature. Dent. Hyg., 62:380–384, 1988.

104. Isokangas, P., et al.: Xylitol chewing gum in caries prevention: A field study in children. J. Am. Dent. Assoc., 117:315–320, 1988.

105. Consensus: Oral health effects of products that increase salivary flow rate. J. Am. Dent. Assoc., 116:757, 1988.

106. Council on Dental Materials and Devices: Pit and fissure sealants. J. Am. Dent. Assoc., 93:134, 1976.

107. Ripa, L. W., et al.: Preventing Pit and Fissure Caries: A Guide to Sealant Use. Massachusetts Dept. of Public Health, Massachusetts Health Research Institute, Inc., 1986.

108. Ripa, L. W.: The current status of pit and fissure sealants: A review. Can. Dent. Assoc. J., 5:367, 1985.

109. Horowitz, H. S., Heifetz, S. B., and Poulsen, S.: Retention and effectiveness of a single application of an adhesive sealant in preventing occlusal caries: Final report after five years of study in Kalispell, Montana. J. Am. Dent. Assoc., 95:1133–1139, 1977.

110. Silverstone, L. M.: Fissure sealants: Laboratory studies. Caries Res., 8:2–26, 1974.

111. Silverstone, L. M.: Operative measures for caries prevention. Caries Res., 12(Suppl. 1):103–112, 1978.

112. Hicks, M. J., and Silverstone, L. M.: The effect of sealant application and sealant loss on caries-like formation in vitro. Pediatr. Dent., 4:111–114, 1982.

113. Frazier, P. J.: Use of sealants: Societal and professional factors. J. Dent. Educ., 48(Suppl. 2):80–95, 1984.

Chapter 4

THE BEGINNING: PRENATAL, INFANT, AND EARLY CHILDHOOD DENTAL HEALTH

The infant comes into the world bringing formidable capabilities to establish human relatedness. Immediately he is a partner in shaping his first and foremost relationship.

Daniel Stern
1977

As early as the first day of life, the human neonate moves in precise and sustained segments of movements that are synchronous with the articulated structure of adult speech.

W. Condon and L. Sander
1974

GROWTH AND DEVELOPMENT

The life of a child from conception to age 3 years is clearly the most profound period of a human being's growth and development. Growth is synonymous with size, whereas development relates to an individual's cognitive, psychomotor, and affective levels of functioning.[1,2]

Prenatal

The prenatal period extends from conception to birth (40 weeks). During the first 8 weeks of intrauterine life, the zygotye (fertilized ovum) is often termed the *embryo*. It is at this stage that rapid differentiation of cells into major organs with a human form occurs. From the eighth to the fortieth weeks of gestation the embryo becomes known as the *fetus*. Early in this period, the circulatory system attains maturity, while other organ systems follow developmentally. Fetal respiration might begin as early as the eighteenth week in utero, but the alveoli cannot be considered functionally developed to permit survival until approximately the twenty-eighth week.[3]

Although neurologic activity is first noted at 8 weeks' gestation, it is not until approximately the fourteenth week that flowing movements of the fetus can be produced on stimulation of all areas except the posterior portion of the head, back, and the vertex. The mother first perceives movement at this time. The fetus might also show signs of swallowing by the fourteenth week; sucking action to gain nourishment is attempted at 29 weeks.[3]

Infancy

The span of time from birth through the second year of life is referred to as infancy.[4] The average newborn infant weighs 3.4 kg, is 51 cm long, and has a head circumference of 35 cm. The full-term infant will usually double his birth weight in less than 6 months and triple it by his first birthday.[3]

A newborn can turn his head from side to side when placed prone on a flat surface. By 4 weeks he can lift his head above the surface, and at about 8 weeks he can smile and coo. Visual fixation on light or a bright object usually occurs hours or days after birth, but the infant's ability to follow it through a 180° arc is often accomplished prior to 3 months of age. By 12 weeks, the infant has some head control when pulled from a supine to a sitting position, but control is generally irregular when the infant is upright, resulting in head-bobbing until approximately 4 months. The grasp reflex becomes more discriminatory at 12 weeks, as hand-eye coordination improves. By 6 months the infant is rolling over and can sit alone.[3]

Vowel sounds and imitative behavior are also observed at approximately 6 months of age; if the parent taps the high chair tray, so might he. Repetitive consonant sounds are initiated, e.g., ba-ba, da-da, at approximately 8 months, along with maintenance of a standing position. Crawling, waving bye-bye, and clapping hands are usually accomplished by 9 months. Walking most often follows and is mastered in most cases by 15 months of age.[3]

During the second year of life (12 to 24 months) there is a decline in the rate of growth (the infant gaining only about 2.3 kg in mass and 13 cm in height), but an acceleration in development. At 1 year, the infant is beginning to enjoy his environment through nursery rhymes, pat-a-cake, and simple repetitive play, e.g., rolling a ball back and forth. By 18 months, the infant can run stiffly, climb stairs, begin stacking blocks, and has a vocabulary of about 10 words. Between 18 and 24 months toilet needs are often verbalized.[3]

Although the infant continues imitative behavior through his second year of life, he becomes increasingly aware of those around him, particularly siblings, and he chooses solitary play. Possessive behavior emerges as he reacts to their desire to engage in play with him and with what he feels are his objects. Normally, by his second birthday the infant will be able to put three words together. How remarkable to think that in 33 short months a single ovum becomes fertilized and develops into a living, breathing human being with needs, emotions, and the ability to walk, talk, and play.

Early Childhood

At 2 years the stage known as early childhood begins and continues to age 6.[4] During this third year of life, the child begins to become interested in play activities that involve other children. By 3 years he begins to share, is anxious to please, responds to verbal guidance, and is highly imaginative. He can also give his name and age and can identify his sex as boy or girl when asked.

Steady weight and height gain of about 2 kg and 6.5 to 9 cm respectively per year usually occur during the third, fourth, and fifth years of life.[3]

Refined motor control allows the 3-year-old to ascend steps with alternating feet; at age 4 he can descend steps by alteration. By 5 most children can hop on one foot and begin to skip.[3]

OROFACIAL GROWTH AND DEVELOPMENT

Development of the head and oral cavity is highly complex and one of the most miraculous examples of growth and development known to man. Therefore, the dental health of the pregnant mother and fetus, infant, and preschooler cannot be overemphasized. Conditions such as cleft lip and palate, caries, periodontal disease, bad oral habits, malocclusions, and developmental interferences creating dental anomalies such as missing teeth, poorly shaped and formed teeth can all occur during these formative years.

Embryonic Development of the Head and Neck

Observable growth of the face begins about the fourth week in utero with the development of the branchial arches. They include one frontonasal process, two maxillary processes, and two mandibular processes that surround the entrance into the oral cavity or stomatodeum.[5] These depressions and protuberances are rapidly transformed into the features of a face by the seventh month of fetal life (Table 4-1).[1]

As the maxillary processes migrate to the midline they join the lateral nasal fold of the frontonasal process, forming a shelf on the medial side of each of the maxillary processes. These shelves unite at the midline and normally complete the fusion by the eighth week in utero, giving rise to the lip, alveolar ridge, and the hard and soft palate. Failure of these processes to fuse results in oral or facial clefts or both.[1] The degree of clefting depends on the stage of embryonic development when the congenital malformation takes place.

Growth of the lateral and medial nasal processes is responsible for the development of the bridge of the nose during the seventh and eighth weeks of intrauterine life.[6] In addition, the eyes position more anteriorly during this period (Fig. 4-1).[5]

The mandibular processes fuse at the midline before the maxillary and nasal processes do. The mandible of the embryo is larger than the maxilla until the fetal stage, when the reverse becomes true, resulting in micrognathia, which is common at birth.[1]

Overall head size accounts for approximately half of the embryo's total body length. By the fifth month of gestation, the head size decreases to a proportion of one-

Table 4-1. Developing Structures of the Head and Face

Structure	Initiation (Weeks in Utero)
Neural plate	2
Buccopharyngeal membrane	2
Mandibular arch initiation	3
Hypoglossal muscles (tongue)	5
Medial and lateral nasal processes	5
Lens of the eye	5
Retina	5
External carotid artery	6
Eustachian tube	6
Larynx	6
Maxillary process	6
External auditory meatus	7
Nasal septum	8
Two palatal shelves fuse together	8
Palatal shelves fuse with nasal septum	10
Ossification of craniofacial skeleton	10
Eyelids completely formed and closed	10
Eyelids open	28

From Pinkham, J. R., et al.: Pediatric Dentistry: Infancy Through Adolescence. Philadelphia, W. B. Saunders, 1988, p. 114.

third and at birth it is one-fourth the length of the infant's body.[1]

At birth, the infant's face appears very similar to those of other newborns. The cranium, forehead, and eyes are large in comparison to the small nose, mouth, ears, mandible, and retruded, virtually nonexistent chin. Although the face is nearly as wide as that of an adult, only 40% of facial height is completed at birth.[7] Vertical growth drastically escalates during the first 3 years of life. Miraculously, this uniform-looking infant face develops into a unique child and adolescent face with distinct and explicit characteristics.

Stages of Tooth Development

Odontogenesis, or the formation of the primary dentition, begins as early as 6

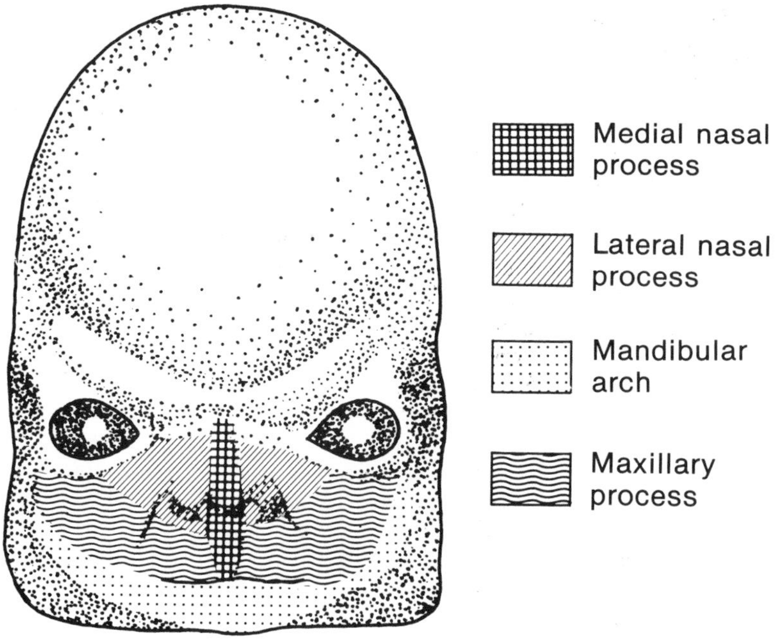

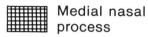
Medial nasal process

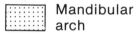
Lateral nasal process

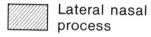
Mandibular arch

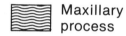
Maxillary process

Figure 4-1. Development of the human face; embryo 18 mm long, eighth week. From Orban, B. J.: Oral Histology and Embryology. 4th Ed. St. Louis, C. V. Mosby, 1957; modified from Sicher, H., and Tandler, J.: Anatomie für Zahnärtze [Anatomy for dentists], Berlin, Julius Springer Verlag, 1928.

weeks in utero with a thickening of the epithelium in the areas where future dental arches will form. These epithelial enlargements represent the dental lamina for each tooth germ. By 8 weeks, 10 spherical zones can be found on both the mandible and the maxilla, delineating the positions of the future primary teeth. At approximately $3\frac{1}{2}$ months in utero, the first permanent molar tooth germ begins formation.[1]

Intially each tooth germ is bud-shaped, formed from ectoderm. As it develops it evolves into a cap shape, incorporating mesoderm into its structure. Ectoderm is responsible for the dental or enamel organ, which consists of four layers of epithelial cells: outer enamel epithelium, stellate reticulum, stratum intermedium, and inner enamel epithelium. The inner enamel epithelium gives rise to ameloblasts. The basement membrane, which separates ameloblasts from the mesoderm, defines the boundaries of the dentinoenamel junction (DEJ). The mesoderm within the concavity of the final bell stage is responsible for the dental papilla, which produces pulp and dentin. The mesoderm surrounding the bell is known as the dental sac. It gives rise to cementum, periodontal ligament, and some alveolar bone (Fig. 4-2).

Although tooth development is a continuous process, the tooth germ undergoes six physiologic stages of development similar to those of other calcified tissues. They are:

Initiation
Proliferation
Histodifferentiation
Morphodifferentiation
Apposition
Calcification

DEVELOPMENTAL ANOMALIES OF ENAMEL AND DENTIN

A variety of disturbances associated with the developmental stages of tooth development can generate clinical aberrations of enamel and dentin. Since specific teeth (e.g., primary, permanent, maxillary, mandibular, central, lateral) and specific parts of the teeth (e.g., crown or roots) develop at different periods of time, the teeth so affected, the location of the defect on the tooth, and the anomalies that result depend on the type of interference (systemic or

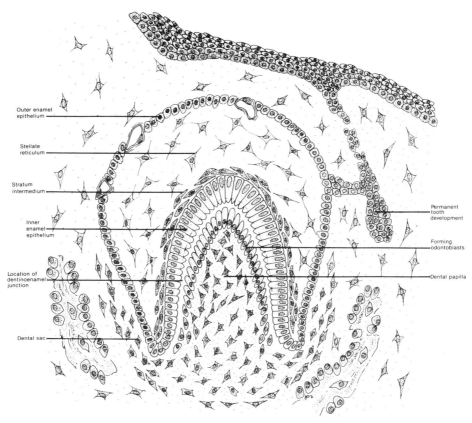

Outer enamel epithelium

Stellate reticulum

Stratum intermedium

Inner enamel epithelium

Location of dentinoenamel junction

Dental sac

Permanent tooth development

Forming odontoblasts

Dental papilla

Figure 4-2. Bell stage of odontogenesis, immediately before the onset of dentin and enamel formation. Original drawing courtesy of D. Overman, Ph.D., West Virginia University.

local) and the stage of the tooth's development at the time the disturbance took place. An interference in utero will affect the primary teeth predominantly, but if the insult occurs after the first year of life only certain permanent teeth will show signs of aberrant development. Conversely, once a malformation is noticed, it becomes quite challenging for the dental health educator to investigate the origin of the medical or dental disturbance and approximate the prenatal or postnatal age at which it occurred.[8] Knowledge of the chronology of both dentitions is invaluable (Table 4-2).[9]

Initiation

Formation of the dental lamina and the subsequent tooth germ starts with the initiation phase, often referred to as the bud

stage. Interferences in development at this point, such as cleft palate, radiation exposure to the pregnant mother, or congenital ectodermal dysplasia, can result in the complete absence (anodontia) or partial absence of teeth (oligodontia) (Fig. 4-3).

Heredity also plays a major role in hypodontia. A missing succedaneous permanent tooth can be correlated approximately 30% of the time with absence of its primary tooth counterpart, because they develop from the dental lamina proper on the lingual aspect of the primary tooth germ.[10] Permanent molars arise from the posterior or distal extension of the dental lamina of the second primary molar.[1]

A developmental disturbance creating excessive cellular activity during this stage can result in the development of supernumerary teeth. Excess teeth affect 0.2 to 4.5% of the population and rarely involve the primary

Table 4-2. Chronology of the Human Dentition

Tooth	Hard Tissue Formation Begins	Amount of Enamel at Birth	Enamel Completed	Eruption	Root Completed (years)	Exfoliation (years)
PRIMARY DENTITION						
Maxillary						
Central incisor	3½ mo in utero	Five-sixths	1½ mo	7½ mo	1½	6–7
Lateral incisor	4 mo in utero	Two-thirds	2½ mo	9 mo	2	7–8
Canine	4½ mo in utero	One-third	9 mo	18 mo	3½	10–12
First molar	4 mo in utero	Cusps united	6 mo	14 mo	2½	9–11
Second molar	4½ mo in utero	Cusp tips still isolated	11 mo	24 mo	3	10–12
Mandibular						
Central incisor	3½ mo in utero	Three-fifths	2½ mo	6 mo	1½	6–7
Lateral incisor	4 mo in utero	Three-fifths	3 mo	7 mo	1½	7–8
Canine	4½ mo in utero	One-third	9 mo	16 mo	3½	9–12
First molar	4 mo in utero	Cusps united	5½ mo	12 mo	2¼	9–11
Second molar	4½ mo in utero	Cusp tips still isolated	10 mo	20 mo	3	10–12
PERMANENT DENTITION						
Maxillary						
Central incisor	3–4 mo	—	4–5 yr	7–8 yr	10	
Lateral incisor	10–12 mo	—	4–5 yr	8–9 yr	11	
Canine	4–5 mo	—	6–7 yr	11–12 yr	13–15	
First premolar	1½–1¾ yr	—	5–6 yr	10–12 yr	12–13	
Second premolar	2–2¼ yr	—	6–7 yr	10–12 yr	12–14	
First molar	At birth	Sometimes a trace	2½–3 yr	6–7 yr	9–10	
Second molar	2½–3 yr	—	7–8 yr	12–13 yr	14–16	
Third molar	7–9 yr	—	12–16 yr	17–21 yr	18–25	
Mandibular						
Central incisor	3–4 mo	—	4–5 yr	6–7 yr	9	
Lateral incisor	3–4 mo	—	4–5 yr	7–8 yr	10	
Canine	4–5 mo	—	6–7 yr	9–10 yr	12–14	
First premolar	1¾–2 yr	—	5–6 yr	10–12 yr	12–13	
Second premolar	2¼–2½ yr	—	6–7 yr	11–12 yr	13–14	
First molar	At birth	Sometimes a trace	2½–3 yr	6–7 yr	9–10	
Second molar	2½–3 yr	—	7–8 yr	11–13 yr	14–15	
Third molar	8–10 yr	—	12–16 yr	17–21 yr	18–25	

From Logan, W. G. H., and Kronfeld, R., Chronology of the Human Dentition. J.A.D.A., *20:*379–427, 1933; slightly modified by McCall and Schour, and revised by Kraus, 1959. Copyright of the American Dental Association. Reprinted with permission.

dentition.[11] The most common site of occurrence is the maxillary anterior region between the central incisors. This is known as a mesiodens.[6] Predeciduous or natal teeth are supernumerary teeth that are present at birth. The frequency of this condition is 1 in 4000, and it is most likely attributed to the tooth germ involved developing in a more superficial position.[12] It usually affects mandibular incisors; their mobility appears to be related to their attachment in soft tissue and the absence of roots.[3] The crowns are defective and removal is generally recommended, particularly if looseness poses

the threat of aspiration. In contrast, primary teeth that erupt prematurely (during the first few weeks of life) are known as neonatal teeth. This occurs in approximately 1 in 2000 births.[3,13] These teeth are usually normal primary teeth and should be retained. A radiograph should be taken to confirm the differential diagnosis.

Proliferation

The proliferation stage is characterized by rapid multiplication of the epithelial cells

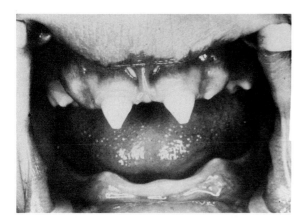

Figure 4-3. Ectodermal dysplasia. Courtesy of the Dental Training Project, Long Island Jewish Hillside Medical Center.

from the initiation stage, forming a cap-like appearance. Interference in development at this time can cause the formation of teeth with more or fewer cusps or roots than the norm. Anomalies such as fusion or gemination can occur. Fusion involves the union of two normally separate tooth germs, leading to a single large tooth (Fig. 4-4); in gemination a single tooth incompletely divides into what appears to be two teeth with two separate pulp chambers and one pulp canal (Fig. 4-5).

Histodifferentiation

Differentiation of cells of the developing tooth into specialized components is the function of this stage; it is often referred to as the bell stage. As discussed previously, cells of the inner enamel epithelium become ameloblasts and peripheral cells of the dental papilla become odontoblasts. An interference during the histodifferentiation stage of development can affect the structural framework of the enamel or dentin matrix.

Amelogenesis imperfecta, occurring in 1:14,000 to 1:16,000 births, manifests as teeth void of enamel or covered with brittle enamel that readily detaches itself from the dentin. Dentinogenesis imperfecta has a frequency of 1:8000 and produces an atypical dentin which obliterates pulp chambers and root canals. The teeth appear opalescent in color and are highly susceptible to wear. The roots of affected teeth are short and blunted.[6,14]

Morphodifferentiation

During morphodifferentiation, the specialized cells arrange themselves in a manner that dictates the final shape and size that a particular tooth will take. Anomalies associated with an interference during the morphodifferentiation stage can manifest clinically as peg-laterals, microdontia, macrodontia, dens-in-dente, taurodontism, and dilaceration (Figs. 4-6, 4-7, 4-8).[3] Syphilis during pregnancy can act as an interference affecting the shape and size of the teeth de-

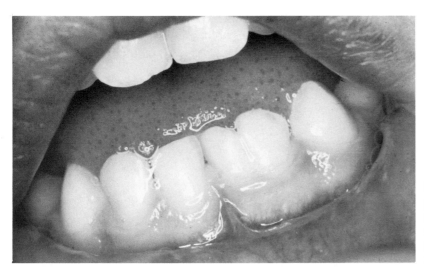

Figure 4-4. Fusion of the primary mandibular left central and lateral incisors. Courtesy of J. E. Bouquot, D.D.S., M.S., West Virginia University.

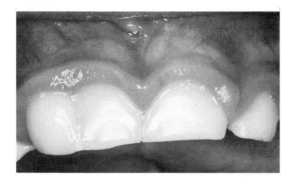

Figure 4-5. Gemination of the primary maxillary right central incisor. Courtesy of D. Holmes, D.D.S., M.S., West Virginia University.

veloping at that time, such as seen in Hutchinson's incisors and mulberry molars. (Figs. 4-9, 4-10).[1]

Apposition

The appositional stage involves the deposition of enamel matrix by ameloblasts and

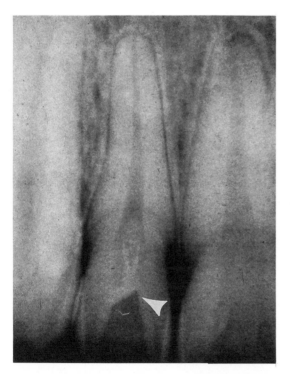

Figure 4-6. Radiograph depicting dens-in-dente of a maxillary lateral incisor. Courtesy of J. E. Bouquot, D.D.S., M.S., West Virginia University.

dentin matrix by odontoblasts. Interferences during this developmental stage can cause hypoplasia or a deficiency in the amount of enamel or dentin formed. Clinical manifestations of hypoplastic tissue include linear depressions, pits, and a thinning of the crown (Fig. 4-11). Such interferences consist of a variety of disorders, both systemic and local, which, depending on the time they occur, can very obviously affect the enamel and dentin of the primary and permanent teeth. Enamel hypoplasia of the primary teeth has been found to occur if the systemic interference curtailed ameloblastic activity prenatally or early during postnatal development. Half of the children who suffer from cerebral palsy[15], phenylketonuria[16], kernicterus following hemolytic disease[17] or whose mothers were infected with rubella during their pregnancy[18] experience enamel hypoplasia of the primary dentition.[6] Systemic disturbances occurring during the first year of life, such as prematurity, vitamin A deficiency, rickets, asthma, and exanthematous fevers, can disrupt the enamel formation of the permanent dentition. Individuals with Down and Hurler syndromes, epidermolysis bullosa, and hypo- or pseudohypoparathyroidism all experience enamel hypoplasia as a consistent dental characteristic.[1] (See Chapter 8.)

Hypoplasia can also be the result of a local insult, e.g., periapical infection or trauma. Severely decayed primary teeth can abscess, transmitting an infectious exudate through the apex of the tooth, thus damaging the permanent tooth developing in the immediate area. The permanent tooth may erupt defective or hypoplastic. Traumatization of a primary tooth through a fall or an accident can transmit impulses to the developing permanent tooth, resulting in an interference in the deposition of enamel matrix by ameloblasts. The permanent teeth of primary precursors affected in such a localized manner have been referred to as Turner teeth[8] (Fig. 4-12).

Hereditary enamel and dentin defects, e.g., amelogenesis and dentinogenesis imperfecta, can also arise during this developmental period. They are usually associ-

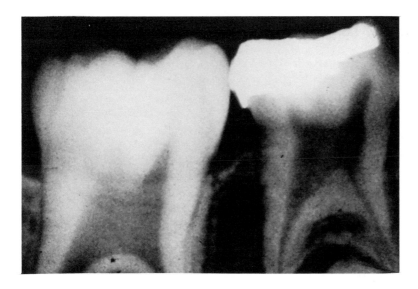

Figure 4-7. Radiograph depicting taurodontism of the primary molars. Note the elongated pulp chambers, defined pulp horns, and short stunted roots. Courtesy of J. E. Bouquot, D.D.S., M.S., West Virginia University.

ated with both the primary and permanent dentition, and the defective surface can involve the entire crown of many or all of the teeth.[6]

Calcification

The next stage in tooth development is calcification or mineralization. During this period, hydroxyapatite crystals are precipitated into the enamel matrix. An interference at this point can result in hypocalcification. This condition is characterized by a sufficient amount of enamel but a deficiency in its mineral content. The resultant enamel is immature. All or portions of the enamel crown can be affected. Clinically, hypocalcified or hypomineralized areas of enamel manifest as white opaque spots on the teeth.

A systemic factor that can be responsible for such a disturbance during this developmental stage is the ingestion of excess fluoride. The mottled enamel that results appears as opaque white with yellow spots or

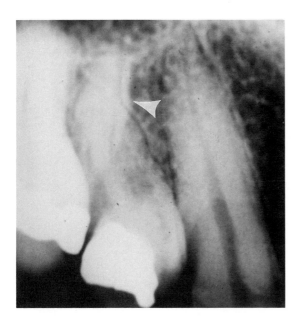

Figure 4-8. Dilaceration of the root of a maxillary premolar. Note the obvious bending of the root.

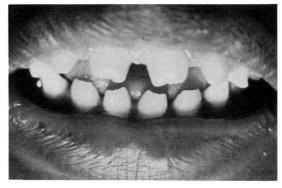

Figure 4-9. Congenital syphilis: Hutchinson's incisors. From Dreizen, S.: The Mouth in Medicine. New York, McGraw-Hill, 1971.

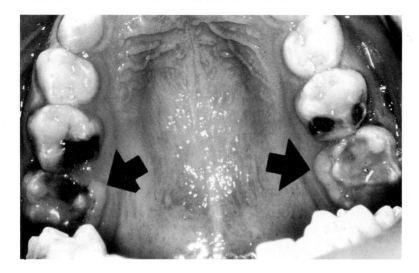

Figure 4-10. Congenital syphilis: mulberry molars. Courtesy of D. Nash, D.M.D., Ed.D., University of Kentucky.

bands. Brown or black bands form in more severe cases of fluorosis.[6] Local factors e.g., periapical infection or trauma and the hereditary condition amelogenesis imperfecta, also impede the calcification process of the enamel.

Tetracycline

Often antibiotics are prescribed to treat the symptoms of a systemic illness, and mothers need to be informed regarding the effect of tetracycline on their children's teeth. Tetracycline should be avoided dur-

ing the developmental period because it is well documented that prenatal as well as postnatal ingestion up to age 8 can lead to permanent discoloration of the teeth. The larger the dosage of the drug relative to body weight, the darker the pigmentation, which ranges from yellow to brown and from gray to black.[14] The ability of tetracycline to intrinsically stain primary and permanent teeth is the result of its reaction with calcium, forming tetracycline-calcium-orthophosphate compounds. Those teeth calcifying at the time the tetracycline is ingested have the drug incorporated in them.[12] Tetracycline-pigmented teeth can also be hy-

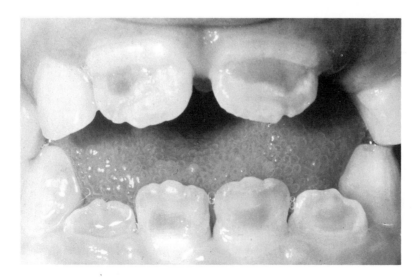

Figure 4-11. Hypoplasia of enamel. Note the pits and linear depressions. Courtesy of D. Holmes, D.D.S., M.S., West Virginia University.

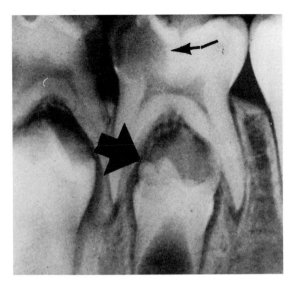

Figure 4-12. Radiograph illustrating Turner's tooth. Chronic apical infection from a carious mandibular second primary molar resulting in severe enamel hypoplasia of the developing succedaneous premolar tooth. Courtesy of P. Pullon, D.D.S., M.S., Palm Beach, FL.

poplastic. The hypoplasia might be related to the illness for which the drug was given rather than the tetracycline itself.[14]

MATERNAL ORAL HEALTH

Pregnant women have been revered throughout history for their beauty and the delicacy of their condition. Pregnancy is a very delicate balance between a mother and child. Because of the unique physiologic communication system that exists during pregnancy, each pregnant woman should strive for optimum health and avoid exposure to potentially harmful conditions or substances as soon as she is aware that she is pregnant. All expectant mothers should receive a dental examination, preventive dental counseling, and any necessary dental treatment as part of their total obstetrical health program.

Prenatal Preventive Counseling

Preventive dental counseling must begin with the mother-to-be, or even better, the woman considering pregnancy. Pregnancy is a time of many changes, resulting in curiosity and a desire to learn. A dental health educator should take advantage of this time. Whether providing one-to-one counseling during a series of dental office visits or speaking to a group of parents during their Lamaze classes, the prenatal educational program should be individualized as well as comprehensive. Table 4-3 is an excellent model program for prenatal and early childhood dental counseling.[1,19] The information gained through counseling must be put into life-long practice to be effective. Both parents need to be knowledgeable regarding the causes of dental disease and need to be motivated to adopt good nutritional and oral hygiene practices themselves so that they can pass them on to their children.

Nutrition

Healthy dietary habits throughout the childbearing years enhance a woman's response to the increased physiologic demands on her during menstruation and pregnancy. If a woman is healthy when she becomes pregnant, her unborn child has a better chance of developing into a healthy baby.

The significance of the pregnant mother's diet became evident during World War II when women were forced to exist on little food. Studies of infants born during this era concluded that a poor maternal diet retarded fetal growth and increased the risk of miscarriage, prematurity, and prolonged labor.[20,21]

A 5- or 7-day diet diary can assess the nutritional status of the individual by analyzing her nutritional strengths and weaknesses. The health of the baby's developing teeth and oral tissues depends on the availability of calcium, phosphorus, and vitamins A, C, and D. As a rule of thumb, the pregnant woman needs approximately 1500 mg of cal-

Table 4-3. A Model Program for Prenatal and Early Childhood Dental Counseling

Purpose
1. To educate parents about their child's dental development
2. To educate parents about the mother's role in fetal development and her oral health needs during pregnancy
3. To educate parents about the importance of the primary teeth
4. To educate parents about dental disease
5. To secure a proper oral environment for the life-long habitation of the permanent teeth through prevention education

Methods
1. Education in development, prevention, and disease
2. Demonstration of oral hygiene procedures
3. Counseling in attitudes and motivation
4. Evaluation of learning, acceptance, and needs

Content
1. Orofacial development of child
   a. Embryonic development of the head and neck
   b. Stages of tooth development
   c. Anomalies of enamel and dentin
      (1) Exposure to disease
      (2) Trauma
2. Oral health needs during pregnancy
   a. Nutrition
   b. Myths and misconceptions about pregnancy and dental caries
   c. Prenatal fluoride
   d. Oral hygiene
   e. Pregnancy gingivitis
   f. Habits (smoking, alcohol, drugs)
   g. Dental treatment
3. Oral health needs after birth
   a. Breast-feeding versus bottle
   b. Nutrition
   c. Nursing bottle caries
   d. Oral hygiene
   e. First visit to the dentist
   f. Fluoride

Adapted from Pinkham, J. R., et al. (Eds.): Pediatric Dentistry: Infancy through Adolescence. Philadelphia, W. B. Saunders, 1988, p. 158.

cium per day, increasing to 2000 mg daily during lactation. Phosphorus is required in the same amounts. If the supply of calcium is adequate, the phosphorus needs will also be met because these minerals are located in similar foods. Calcium and phosphorus are the principal elements found in enamel and dentin. Vitamins, particularly C and D, aid in depositing these minerals in enamel and dentin by fostering their absorption. Vitamin A is required for the differentiation and maintenance of ameloblasts and odontoblasts. Healthy gingival tissues are also achieved through adequate levels of vitamins A and C. Table 4-4 lists foods high in these nutrients.[8,22]

Dental Caries

The basic four food groups provide the framework for a well-balanced diet. Calcium supplements and an adequate intake of milk and dairy products are essential for tooth and bone formation. It is important to advise the pregnant mother that the common belief that she will lose a tooth for every child is a myth. If her nutritional stores are sufficient, the fetus should not extract calcium from her body and will not withdraw calcium from her teeth. If the dietary source of calcium is insufficient to maintain the maternal serum calcium level, then the calcium stored in her bones will be drawn upon. Teeth, unlike bone, do not act as calcium reservoirs.[23] Minerals within a normal erupted tooth cannot be removed through the pulp.

Dental caries in the expectant mother might instead be due to the fact that she has neglected her oral hygiene because morning sickness has interfered with routine plaque-control procedures; or her gag reflex is easily stimulated by brushing and flossing; or she has increased her consumption of sucrose, blaming this dietary change on a craving for sweets. Dental caries susceptibility is not the result of pregnancy; it involves a possible lapse in home care habits or the continuation of poor habits. People neglect their teeth because dental health is not a priority (e.g., avoiding the sick sensation associated with brushing might have replaced the need for clean teeth) or they lack the dietary and oral hygiene information to behave differently. Understanding and support for the pregnant patient is as essential as encouraging proper oral hygiene care and a diet low in fermentable carbohydrates.[24]

Table 4-4. Good Sources of Vitamins and Minerals Involved in Tooth Formation

Calcium	Phosphorus	Vitamin A	Vitamin D	Vitamin C
Milk	Milk	Dark green leafy	Milk	Raw, frozen, or
Nonfat dry milk	Cheese	vegetables:	Egg yolk	canned citrus fruits:
Cheese	Egg yolk	Spinach	Fish	Oranges
Turnip greens	Meats	Turnip tops		Grapefruit
Pink salmon	Fish	Chard		Lemons
Kale	Poultry	Beet		Strawberries
Broccoli	Whole grains	Greens		Cantaloupe
Orange		Green-stemmed		Pineapple
Egg		vegetables:		Vegetables:
		Broccoli		Broccoli
		Asparagus		Brussels sprouts
		Yellow vegetables:		Spinach
		Carrots		Kale
		Sweet potatoes		Green peppers
		Winter squash		Cabbage
		Pumpkins		Turnips
		Yellow fruits:		Potatoes
		Apricots		Sweet potatoes
		Peaches		
		Cantaloupes		

Prenatal Fluoride

In 1966, the United States Food and Drug Administration banned advertising that claimed dental caries prevention in the unborn children of pregnant women taking fluoride supplements.[12] The American Dental Association National Institute of Dental Research Symposium in 1980 concluded that some degree of caries prevention is afforded the primary teeth in utero if the pregnant woman receives systemic fluoride supplementation.[25] Six studies[26-31] showed a 9 to 35% benefit for the primary teeth with maternal ingestion of 1 mg/day of fluoride, yet controversy and discussion still prevail. The questions remain—what role does the placenta have in regulating fetal fluoride intake, and what is the optimum fluoride dosage for prenatal use?

Professionals during the 1930s through 1960s believed the placenta acted as a barrier, preventing the passage of fluoride to the fetus. It is now believed that fluoride passes through the placenta in physiologic concentrations.[32-34] If fluoride is excessive, only a partial transfer is permitted due to dilution by maternal circulation, renal ex-

cretion, and maternal bone absorption.[25] Due to the maternal loss of fluoride, 2 mg of fluoride daily is considered a conservative dosage during pregnancy for women in fluoridated and nonfluoridated communities. It is suggested that fluoride supplementation begin by the 10th and 12th week of gestation. Supplemental fluoride should be taken on an empty stomach, and one should refrain from eating for 30 minutes and from taking calcium for at least 1 hour after ingestion.[25]

Many remain skeptical about the significance of prenatal fluoride because the portion of the primary dentition that is mineralized in utero is less caries-susceptible than the remaining tooth structure, which is mineralized after birth.[12] Further investigation is necessary regarding the cariostatic benefits of this practice.[1]

Periodontal Disease and Oral Hygiene

Pregnant women need to be cognizant of the effect of plaque on their own oral tissues. The gingival response to plaque is exaggerated by hormonal changes, e.g., the production of prostaglandins associated with pregnancy.[35] In studies, from 36 to 100% of pregnant women experience the phenomenon known as pregnancy gingivitis.[36-38] Loe, in 1965, described these gingival changes at the clinical level as inflammatory, seen as early as the second month of gestation, reaching maximal severity by the eighth month if untreated, and decreasing after parturition.[38] About 2% of pregnant women develop what is known as a pregnancy tumor. This highly vascular type of pyogenic granuloma is a benign lesion referred to specifically as a granuloma gravidarum.[39] It involves an overgrowth of connective tissue usually located on the maxilla on the gingival papilla between the lateral incisor and the canine (Fig. 4-13). The condition arises as a result of poor oral hygiene compounded by the hormonal and vascular changes in the pregnant woman's body. The mass is usually painless unless it becomes so large that it interferes with occlusion and mastication. Continuous meticulous oral hygiene usually causes the granuloma to regress in size, but referral to a dentist is warranted.

Substance Use and Abuse

Nutritional intake during pregnancy and lactation is vital to the mother's total health as well as the health of her child, and consumption of drugs, alcohol, and tobacco can be hazardous.

Use of legal or illegal drugs must be avoided. If drugs are found to be necessary on consultation with a physician or dentist, only those proved safe during pregnancy should be prescribed. Countless developmental anomalies can result from maternal drug use.

The detrimental effects of alcohol on the unborn child can be equally frightening. Excessive alcohol consumption by the mother during pregnancy can result in fetal alcohol syndrome (FAS), now recognized as a leading cause of mental and/or physical disabilities.[40] Mothers who drink more than 45 ml of alcohol per day face twice the risk of abstinent or moderately drinking mothers of having a child with an abnormality.[41]

The craniofacial defects commonly observed in individuals with FAS include short palpebral fissures; short, depressed midface with flat nasal bridge; short philtrum and thin upper lip; epicanthal folds and bilateral ptosis; microcephaly; and cleft palate.[42]

Over the past few years there has been a major concern over the increasing prevalence of smoking among women 20 to 24 years of age, many of whom are pregnant.[43] The risk of maternal cardiovascular disease, particularly hypertension, increases during pregnancy. General dietary and nutritional stores are depleted from smoking, which can

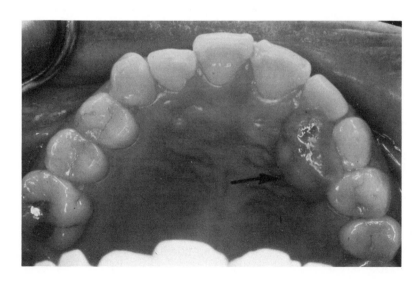

Figure 4-13. Pregnancy tumor: a palatal lesion is located between the maxillary lateral incisor and canine. Courtesy of R. I. Hart, D.D.S., West Virginia University.

affect the mother's oral tissues, increasing the frequency and severity of periodontal disease. The risks of spontaneous abortion and premature birth of an infant with measurable growth deficiencies are much greater for a smoker.[44,45] Studies suggest that there is a strong relationship between low birth weight and enamel hypoplasia in the primary dentition.[46]

Cigarette smoking and drug use are also believed to be instrumental in causing sudden infant death syndrome (SIDS), by inhibiting fetal circulation. A reduction in oxygen to the brain via the bloodstream interferes with the infant's proper breathing.

Dental Treatment During Pregnancy

During the first 2 months of the first trimester many women are unaware or unsure that they are pregnant. It is important to question women of childbearing age during their medical history or recall history update prior to treatment.[24] If there is a possibility that the patient is pregnant, diagnostic radiographs should be postponed and only emergency treatment provided. A routine prophylaxis and examination are permissible during the first trimester. Needless to say, a plaque-control program is a requirement during the entire gestation period. The second trimester (fifth or sixth month) is a more suitable time for providing dental care because organogenesis is essentially complete. Radiographs with adequate protection and use of a high-speed film are allowed.[35] Later in pregnancy, care becomes more difficult because of patient discomfort. By the third trimester the fetus is large enough to put pressure on the major abdominal veins, blocking the blood return from the inferior vena cava when the patient is in a reclined position. Hypotension and syncope can occur if the patient is supine for too long.[24]

Routine restorative treatment can be provided with a local anesthetic during the second and third trimesters, but nitrous oxide and general anesthesia are contraindicated during the entire pregnancy.[24]

ORAL HEALTH NEEDS OF THE INFANT

Freud described the mouth as the center of nutritional, relational, and erogenous gratification. From birth, it is through the mouth and through contact with the mother during feeding that the infant becomes aware of his environment. He discovers pleasure from the warm milk passing over his gingivae during suckling. The baby imitates this behavior by digital nonnutritive sucking, which allows him a sense of his mother even in her absence. The mouth occupies an important place in the initiation of an individual's physical, social, and emotional functioning.[47]

Breast-Feeding vs. Bottle-Feeding

The suckling instinct is satisfied to a greater degree by breast-feeding than by bottle-feeding. Although jaw size and relationship are primarily predicted by genetic factors, suckling rather than sucking behavior reinforces proper jaw position and exercises the mandible. Certainly, to determine breast-feeding's effect on craniofacial growth and development patterns, the duration and consistency of the feeding practice would need to be analyzed.[48] A longitudinal study conducted at the University of Iowa showed no significant change in arch parameters among infants during the first 18 months of life whether they were breast-fed or used conventional feeding nipples and pacifiers.[49] As the infant breast-feeds, the mouth remains fairly closed with the gum pads apart, the tongue moves forward, keeping in constant contact with the lower lip, and the mandible moves up and down and back and forth in a rhythmic motion. This movement not only strengthens the musculature but reduces the risk of ear and respiratory infections by assisting with the opening and drainage of the eustachian tubes and pharynx. The conventional bottle nipple only requires the infant to suck because it contacts only the mucous membrane of the lips. The mouth is open wider, placing a greater demand on the lips and buccinator muscle for sucking. Consequently, little movement of the mandible is necessary. The intensity of the sucking action itself is also decreased because of the large hole at the end of the artificial nipple, which increases the flow of milk to the back of the infant's throat[3] (Fig. 4-14).

Between 1921 and 1984, the number of breast-fed infants increased by 38% and formula-fed babies decreased by 32%.[50] Breast milk offers several advantages over bovine milk or formula. Although breast milk contains little vitamin D, it is the most effective food for meeting the newborn's nutritional needs if the mother is well nourished. Lactation requires the mother to consume an additional 1000 calories daily by increasing her intake of dairy products, fruits, and vegetables. The colostrum in breast milk provides the infant with maternal antibodies and macrophages beyond the first 6 months of life, giving him considerable protection against infection.[12,51] Breast-feeding also seems to allow the infant control of his own intake of milk, reducing the possibility of overfeeding by the mother.[12]

Nursing Bottle Mouth Syndrome

Once the teeth have erupted they are susceptible to dental caries. One of the first major conditions that can jeopardize the health of the primary teeth after birth is an entity known as nursing bottle caries, baby bottle syndrome, nursing bottle mouth syndrome (NBMS), or bottle mouth caries.

Nursing bottle mouth syndrome is the development of rampant carious lesions in a child who has been put to bed at night or at nap time with a bottle of milk or sweetened liquid. It can also occur in breast-fed children if they are allowed to fall asleep while nursing and retain some of the milk in their mouths.

The major contributing factor to this problem is the prolonged amount of time the child spends nursing each day. If the child falls asleep with a partially full bottle containing a fermentable carbohydrate liquid (e.g., sucrose in soda, lactose in milk) in his mouth, the nipple will continue to drip, causing the liquid to stagnate on the teeth. The carbohydrate-containing liquid offers an excellent substrate for acidogenic microorganisms.[14]

Other contributing factors include (1) a decrease in swallowing during sleep, which prevents clearance of the liquid from the mouth; (2) a reduction in salivary flow during sleep, which compromises buffering capacity; (3) a more viscous saliva in children, which enhances plaque adherence on the teeth; and (4) a warm oral environment during sleep, which provides a culture medium for bacterial growth.[52]

The pooling of liquid, predominantly over the smooth surfaces of the primary maxillary incisors, increases their risk of decay (Fig. 4-15). The tongue lies over the mandibular teeth during feeding, protecting them from repeated acid attacks.[52] The other maxillary teeth are involved to varying degrees depending on the child's sucking habits.[53] Demineralization usually appears clinically by 2 to 4 years of age. It can appear unilaterally if the child habitually sleeps on one side.[52]

Early recognition and treatment are necessary to save the child's teeth, but preven-

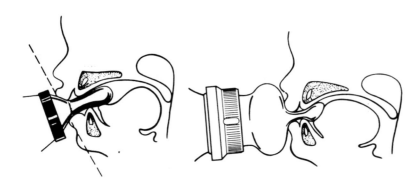

Figure 4-14. Comparison of the oral musculature during feeding with a conventional nipple and a nipple that closely resembles the mother's nipple. Note the position of the lips and tongue.

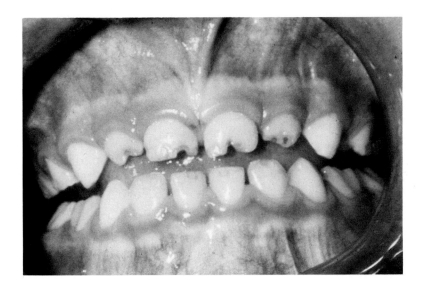

Figure 4-15. Nursing bottle caries.

tion is the key. The dental health educator should begin parental education early to avoid the hazards of NBMS by recommending the following preventive measures: (1) hold the child while feeding, so if he falls asleep feeding can be discontinued and the child can be placed in bed; (2) put the child to bed without a bottle or with a bottle filled with plain water only; (3) avoid dipping a pacifier in a sweetened liquid or honey; (4) clean plaque from the child's teeth with wet gauze or a washcloth as soon as the first tooth erupts; (5) consult with a pediatric dentist or physician to assess the child's particular need for a fluoride supplement; (6) become knowledgeable about the sugar content in a variety of commercial formulas and baby food; and (7) discontinue nursing as soon as the child can drink from a cup, preferably by his first birthday.

Oral Hygiene

Parents should begin cleansing their child's teeth as soon as the first tooth erupts. Gentle wiping of the teeth with a wet gauze or a soft damp washcloth wrapped around the finger is recommended, particularly after feeding (Fig. 4-16). The alveolar ridges where teeth will later erupt, the tongue, the vestibule, and the palate should also be swabbed to remove milk or food residue.

When the child reaches about 18 months of age, a soft-bristled toothbrush with a small head should be used. A small amount of fluoridated toothpaste, if any, is recommended because of the difficulty children have with expectorating. Flossing should be initiated after the eruption of the first permanent molars. Due to the primate or natural spacing between the primary lateral

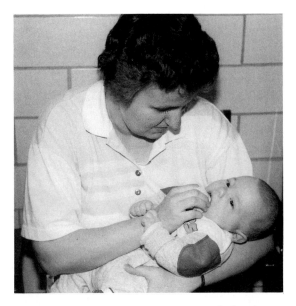

Figure 4-16. A parent can accomplish plaque control on an infant by cradling the baby with one hand and wiping the teeth and gingivae with the other.

and cuspid on the maxilla and the primary cuspid and first molar on the mandible, toothbrushing alone is usually sufficient for interproximal plaque removal prior to that time (Fig. 4-17).

For the child to become accustomed to and enjoy home care it must begin early in infancy and practiced daily. The dental health educator must not only teach the parents how to perform plaque removal, but also advise them on where and how to position their child to see and reach all areas of the mouth and teeth. Bathrooms are crowded, and the surfaces are dangerous. For an infant a dressing table is ideal. As the child becomes bigger, he can lie across the sofa with his head on a parent's lap, or he can be cradled between both parents seated facing each other. Oral hygiene can become a family ritual, rewarding for the child and his parents. Although bedtime is preferable, the time of the day for oral hygiene should be consistent and coordinated with the child's most receptive behavior.[52] (See Chapter 8 for patient positioning techniques.)

First Dental Visit

Early orientation of the infant to oral hygiene at home prepares the child for his first dental visit. The first appointment should be a pleasant one, allaying any apprehensions the child might feel. Ideally the child should be between 6 and 12 months of age when he first visits the dentist.[52,54] The purpose of this initial visit is to evaluate the soft tissue, existing dentition, and jaws for proper formation and alignment of structures.[53] If there has been no prenatal dental counseling, a series of visits should be scheduled to discuss eruption times, oral hygiene measures, the possible need for fluoride supplementation, nursing bottle mouth syndrome, and any questions the parents have concerning their child's teeth such as teething or thumbsucking. The dental health educator must remember step-by-step learning and not to overwhelm the parents with facts. It is advisable to establish routine appointments for just such discussions and evaluations of the preventive dental health program prescribed.

Fluoride

Breast milk and cow's milk contain only trace amounts of fluoride. Prior to 1980 the concentration of fluoride found in formulas varied greatly (Table 4-5).[52] Because of the high concentrations of fluoride in some of the formulas tested it was suggested that fluoride supplementation not be prescribed for children drinking formulas during the first 6 months of life.[55] Subsequently formula manufacturers agreed to lower the fluoride content of their products to less than 0.15 ppm. Such a reduction reduced the risk of fluorosis for the child. In light of these events fluoride supplements are important for those children who do not reside in water fluoridated communities or those who do, but rely on breast-feeding, cow's milk, or formulas prepared with fluoride-deficient

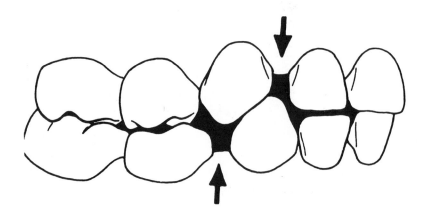

Figure 4-17. Primate space.

water as their primary or only source of fluid intake. When additional foods or fluoridated water is added to the child's diet the mother should be instructed to discontinue giving the fluoride supplements to her child.[1]

If the parents are unsure if their water supply is fluoridated, the local or state health department will test a sample of their water and provide their dentist with the exact concentration of fluoride. Health de-

Table 4-5. Examples of the Variations of Fluoride Content of Human Milk, Cow's Milk, Milk-Based Formulas, and Soy-Based Preparations

Source	Type	F Concentration (mg/ml)
Human milk	—	0.016
Whole cow's milk	—	0.019
2% milk	—	0.018
Skim milk	—	0.018
Chocolate milk	—	0.020
Evaporated milk	—	0.037
Similac	Ready-to-feed	0.12
Similac	Concentrate	0.68
Similac with iron	Concentrate	0.60
Similac Advance	Ready-to-feed	0.14
Similac Advance	Concentrate	0.18
Enfamil	Ready-to-feed	0.70
Enfamil	Concentrate	<0.10
Enfamil with iron	Ready to feed	0.78
Enfamil with iron	Concentrate	0.13
SMA	Ready-to-feed	0.27
SMA	Concentrate	0.33
Isomil	Ready-to-feed	0.43
Isomil	Concentrate	<0.10
ProSobee	Ready-to-feed	0.59
ProSobee	Concentrate	<0.10
Nursoy	Ready-to-feed	0.38
Nursoy	Concentrate	0.26

From Wei, S. H. Y., Fomon, S. J., and Anderson, T. A.: Nutrition and dental health. In The Food That Stays: An Update on Nutrition, Diet, Sugar, and Caries. Edited by E. A. Sweeney. New York, Medcom, 1977, p. 19.

Table 4-6. Supplemental Fluoride Dosage Schedule (in Milligrams F per day*) According to Fluoride Concentration of Drinking Water

Age (years)	Concentration of Fluoride in Water (ppm)		
	<0.3	0.3 to 0.7	>0.7
Birth to 2	0.25	0	0
2 to 3	0.5	0.25	0
3 to 14†	1.0	0.5	0

* 2.2 mg NaF contains 1 mg F.
† The American Academy of Pediatrics recommends providing tablets through at least age 16.

From Accepted Dental Therapeutics, 40th Ed, Chicago, American Dental Association, 1984.

partments are also helpful in providing information regarding school fluoridation levels and the types of fluoride programs available to schoolchildren.

Supplements can be as effective as water fluoridation if parents comply with the prescribed regimen for their child. Most dietary supplements contain sodium fluoride. Liquid preparations are ideal for very young children because the drops can be placed directly on the teeth before being swallowed. Although the fluoride supplement can also be placed in food or drink, it might not be as topically effective.[1] By age 3, children should be encouraged to chew, swish, and swallow the supplement in tablet form.

The dosage prescribed is determined by the child's age and the fluoride content of his drinking water. Table 4-6 lists the currently recommended daily dosage schedule for fluoride supplementation.[56]

Importance of the Primary Teeth

Waiting and watching for a first tooth is a major event for parents. Too often after the primary teeth erupt, they are ignored because of the knowledge that they will be exfoliated and replaced by the permanent dentition. The primary teeth serve a vital role in the child's development and must be provided all the necessary care to remain healthy until they are lost.

A severely decayed or traumatized primary tooth creates an unhealthy environment for the developing succedaneous permanent tooth, which can result in a "Turner's tooth," as previously discussed. To compound the problem, if the primary tooth must be extracted or is lost prematurely due to caries or trauma, the adjacent teeth can drift laterally to fill the vacant space. The result is often malocclusion due to insufficient space maintenance for the permanent tooth, often blocking its eruption.

Speech and mastication, two essential functions, can also be adversely affected by early loss of primary teeth. It is not a simple task to pronounce "s" and "th" words or eat an ear of corn or an apple without using the maxillary incisors. Peer ridicule because of a child's premature toothless appearance can be damaging to the child's self esteem. Many children, even at a very young age, learn to judge one another on the basis of esthetics. To have a toothless smile at 7 is deemed acceptable because virtually everyone else in the class is also missing front teeth, but being different can be a difficult experience.

Teething

The approximate time that the teeth will erupt is relatively predictable (Table 4-2). Parents should be advised when to begin looking for particular teeth and be alerted to the common signs and symptoms of teething.

Teething is a natural process and not an illness. Approximately 40% of children have no symptoms associated with teething.[57] Yet some children do experience difficulty during this period, and it can become a time of anxiety for parents as well.[1] Because the infant cannot isolate the area of pressure in his body at this young age, he might display one or more of the following systemic and local symptoms: excessive salivation or drooling, extreme irritability, disturbed eating patterns, disturbed sleeping patterns, a desire to chew, and a slight elevation in temperature.

Wide disagreement exists as to whether specific problems such as vomiting, diarrhea, high fever, rash, and rhinitis are ac-

tually caused by teething.[58,59] Because the level of maternal antibodies derived from the placenta declines at 5 to 6 months of age, it is plausible that the infant could become ill at approximately the same time the first tooth erupts.[2,12] If such problems arise in conjunction with teething, the dental health educator should recommend a consultation with a physician.

Intraorally, at the location where the tooth is about to erupt, the alveolar mucosa might appear inflamed and bulbous. Recommended treatment is palliative and includes (1) keeping the area clean and free of food debris to reduce eruption gingivitis, (2) acetaminophen for a slight fever of short duration, (3) a chewable object such as a teething ring to apply pressure to the area (rather than a teething cookie, which might contain sugar; also, large pieces can be broken off and aspirated), (4) a topical anesthetic (e.g., Baby Anbesol, accepted by the ADA Council on Dental Therapeutics) to relieve local irritation (a teething ring filled with cold water or a cool spoon rubbed gently across the alveolar ridge can also numb the area to allay discomfort), and (5) mild sedation for the extremely irritable child.[2] Some people believe lancing the gingiva will expedite the tooth's eruption. This is a myth. The parents should be reassured and advised that treating their child with tender loving care (TLC) is usually the best medicine.[1,57]

Digit Sucking and Pacifiers

Non-nutritive sucking behavior is generally considered normal during prenatal and infant development. Although thumbsucking activity in infants has not been correlated with the type of feeding used, it has been related to the length of time spent feeding[60-62] and the presence of tension during feeding[2] Many children never adopt this habit, and some suck their thumb only when overtired or bored. Prolonged thumbsucking during childhood can be a more complex issue related to emotional starvation or a fear of someone or something. Thumbsucking provides comfort and a feeling of security.

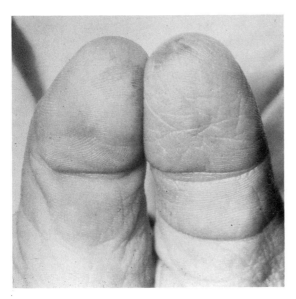

Figure 4-18. Digital thumbsucking habit. Compare the sucked (as viewed on the right) and unsucked (left) thumbs; note the differences in skin texture.

"The point at which non-nutritive sucking becomes a habit and is not considered normal is unclear."[1] Thumb, digit, and pacifier sucking are the most common, but multiple finger and knuckle sucking also occur (Fig. 4-18). A major study indicated that the average age for a child to cease a digit-sucking habit was 3.8 years, although some children continued the habit up to 15 years of age.[62]

The clinical manifestations of a digital sucking habit are proportional to the duration, intensity, and frequency of the habit. Possible oral effects include anterior openbite and overjet, labial flare of the maxillary anterior teeth, high palatal vault, posterior crossbite, and lingual inclination of the mandibular anterior teeth (Fig. 4-19). Secondary oral habits such as lip-sucking, mouth-breathing, tongue-thrusting, and speech problems can become part of the child's behavior pattern due to a malocclusion created by the primary digital sucking habit.[6] In most cases, if non-nutritive sucking is discontinued prior to the eruption of the permanent teeth, any deleterious tooth movement usually resolves itself.[1]

It is possible for a child to cease the digital habit naturally when passing from the sucking to the chewing phase, or the digit can be replaced with a pacifier. Terminating a pacifier habit might be less difficult than terminating the digit habit because parents can control when the pacifier is used and can wean the child gradually. Nuk-Sauger, the first manufacturer to create a pacifier that resembled the mother's nipple, claims that its product is less detrimental to the dentition than the thumb or a conventional bottle nipple or pacifier (Fig. 4-20).[63] As with breast-feeding, these statements cannot yet be substantiated. Pacifier users consistently exhibit anterior openbite due to the reduction in vertical growth of the incisors; full eruption is impeded because the anterior teeth rest on the pacifier.[64]

The first step in correcting a persistent habit that has affected the child's occlusion is for the dental health educator to take a case history to determine the cause. Corrective appliances e.g., palatal crib (Fig. 4-21) are only indicated when the child is willing to break the habit and needs a reminder to help him accomplish his goal. Parental ridicule and punishment are contraindicated. A reward system mutually agreeable to the parents and child is sometimes effective. Some dentists request that the parents ignore the habit and schedule the child to meet with them regularly while keeping a diary of their habit. When the underlying cause is more complex, the dental health educator is obligated to refer the family to a physician or a counselor for treatment before dental manipulation is conducted.[14]

Emergency Treatment

Parents sometimes bring a young child to the dental office with mouth pain of a non-traumatic nature. Usually these emergency visits are associated with nursing bottle caries or acute herpetic gingivostomatitis. Most of the dental emergencies of children 1½ to 2½ years of age, however, are the result of trauma to the primary dentition or the soft tissue related to falls.[1] These incidents are further complicated for the child with a chronic seizure disorder. (See Chapter 8.)

The teeth most commonly injured are the

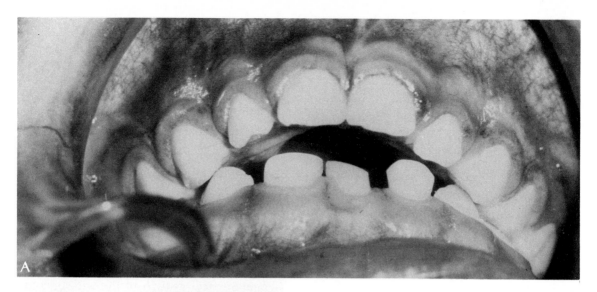

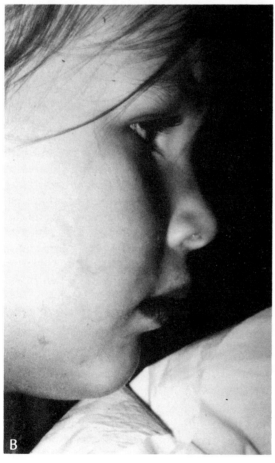

Figure 4-19. Oral manifestations of a thumb-sucking habit. A. Anterior openbite. B. Retrognathic profile.

maxillary central incisors, particularly in children with class II malocclusions. Anatomically, the apicies of the primary incisors are in close proximity to the developing permanent anterior teeth. A primary tooth with an intrusion injury should be radiographed the same day to assess whether the intruded incisor is contacting the permanent tooth bud. If they are touching, the primary tooth should be extracted. Such an injury can (1) interfere with the development of the enamel of the permanent tooth, resulting in hypoplasia or hypocalcification, or (2) alter the path of development of the crown, causing dilaceration or ectopic eruption. If the primary and permanent teeth do not contact,

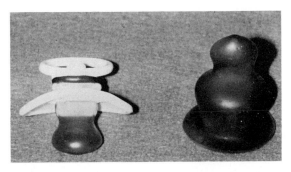

Figure 4-20. Orthodontic pacifier and bottle nipple.

the primary tooth should be allowed to re-erupt. This process takes approximately 2 to 6 months.[1]

Because the alveolar bone in a young child has large marrow spaces, it is relatively spongy and pliable. Consequently, extrusion and lateral luxation injuries are the most common. It is usually recommended that the injured primary tooth be extracted to prevent aspiration due to the child's age and to decrease the risk of further damage to the developing permanent tooth.[1]

Another major cause of dental injuries in young children is automobile accidents, which can result in the avulsion of a primary tooth. Premature loss of a primary tooth can not only damage but delay the eruption of the permanent tooth by 1 to 2 years. If a primary tooth has been avulsed it should not

be reimplanted. Appliances can be fabricated to satisfy parents concerned about their child's appearance.[1]

Electric burns occur most frequently between 18 and 24 months of age. These burns are commonly caused when a child chews on the live end of an electric cord. The saliva acts as a conductor and completes the circuit with the child's mouth. Extensive tissue damage involving the commissure of the lip can be disfiguring, impede function, and reduce the size of the oral stoma.[1]

The construction of a burn appliance within 10 days of the injury has been shown to prevent contracture of the healing tissue and provides a good cosmetic result when worn daily for a period of 6 to 8 months and 12 hours per day for an additional 6 months (Fig. 4-22). After splint therapy is completed the child should be evaluated by a plastic surgeon. Often no surgery is required if the appliance is worn religiously.[1,14]

Child abuse is also responsible for dental trauma. Over half of abused children experience head and neck injuries. (This topic is discussed in further detail in Chapter 5.) *Radiographs.* If radiographs are indicated for a dental emergency, the infant is usually seated on a parent's lap. The parent stabilizes both the child and the film.[1] It is imperative that both parent and child wear lead aprons that include thyroid collars for protection. The dental health educator

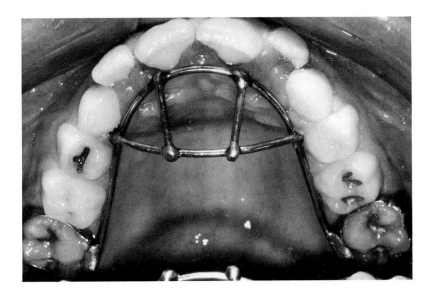

Figure 4-21. Palatal crib appliance. Courtesy of D. Holmes, D.D.S., M.S., West Virginia University.

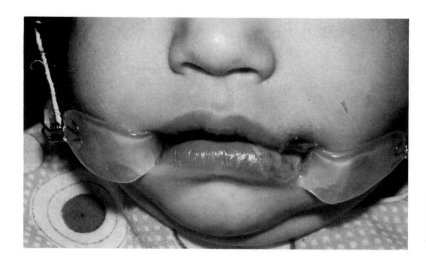

Figure 4-22. Burn appliance. Courtesy of D. Holmes, D.D.S., M.S., West Virginia University.

should have a parent or a significant other hold the child to accomplish the procedure and should work as rapidly as possible and talk to the youngster to help him understand what is about to occur.[1] This is probably the infant's first dental visit, and the dental health educator should be caring to ensure that it is a pleasurable one.[65]

ORAL HEALTH CONCERNS DURING EARLY CHILDHOOD

The preschool years are the why and how come years. This age group undergoes enormous social growth.[1] Piaget categorizes early childhood as the preoperational stage. During this stage, development has progressed from the sensorimotor representation of the infant to 2-year-old, to prelogical thought and solution to problems.[66]

Preschoolers eagerly strive for independence. Wanting to feed themselves, wash and dress themselves, brush their own teeth, and lace their shoes are all important in their quest to gain self-control. The parents play a major role in a preschooler's life. Anyone who observes a child playing will note that the images they portray are centered around the values of their adult models. Likewise, if parents believe dental health is important and establish good dental health practices early, the chances that their child will de-

velop these same attitudes and habits are greatly increased.[67-71]

Nutrition and Dental Caries

Most preschoolers do not appear to be as interested in eating as they were as infants. The loss of appetite might be related to a decrease in the growth rate during early childhood. Instead of trying to coerce the young child to eat, parents should be advised to emphasize proper eating habits. Selective eaters develop because parents tend to be more permissive concerning their young child's eating habits, just as long as they eat. A 2-year national nutrition survey of preschoolers showed an inverse relationship between age and willingness to try new foods (Table 4-7).[72] In addition, preschoolers tended to dislike foods that were disliked by their older siblings.[67] Serving a

Table 4-7. Reactions of Children to New Foods

Age (yr)	Willingness to Try New Foods (%)	Flatly Refuse New Foods (%)
1–2	77	6
2–4	68	14
4–6	60	18

From Owen, G. M., et al.: A study of nutritional status of preschool children in the United States, 1968–70. Pediatr., 53:597, 1974.

Table 4-8. Relative Cariogenicity of Various Sugars

Sugar	Cariogenicity
Sucrose	High
Lactose	Medium
Glucose	Medium
Maltose	Medium to low
Fructose	Medium
Sorbitol	Low
Mannitol	Low
Xylitol	Low
Starch	Low

From Ehrlich, A.: Nutrition and Dental Health. New York, Delmar Publishers, 1987, p. 187.

child a variety of healthful foods at an early age might reduce the chances of developing a picky eater.

Snacking is also an area of concern because most snacks that are appealing to children are high in sodium, fat, and fermentable carbohydrates. Although sucrose is one of the major carbohydrates responsible for acid production, other simple (refined or fermentable) carbohydrates also have cariogenic potential. Polysaccharides or complex carbohydrates such as starch are less cariogenic because they must be broken down into simple sugars before bacterial plaque can utilize them to form acid and lower the pH in and around the tooth (Table 4-8).[51] Parents, teachers, and sitters need to be made aware of "good" and "bad" snacks. They must read labels, avoiding sucrose, fructose, glucose, corn sweeteners, honey, and molasses. Raisins, once believed to be an ideal snack, are highly cariogenic in both content and retentiveness. A small box of raisins contains 17 teaspoons of sugar; this is over three times the sugar found in 6 ounces of cola.[73] Foods that are considered low "caries-causers" are cheese, peanuts, yogurt, corn chips, pizza, bologna, raw carrots, celery, popcorn, and pretzels.[22] Remember, if fermentable carbohydrates are going to be eaten they should be consumed with a meal to reduce their cariogenicity. Ideally, raw sugar in the form of cookies, cake, candy, and pies should be limited to special occasions such as birthdays, Easter, Halloween, and Valentine's Day. Consis-

tently restricting a child's intake of simple sugars early will teach him good snacking habits, and he will not expect different from a parent or anyone else.

As mentioned previously, the preschool child is influenced to a large extent by experiences within his family. In-between-meal snacking, physical inactivity, food preferences, and overeating are all habits that are influenced by the actions of other family members. Parents must recognize the role of diet in the prevention of disease, whether it be rickets, cardiovascular disease, cancer, or dental caries, to name a few, and teach their children early through word and deed to develop good eating habits.

Gingivitis

Children accumulate dental plaque quickly, but they experience less gingival inflammation than an adult would with the same amount of plaque collection. The difference appears to be histologic. In childhood gingivitis, lymphocytic infiltrate is dominant, whereas plasma cells are seen in adult gingivitis.[74] Although gingivitis in early childhood is common, it does not, probably due to some immune response, seem to progress to periodontitis (except in rare cases of prepubertal periodontitis, which affects the alveolar bone surrounding the primary teeth). Gingivitis for the most part is temporary and tends to coincide with the eruption of the primary teeth.[75] Although plaque control gives the child a pleasant appearance and establishes an excellent regimen for prevention of future periodontal problems, its primary role for this age group is in reducing habit formation and to assist in reducing of dental caries.

Primary herpetic infections go unnoticed in some preschoolers. When acute symptoms arise, the infection is referred to as acute herpetic gingivostomatitis (Fig. 4-23). Active symptoms usually affect the child between 2 and 6 years of age and manifest intraorally as inflamed gingiva with yellow or white fluid-filled vesicles. These vesicles, usually found on the mucous membranes, will rupture, forming painful ulcers.[14] The

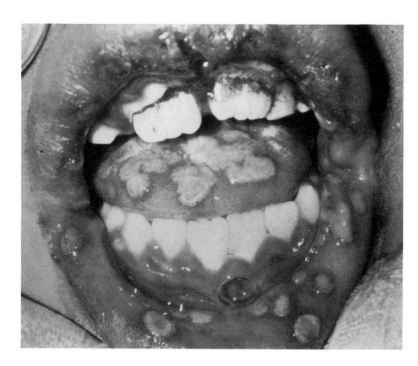

Figure 4-23. Primary HSV1 —acute herpetic gingivostomatitis. Courtesy of D. Nash, D.M.D., Ed.D., University of Kentucky.

child is not able to tolerate acidic foods or beverages and is often tired and irritable. Treatment is discussed in Chapter 9.

Oral Hygiene

A preschooler should be encouraged to brush his own teeth so that he is involved in the process. Prior to age 7, children do not possess the fine motor coordination or the attention span to brush their teeth adequately without assistance. The most effective approach is to have the child brush between meals without supervision. Because plaque removal at bedtime is so critical it is suggested that the child brush, then disclose the remaining plaque, and have the parent finish where the child missed. As the interproximal spaces close with the eruption of the permanent first molars and incisors, flossing becomes necessary. Parents should also be responsible for this activity at bedtime. A plaque removal program at home requires teamwork, with designated responsibilities for both parents and child.

What is the correct technique for cleaning the teeth? The American Dental Association most often recommends circular motions with the toothbrush for the child. The parent can use the modified rolling stroke by placing the toothbrush bristles on the gingiva in an apical direction at about a 45° angle from the tooth. First, gentle rotary or circular motions to stimulate the gingiva are made, followed by a roll or sweep of the brush, occlusally cleansing the entire crown. The circular/sweep sequence is performed several times before moving the toothbrush to the next area. Parents should be advised to brush the way the teeth grow, overlapping at least one tooth when placing the brush on the next area. The occlusal surfaces should be cleaned with a horizontal or scrubbing movement. The tongue should also be brushed with two or three posterior-to-anterior sweeping motions.

Only a small quantity of fluoride dentifrice is needed. Studies reveal that preschoolers tend to swallow the dentifrice used while brushing, a practice that could ultimately cause fluorosis.[76] Dietary fluoride supplementation should be continued during the period of early childhood if the family does not have access to fluoridated drinking water.

BEHAVIOR MANAGEMENT

Guidance of a child's behavior in the dental office is an integral part of his comprehensive care. The dental health educator, the parents, and the child have different roles but are equally involved in making the child's dental experience a favorable one. Figure 4-24 illustrates this relationship. Although parents are primarily involved in the child's care, lifestyles are changing and the effects of the entire family environment need to be considered, e.g., socioeconomic status and number and ordinal position of siblings.[14] Reciprocal communication at all three levels is important.

Most behavior management practices are designed for the preschooler. At this stage a child's behavior is overt, easily observed, with little reservation.[77] In an attempt to gain independence, the preschooler tests authority to see how far his boundaries lie. Most dentists agree that the preschool child is clearly, from a behavioral perspective, the most challenging of all dental patients.[1]

Factors Influencing Dental Behavior

Fear represents the source of the majority of management problems known to the den-

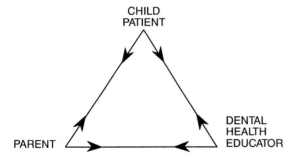

Figure 4-24. Dental health educator–parent–child interaction triangle. Adapted from Wright, G. Z.: Psychological management of children's behaviors. *In* Dentistry for the Child and Adolescent. 5th Ed. Edited by R. E. McDonald and D. R. Avery. St. Louis, C. V. Mosby, 1987, p. 39.

tal health educator. Approximately 16% of elementary schoolchildren describe themselves as highly fearful about dental treatment. Factors that cause the child to fear the dental visit and lead to misbehavior have been related to the child's background.

Dental Problem. Sometimes children arrive at their first appointment aware that they have a dental problem. The knowledge might be the result of pain felt by the child or apprehension conveyed to the child by a parent who notices something wrong with the child's mouth. Whatever the reason, this finding suggests that the dental health educator must alert parents to the value of taking their child to a dentist prior to the development of a dental problem.[14,78]

Parental Anxieties. In the recent past the mother was the one who usually accompanied her child to the dentist. Research indicated, therefore, that maternal anxiety had the most significant effect on the child's behavior in the dental office, particularly if the child was under 4 years of age.[14] Today, because of changing social roles, the anxieties of both parents appear to have a negative effect on the child's behavior. If a parent displays fear or anxiety, misinforms the child about a dental procedure, or uses dental scare tactics (e.g., "Sit still and listen to what the dentist tells you or he'll give you a shot"), the child will have unrealistic, perhaps horrifying expectations about his dental visit.

Medical History. Previous medical appointments and hospital experiences are considerations in a child's medical history. A child's perception of medical care is based on the physician's rapport with the child and the physician's ability to cause pain. Studies confirm that a child who views medical experiences positively is more likely to be a cooperative dental patient.[14,79]

Classifications of Behavior

The child dental patient can be classified according to three categories:[14] Cooperative, lacking in cooperative ability, or potentially cooperative.

Cooperative behavior denotes a reasonably relaxed child who has a good relationship with the dental health educator. Such a child is usually interested in the dental procedure and performs at an acceptable level to allow the professional to function effectively and efficiently.[3]

Lacking in cooperative ability describes very young children who cannot communicate or individuals with disabling conditions that prohibit their cooperation in the usual manner.[3]

The *potentially cooperative* patient is referred to as the "behavior problem." This child has the capability to perform cooperatively, but instead displays one or more of the following behaviors: (1) uncontrolled behavior tantrums characterized by tears, loud crying, and lashing out of the arms and legs; (2) defiant behavior portrayed by a verbal protest (e.g., "I won't" or "I don't want") or nonverbal refusal of care by keeping the lips pressed together and the teeth clenched; (3) timid behavior exemplified by hiding behind a parent or quietly whimpering; (4) tense cooperative behavior that allows dental treatment although the child is highly anxious, perspiring, and holding tightly onto the arms of the dental chair; and (5) whining behavior characterized by constant whimpering during the dental procedure with frequent complaints of pain, yet rarely accompanied by tears.[3]

Behavior Management Strategies

Successful management of the child patient relates to office procedures as well as to the creation of a good relationship between the dental health educator and the child. Although pharmacologic management of a child's inappropriate behavior is effective, it is not always necessary or advisable. It is preferable to practice behavior modification strategies that can lead to recognizable and lasting improvements in a child's behavior.

PREAPPOINTMENT BEHAVIOR MODIFICATION

Preappointment behavior modification entails (1) making a positive initial telephone contact with a parent for appointment scheduling; (2) arranging for the parents and child to come to the dental office for a tour and orientation involving audiovisual or live-patient models depicting the dental team and the first office visit;[14] and/or (3) sending a previsit letter that confirms the appointment and time, expresses appreciation for the parents' interest in the practice, outlines the procedures to be performed during the first visit, and includes other information relevant to the situation.[3]

OPERATORY PROTOCOL

The infant is most often examined while remaining on the parent's lap. Generally, the preschooler should sit by himself in the dental chair with a parent accompanying him in the operatory if he is under 3, mentally or physically disabled, or if it would be advantageous for the mother to observe what is being done, e.g., oral hygiene instructions or how the child is behaving. A parent permitted in the operatory should remain in the background unless asked to participate by the dental health educator.

When appropriate, it is wise to separate the parent from the child for the following reasons:[3]

1. The parent often repeats orders, annoying both the dental health educator and the child.
2. The parent's presence can form a barrier between the dental health educator and the child, preventing the establishment of a trusting, interpersonal relationship.
3. The dental health educator is unable to use voice intonation in the presence of most parents because they become offended.
4. The child divides his attention between parent and dental health educator.
5. The dental health educator divides his attention between parent and child.

Media exposure in the operatory is also an interesting technique for reducing fearful, uncooperative behavior.[80] Listening to tapes or watching television during the appointment can be made contingent on the child behaving in a calm, cooperative manner. If disruptive behavior occurs, television watching can be interrupted for a few seconds. The brief withdrawal of a child from a reinforcing situation is known as time out.

COMMUNICATING WITH CHILDREN

The first objective in the successful management of a young child is to establish communication. This should begin in the waiting area with the dental health educator first positioning himself between the child and parent, starting a conversation with the child, and touching his hand or shoulder to lead him into the operatory. The child should never be asked if he is ready to have his teeth examined. The dental health educator should simply say, "It's time to come with me now, Johnny; we're going to take a look at your teeth." The dental health educator should involve the child in conversation to learn about him as well as to relax him once he is in the operatory. Verbal communication is effective when it begins with compliments and is followed by questions that require explanations by the child.[14]

TELL, SHOW, DO

Tell, show, do is the classical educational method for communicating with children and preparing them to be highly cooperative dental patients.[81] *Telling* consists of explaining to the child exactly what is going to be done or what was done, as is the case with an injection of a local anesthetic. The dental health educator should speak to the child on his own cognitive level and always be truthful. *Showing* involves demonstrating to the child what will be occurring. By using the multisensory approach, the dental health educator can demonstrate the rubber cup polishing technique by allowing the child to see the handpiece, touch the rubber cup as it rotates, smell the flavored prophylaxis paste, and hear the sound that the handpiece makes. *Doing* entails just that. The child should be told what is being done

as it is being accomplished. The dental health educator should not perform any procedures until the child has a clear awareness of what is planned.[1,80,81]

VOICE CONTROL

The use of a more authorative tone with a child is known as voice control. A serious facial expression must be used in conjunction with this technique to be effective. It is usually well received by the misbehaving preschooler.[1]

HAND-OVER-MOUTH EXERCISE

Communication can be re-established with the defiant or hysterical child when the hand-over-mouth exercise (HOME) is used along with voice control. HOME is a method for effectively getting the attention of the 3- to 6-year old. It should not be used with children under 3 or individuals mentally functioning at this age level or below, because they lack the ability to understand the situation.[82] The HOME technique consists of the dental health educator placing his hand over the child's mouth only to muffle the crying and placing his face close to the child's while speaking directly in his ear, "If you want me to take my hand away from your mouth, you must stop screaming and listen to me. I only want to look at your teeth and talk to you." Wait several seconds and repeat the statement, adding, "Are you ready for me to remove my hand?" Usually the child nods and with a final word of caution to remain quiet, the hand is removed. The parent should be advised of this procedure during the office orientation. A consent form should be signed permitting the dental health educator to perform the procedure if necessary. If HOME is required during an appointment it should be noted in the patient's chart along with any other information relevant to the child's behavior. Prior to initiating hand-over-mouth, the dental health educator is advised to just place his face in close proximity to the child's face and employ voice control. Often invading the child's personal space is sufficient to promote desired behavior. Physical restraint that involves restriction of the child's body movements is discussed in Chapter 8.

TERMINOLOGY

To improve the clarity of information given to the preschooler, one must address the child at his level of comprehension. This does not mean either the use of baby talk or speaking above the child's cognitive level by using terminology such as rubber dam or injection.

The following is a list of word substitutes that can be used when explaining dental procedures to children:[3,14]

Dental Terminology	Word Substitute
air	Mr. Wind, breeze
water syringe	water fountain
suction	vacuum cleaner
impression material	pudding, mashed potatoes
anesthetic	sleepy water
rubber dam	raincoat
rubber dam clamp	tooth button
rubber dam frame	coat rack
radiographic equipment	camera
radiograph	picture
caries	sick tooth
explorer	tooth counter
sealant	coat of armor, tooth paint
prophylaxis paste	special toothpaste
fluoride gel	cavity fighter
high speed	whistle
low speed	motorcycle

OTHER RECOMMENDATIONS

Preschoolers should be scheduled in the morning, when they are rested and quiet. If the child gets upset easily, the dental health educator should tell the parent to refrain from feeding the child breakfast. Shorter appointments are also advisable if the child has a particularly short attention span. Play-

ing should not take place in the dental operatory; a child could get hurt, or he could take advantage of the situation.

The child should always be treated as an individual. The dental health educator must remember to praise the child routinely; people react favorably to positive reinforcement. Such items as rings, balloons, and badges should be given to children after the appointment. These gifts should not be used as bribes for good behavior; instead they should be used as tokens of friendship and appreciation for the child's efforts. Sending birthday and valentine cards to children is also a gesture of good will.

Be creative with the design of the dental office. Bright colors, pictures, books, and toys should occupy the reception area. The walls between the reception area and the operatory should be soundproof. A prevention area and a conference room separate from the dental operatories are also recommended.[3]

PEDIATRIC RADIOGRAPHIC ASSESSMENTS

The selection of radiographs for the preschool child is determined by the size of the patient's mouth, the condition of the patient's dentition with regard to development and caries, the child's previous radiographic history, and the patient's degree of cooperativeness.[14]

SIZE

Size zero film, used for pediatric periapical and bitewing radiographs, is usually small enough to ensure a child's comfort. If a child experiences difficulty with the film impinging on the floor of the mouth, the anterior corners of the film should be bent gently. The film can also be inserted in the mouth vertically if it is too large for horizontal placement.[1] Regardless of the size of the child's mouth, anterior occlusal films (size 2) are the easiest radiographs to take of the primary dentition because the child is only required to bite on the film packet.

Intraoral Findings

If the preschool child is asymptomatic and the interproximal surfaces of the primary teeth can be visually examined and no carious lesions exist, no radiographs are necessary.[1] When the preschooler's contacts are closed, two posterior bitewings using size 0 film are indicated to determine the presence of interproximal decay. Extensive caries requires the exposure of a 4-film survey: maxillary and mandibular anterior occlusals and left and right posterior bitewings. Additional periapical radiographs are requested to assess how far the decay process has advanced in an individual tooth, (e.g., pulpal pathosis). Occlusal films are invaluable for evaluating normal permanent tooth development and alignment and the status of a developing permanent tooth when deep caries or trauma affects its primary counterpart.

Radiographic History

The dental health educator should obtain a thorough history of a child's previous x-ray exposures. In 1985, the American Academy of Pediatric Dentistry recommended radiographic exposure "at a rate necessary to maximize detection of abnormalities yet minimize exposure to ionizing radiation."[1] Professionals should request and share existing films with other professionals to avoid duplication and unnecessary exposure. Parents should be advised to keep a radiation record on their child similar to an immunization card that includes date, number, type of radiographs taken, and the individual(s) who requested and exposed them.[83]

Behavioral Considerations

The radiographic procedure should begin by explaining to the child that a picture of his teeth is going to be taken with a special tooth camera. Working rapidly by having the x-ray equipment properly angled and as close to the correct position as possible prior to placing the film in the child's mouth is imperative. Some children, due to gagging or a short attention span, can only retain the film in their mouths for a short period of time. High kilovoltage and short exposure time with fast film is recommended. Talking constantly to the child and explaining each step will establish a rapport with him. The child should focus on an object on the wall directly in front of him and listen for the "horn" or the "bird to sing" to ensure he will not move his head when the film is being exposed. The use of continuous praise will motivate the child to try harder to accomplish the task. If the child is unsuccessful after several attempts, he should be praised for at least one film, exposed or unexposed, and he should be told in a positive manner that the rest of the films will be obtained during his next appointment.[65]

Due to the ease and brevity of occlusal projections, they should be exposed first to establish the child's confidence; this increases the probability that he will allow further radiographs to be exposed.

PEDIATRIC RADIOGRAPHIC TECHNIQUE

Anterior Occlusal

Maxillary. Position the child with the alatragus line (occlusal plane) parallel to the floor. The child must bite on the radiograph to hold it in place. The incisal edge of the arch should border the film. The central x-ray beam is directed over the nose, encompassing the film, at a 60° angle (Fig. 4-25).[65] *Mandibular.* The tube side of the film is placed toward the mandibular incisors. A 60° angle cannot be obtained with the occlusal plane parallel to the floor. Compensate by positioning the child backward with the alatragus line 30° from the floor and the

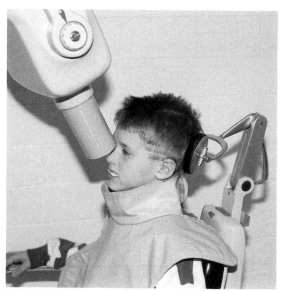

Figure 4-25. Maxillary anterior occlusal exposure technique.

x-ray tube directed upward 30° under the chin, totaling 60° (Fig. 4-26).[65]

Periapicals

The Rinn Snap-A-Ray is a plastic film holder used to secure periapical size 0 film

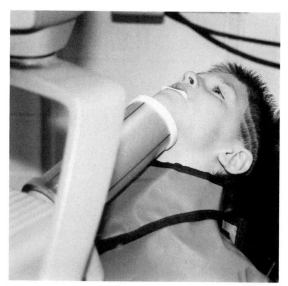

Figure 4-26. Mandibular anterior occlusal exposure technique.

(Fig. 4-27). The child bites on the plastic to stabilize the film. With the alatragus line parallel to the floor, the central x-ray beam should be directed at a 40° vertical angle below the pupil of the eye for a maxillary exposure and at a negative vertical angulation of 10° for a mandibular projection. The horizontal angulation is obtained by referring to the position of the film in the holder protruding from the child's mouth.[65]

Bitewings

Bitewing tabs shaped like a step to prevent irritation of the buccal mucosa are attached to size 0 film to examine the interproximal surfaces of the primary teeth. Because the contact areas of deciduous teeth angle slightly in an anterior-posterior direction, the central beam should be aimed between the embrasures rather than perpendicular to the midline as done for bitewings of the permanent dentition. This will prevent horizontal overlap. The child can smile while biting on the film to assist with orienting the beam. Bitewings should include a view of the distal surface of the canine. A positive vertical angulation of 10° is also recommended[65] (Fig. 4-28).

Lateral Jaw

This radiographic technique involves the extraoral placement of the film packet. This procedure is ideal for the uncooperative child or the developmentally disabled individual who requires a periapical radiograph and will not allow a film to be placed intraorally. (See Chapter 8.)

Panoramic Radiography

These extraoral films result in less radiation exposure to the child and provide excellent coverage of intraoral structures (Fig. 4-29). The main disadvantage of panograms is the loss of image detail. This type of radiographic examination is usually accepted by the nervous or disturbed child as long as

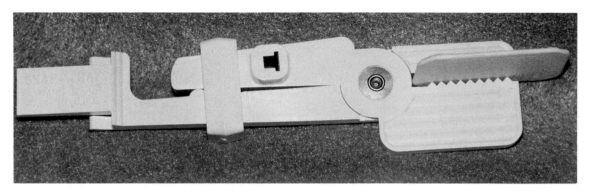

Figure 4-27. Rinn Snap-A-Ray intraoral film holder.

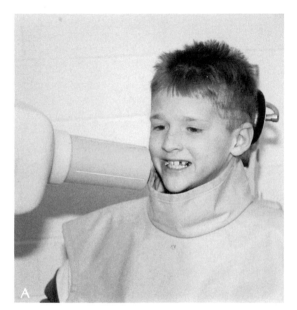

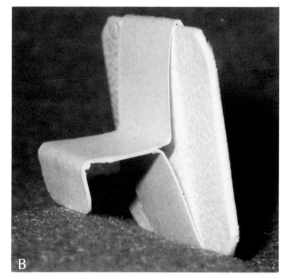

Figure 4-28. A. Bitewing exposure technique. B. Bitewing tab simulating a step on which the child should bite for comfort.

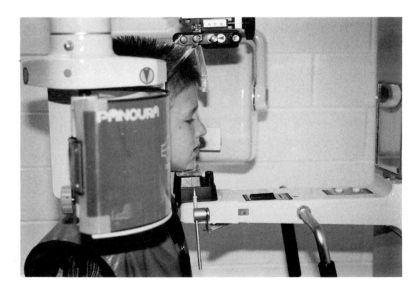

Figure 4-29. Panoramic radiography.

he is able to remain immobile for 15 to 22 seconds.[14]

REFERENCES

1. Pinkham, J. R., et al. (Eds.): Pediatric Dentistry: Infancy through Adolescence. Philadelphia, W. B. Saunders, 1988.
2. Mathewson, R. J., et al.: Fundamentals of Dentistry for Children. Chicago, Quintessence, 1982.
3. West Virginia University, School of Dentistry: Pediatric Dentistry Study Guide. Morgantown, WV, 1988.
4. Lowrey G. H.: Growth and Development of Children. 6th Ed. Chicago, Year Book, 1973.
5. Orban, B. J.: Oral Histology and Embryology. St. Louis, C. V. Mosby, 1957.
6. Loevy, H. T.: Dental Management of the Child Patient. Chicago, Quintessence, 1981.
7. Ranly, D. M.: A Synopsis of Craniofacial Growth. New York, Appleton-Century-Crofts, 1980.
8. Charonko, C. V., and DeBiase, C. B.: Dental health for children: An adult responsibility. J. Prac. Nurs., 34:45-54, 1984.
9. Logan, W. H. G., and Kronfeld, R.: Chronology of the human dentition. J. Am. Dent. Assoc., 20:379-427, 1933.
10. Grahanen, H., and Granath, L.: Numerical variations and their correlations with the permanent dentition. Odont. Rev., 4:348-357, 1961.
11. Brook, A. H.: Dental anomalies of number, form and size: Their prevalence in British schoolchildren. J. Int. Assoc. Dent. Child., 5:37-53, 1974.
12. Wei, S. H. Y. (Ed.): Pediatric Dental Care: An Update for the Dentist and for the Pediatrician. New York, Medcom, 1978.
13. Bodenhoff, J., and Gorlin, R. J.: Natal and neonatal teeth: Folklore and fact. Pediatrics, 32:1078-1093, 1963.
14. McDonald, R. E., and Avery, D. R.: Dentistry for the Child and Adolescent. 5th Ed. St. Louis, C. V. Mosby, 1987.
15. Watson, A. O., Massler, M., and Perlstein, M. A.: Tooth ring analysis in cerebral palsy. Am. J. Dis. Child., 107:370-378, 1964.
16. Myers, H. M., Dumas, M., and Ballhorn, H. B.: Dental manifestations of phenylketonuria. J. Am. Dent. Assoc., 77:586-588, 1986.
17. Miller, J., and Forrester, R. M.: Neonatal enamel hypoplasia associated with haemolytic disease and with prematurity. Brit. Dent. J., 106:93-104, 1959.
18. Gullikson, J. S.: Tooth morphology in rubella syndrome children. J. Dent. Child., 42:479-482, 1975.
19. Sanger, R. G.: Preventive dental health program for the infant. Dent. Hyg., 51:408-412, 1977.
20. Ebbs, J. H., et al.: The influence of improved prenatal nutrition upon the infant. Can. Med. Assoc. J., 126:6-8, 1942.
21. Keys, A. J., et al.: Growth and development. *In* The Biology of Human Starvation. Vol. 2. Minneapolis, University of Minnesota Press, 1950.
22. Nizel, A. E., and Papas, A. S.: Nutrition in Clinical Dentistry. 3rd Ed. Philadelphia, W. B. Saunders, 1989.
23. Cheney, H. G., and Cheney, V. C.: The dental hygienist as a health educator in prenatal care. Dent. Hyg., 48:150-153, 1974.
24. Woodall, I. R., et al.: Comprehensive Dental Hygiene Care. 3rd Ed. St. Louis, C. V. Mosby, 1989.
25. Glenn, F. B., and Glenn, W. D.: Optimum dosage for prenatal fluoride supplementation (PNF): Part IX. J. Dent. Child., 54:445-450, 1987.
26. Arnold, F. A., et al.: Effect of fluoridated public water supplies on dental caries prevalence. Pub. Health Rep., 71:652-658, 1956.
27. Blaney, J. R., and Hill, I. N.: Evanston dental caries study XXIV: Prenatal fluorides—value of waterborne fluorides during pregnancy. J. Am. Dent. Assoc., 69:291-294, 1964.
28. Soricelli, D., Ship, I., and Cohen A.: Effects of fluoridation on dental caries in Philadelphia schoolchildren 1954–1964. Penn. Dent. J., 32:47-51, 1964.
29. Horowitz, H. S., and Heifetz, S. B.: Effects of prenatal exposure to fluoridation on dental caries. Pub. Health Rep., 82:297-304, 1967.
30. Lewis, D. W., Hunt, A. M., and Kowall, K.: Initial dental care time, cost, and treatment requirements under changing exposure to fluoride during tooth development. J. Can. Dent. Assoc., 4:140-144, 1972.
31. Tank, G., and Storvick, C. A.: Caries experience of children one to six years old in two Oregon Communities (Corwallis and Albany). J. Am. Dent. Assoc., 69:749-757, 1964.
32. Martin, D. J.: The Evanston dental caries study. J. Dent. Res., 27:27-33, 1948.
33. Gedalia, I., et al.: The fluoride content of teeth and bones of human foetuses. Arch. Oral Biol., 9:331-340, 1964.
34. Smith, M. C., and Smith, H. V.: The occurrence of mottled enamel on the temporary teeth. J. Am. Dent. Assoc., 22:814-817, 1935.
35. Davis, I.: Prenatal dental care and education for the expectant mother. J. Mich. Dent. Assoc., 70:211-213, 1988.
36. Chaiken, B. S.: Incidence of gingivitis in pregnancy. Quintessence Int., 8:81, 1977.
37. Adams, D., Carney, J., and Dicks, D.: Pregnancy gingivitis: A survey of 100 antenatal patients. J. Dent., 2:106, 1974.
38. Loe, H.: Periodontal changes in pregnancy. J. Periodont., 36:209, 1965.
39. Spouge, J. D.: Oral Pathology. St. Louis, C. V. Mosby, 1973.
40. Barnett, R., and Shusterman, S.: Fetal alcohol syndrome: Review of literature and report of cases. J. Am. Dent. Assoc., 111:591-593, 1985.
41. Olegard, R., et al.: Effects on the child of alcohol abuse during pregnancy. Acta Pediatr. Scand., 275(Suppl.):165-171, 1978.
42. Webb, S., Hochberg, M. S., and Sher, M. R.: Fetal alcohol syndrome: Report of case. J. Am. Dent. Assoc., 116:196-198, 1988.
43. Amler, R. W., and Dull, H. B. (Eds.): Closing the Gap: The Burden of Unnecessary Illness. New York, Oxford University Press, 1987.
44. U. S. Department of Health Education and Welfare: Smoking and Health: A Report of the Surgeon General. Washington, DC, 1979.
45. Bergner, S., and Susser, M. W.: Low birthweight and parental nutrition: An interpretive review. Pediatrics, 46:946-966, 1970.
46. Melander, M., et al.: Mineralization defects in deciduous teeth of low birthweight infants. Acta Paediatr. Scand., 71:727, 1982.
47. Kellerman, M. R.: What are the psychological factors involved in motivating individuals to retain their teeth? Int. Dent. J., 34:105-108, 1984.
48. Sanger, R. G., and Bystrom, E. B.: Breast-feeding: Does it affect oral facial growth? Dent. Hyg., 56:44-47, 1982.
49. Bishara, S. E., et al.: Influence of feeding and non-nutritive sucking methods on the development of the dental arches: Longitudinal study of the first 18 months of life. Pediatr. Dent., 9:13-21, 1987.

50. Martinez, A., and Kreiger, F. W.: 1984 milk-feeding patterns in the United States. Pediatrics, 76:6, 1985.
51. Ehrlich, A.: Nutrition and Dental Health. New York, Delmar, 1987.
52. Sweeney, E. A. (Ed.): The Food That Stays: An Update on Nutrition, Diet, Sugar, and Caries. New York, Medcom, 1977.
53. Harris, N. O., and Christen, A. G.: Primary Preventive Dentistry. 2nd Ed. East Norwalk, CT, Appleton & Lange, 1987.
54. Goepferd, S. J.: An infant oral health program: The first 18 months. Pediatr. Dent., 9:9-12, 1987.
55. Johnson, J., and Bawden, J. W.: The fluoride content of infant formulas available in 1985. Pediatr. Dent., 9:33-37, 1987.
56. Council on Dental Therapeutics: Supplemental fluoride dosage schedule. *In* Accepted Dental Therapeutics. 40th Ed. Chicago, American Dental Association, 1984.
57. Carpenter, J. S.: The relationship between teething and systemic disturbances. J. Dent. Child., 45:381, 1978.
58. Honig, J. J.: Teething—are today's pediatricians using yesterday's notions? J. Pediatr., 88:415-417, 1975.
59. VanDerHorst, R. L.: On teething in infancy. Clin. Pediatr., 12:607-610, 1973.
60. Klackenburg, G.: Thumbsucking: Frequency and etiology. Pediatr., 4:418-423, 1949.
61. Yarrou, L. J.: The relationship between nutritive sucking experiences in infancy and non-nutritive sucking in childhood. J. Genet. Psychol. 84:149-154, 1954.
62. Traisman, A. S., and Traisman, H. S.: Thumb and finger sucking: A study of 2,650 infants and children. J. Pediatr., 52:566-577, 1958.
63. Nuk-Sauger Preventive Orthodontic Progress Manual. Rocky Mountain Dental Products. Denver, Colorado.
64. Larrson, E.: The effect of dummy-sucking on the occlusion: A review. European J. Ortho., 8:127-130, 1986.
65. Bean, L. R., and Isaac, H. K.: X-ray and the Child. Dent. Clin. North Am., 17:13-24, 1973.
66. Piaget, J., and Inhelder, B.: The Psychology of the Child. New York, Basic Books, 1969.
67. Holt, R. D., et al.: Dental Health education through home visits to mothers with young children. Community Dent. Oral Epidemiol., 11:98-101, 1983.
68. Doshi, S. B.: A study of dental habits, knowledge, and opinions of nursing mothers. J. Can. Dent. Assoc., 6:429-432, 1985.
69. Rayner, J. F.: Socioeconomic status and factors influencing the dental health practices of mothers. Am. J. Pub. Health, 60:1250-1257, 1970.
70. Chambers, D. W.: Patient motivation and education. *In* Pediatric Dentistry: Scientific Foundations and Clinical Practice. Edited by R. E. Stewart. St. Louis, C. V. Mosby, 1982.
71. Faigel, H. C.: Getting parents to follow advice: The art of communication. Clin. Pediatr., 13:403-405, 1974.
72. Owen, G. M., et al.: A study of nutritional status of preschool children in the United States, 1968–70. Pediatr., 53:597, 1974.
73. Bowes, A., and Church, C. F.: Food Values of Portions Commonly Used. 8th Ed. Philadelphia, College Offset Press, 1956.
74. Ranney, R., et al.: Pathogenesis of gingivitis and periodontal disease in chidren and young adults. Pediatr. Dent., 3:89, 1981.
75. Weddell, J. A., and Klein, A. I.: Socioeconomic correlation of oral disease in six-to-thirty-six month children. Pediatr. Dent., 3:306-310, 1981.
76. Barnhart, W. E., et al.: Dentifrice usage and ingestion among four age groups. J. Dent. Res., 53:1317, 1974.
77. Stone, L. J., and Church, J.: Childhood and Adolescence. 3rd Ed. New York, Random House, 1975.
78. Wright, G. Z., and Alpein, G. D.: Variables influencing children's cooperative behavior at the first dental visit. J. Dent. Child., 38:60-64, 1971.
79. Wright, G. Z., Starkey, P. E., and Gardner, D. E.: Managing Children's Behavior in the Dental Office. St. Louis, C. V. Mosby, 1983.
80. Ingersoll, B. D.: Patient Management Skills for Dental Assistants and Hygienists. East Norwalk, CT, Appleton-Century-Crofts, 1986.
81. Addleston, H. K.: Child patient training. Fort. Rev. Chicago Dent. Soc., 38:7-9, 27-29, 1959.
82. Levitas, T. C.: HOME—hand over mouth exercise. J. Dent. Child., 41:178-182, 1974.
83. Nowak, A. J., et al.: Summary of the conference on radiation exposure in pediatric dentistry. J. Am. Dent. Assoc., 103:426-428, 1981.

Chapter 5

THE ELEMENTARY SCHOOL CHILD

*The wisest of our children will not be those
who merely enjoy the spectacle; it will be those
who climb out of the pit upon the stage and
lose themselves in action.*

Will Durant

The transition of the child from home to school presents new physical, cognitive, and emotional concerns related to dentistry. Involvement in a child's dental health throughout his school years offers an opportunity for long-term communication and the development of sound dental practices. The dental health educator therefore plays a key role in the success of a school-based dental health program. From teaching the children and parents, to serving as a resource person and inservice educator to teachers, and to providing dental services, the challenges for the dental professional are limitless. The full benefits of dental health instruction in changing knowledge, attitudes, and behavior are gained when a sizeable commitment is given to the program at all levels. (Program development is discussed in detail in Chapter 11.)

PHYSICAL, COGNITIVE, AND EMOTIONAL GROWTH AND DEVELOPMENT

Late childhood refers to the period of a child's life between 7 and 12 years of age.[1]

Remarkably, by this stage, a child's body proportions are very similar to those of an adult, with the exception of the length of the arms and legs. Other growth and development changes that occur in this age group include an increase in blood pressure, a decrease in pulse rate, and an increase in muscle tissue and skeletal mineralization.[2]

According to Piaget, children ages 7 to 12 have reached the third major stage of cognitive development, the concrete operational phase. During this period of development a child acquires the ability to understand relativity and the differences between mass, length, weight, and number.[3]

A greater degree of emotional satisfaction during this period is derived from peer approval due to the transition from home to school. Issues such as style of clothes and facial appearance seem insignficant to a preschooler, but they become of increasing concern to the child by approximately his eighth year, when body image begins to become an emotional part of his existence.[2] An awareness of individual differences also originates during late childhood. Children tend to become critical of themselves and others, often perceiving themselves the way they believe their peers perceive them. A lack of acceptance can be emotionally damaging to a child if he does not have role models or significant others to boost his self-esteem.

Orofacial Growth and Development

By age 12, approximately 90% of facial growth has been completed.[2] Between ages 6 and 7 all four first permanent molars have begun to erupt. Parents and children frequently do not notice the eruption of the first permanent molars, because they appear posterior to the second primary molars, requiring no teeth to be lost to indicate where they will emerge.

The exfoliation of the mandibular and maxillary primary incisors with subsequent eruption of the permanent central and lateral teeth also happens during late childhood. In comparison, the permanent incisors are larger and must erupt in a more confined area than their primary predecessors. The growth of the permanent incisors is slow but continuous, and these teeth often erupt in an inclined position, which accounts for their labial flare. This minor asymmetry in the anterior segment is often referred to as the "ugly duckling stage."[4]

A greater awareness seems to accompany the eruption of the central incisors. Parents frequently question why they are so large, rotated, or appear yellow. Parents (and children, if they display an interest) need to be informed that permanent teeth only look different because of their proximity to the very small, white primary teeth.

THE CHILD DENTAL PATIENT

The child patient between 7 and 12 years of age provides the dental health educator with minimal behavioral entanglement. For the most part the child can be reasoned with and offers logical communication. At the beginning of this period of development, the child continues to be dependent on his parents while experiencing the challenges of a new environment—the school. By the conclusion of this growth period, he has achieved partial independence from his parents and is ready to embark on adolescence.[2,5]

Dental Caries Assessment

The prevalence of dental caries in the 5- to 17-year-old age bracket is discussed in Chapter 3. The topography of the occlusal surfaces of molar and premolar teeth makes them highly susceptible to decay during childhood. Approximately one-third of children under 3 have sustained dental caries in the primary dentition, 67% of these lesions affecting the occlusal surface. Sixty-five percent of the occlusal surfaces of permanent first molars in 12-year-olds have either been restored or are currently decayed.[2]

Periodontal Disease Evaluation

The greatest increase of gingivitis is often seen in the 6- to 7-year-old, with the eruption of the first permanent teeth. By age 9, a relatively high percentage of children begin to form supragingival calculus.[6] It is at this point that bacterial deposits (plaque and calculus) might be more significant in the initiation of gingivitis. In a study of almost 3000 children living in a naturally fluoridated community, approximately 90% of 8- to 18-year-olds experienced inflammation of one or more gingival papillae or margins.[7] (See prevalence reports in Chapter 3.)

A thorough examination of patients in this age group involves both a periodontal probing and a gingival index to assess inflammation.[2] Gingivitis associated with poor oral hygiene is usually mild in late childhood and can be resolved with an oral prophylaxis and effective daily plaque removal.

Radiographic Appraisal

The basic pediatric radiographic survey must be modified when a child makes the transition from the primary to the mixed dentition stage. The number and type of films exposed on a school-age child should be determined by the size of the tooth-bearing areas; the adequacy of tissue coverage by the size of the films tolerated; and the needs of the child, e.g., developmental dental anomalies, delayed eruption, and pathosis of the hard and soft tissues, which includes dental caries.

No particular radiographic survey is considered best. A variety of film combinations are possible as long as the films that are taken sufficiently expose all tissue areas. Normally a 12-film survey accomplishes this goal (4 posterior periapicals, 6 anterior periapicals, and 2 posterior bitewings). The addition of a panoramic film further extends the plane of vision to include the maxillary region and the entire mandible showing the temporomandibular joint (TMJ).

Because of the small size of the oral cavity, the school-age child might require placement of the anterior periapical film in a more posterior palatal position to obtain proper orientation. Cotton rolls can be attached to the film to help fill the palatal space and keep the film from moving. The developing teeth can be viewed by increasing the vertical angulation of the cone when exposing posterior periapical films. Larger, size 2 films can be used for bitewings instead of the size 0 films, used to take bitewings on the preschooler.

Lateral cephalometric head films are taken to analyze the relationship between the skeleton and the teeth. These diagnostic films are usually requested when significant craniofacial disproportions are noted and orthodontic treatment is being contemplated.[2,8]

PREVENTION OF DENTAL DISEASE

The preventive home care program established for a child age 7 to 12 should continue under parental supervision. As the child progresses toward adolescence, the parents' role in the surveillance of their child's oral hygiene practices diminishes.[2]

As the child advances from the primary dentition stage to the mixed dentition stage, the need for dental office preventive procedures increases. The possibility of buccal pit, lingual pit, or occlusal decay might suggest the need for sealants, continued fluoride supplementation if appropriate, and biannual professional fluoride applications for smooth-surface protection. A routine oral prophylaxis might also be warranted due to the deposition of calculus. Because the child spends approximately 8 hours per day in school and might prepare his own snack or dinner on returning home, nutritional counseling can also be a consideration.

Traumatic injuries to the head and oral cavity are also common in this age group. Playground accidents, bicycle riding incidents, and facial trauma associated with child abuse occur and must be treated. The scars from these episodes or any form of orofacial disfigurement can be both external and internal.

The dental health educator is responsible for providing information about the need for care, the benefits, the anticipated surgical and nonsurgical restorative options, and the maintenance procedures required that will give the child a positive body image at the time when appearance is such a critical facet of his emotional growth. Orthodontics is often a part of the treatment needs of a child in the latter years of late childhood.

Oral Hygiene

Plaque removal sessions at home with the parent(s) and the school age child are similar to those discussed for the preschooler. Through approximately 9 years of age, plaque removal procedures before bedtime should involve the child brushing his own teeth as instructed, followed by the parent disclosing the teeth. Parents can promote learning by showing the child the stained areas where plaque remains and how these areas can be effectively cleansed. At this point, instead of the parent removing the plaque as is done with the preschooler, the parent should supervise while the child attempts to do so himself. It should be stressed that proper brushing of the teeth and tongue entails at least 3 minutes. A fluoride dentrifice can be used safely because of the child's ability to expectorate at this age. Soft, multi-tufted nylon toothbrushes should be selected that are appropriately sized and contoured for the child's mouth.

The routine exfoliation and eruption of teeth that occurs during this developmental period might make a child hesitant to thoroughly brush some areas due to their degree of soreness. Gentle manipulation of the toothbrush to remove plaque and food debris is usually all that is necessary to maintain gingival health.[2]

By age 10, most children have the fine motor coordination necessary for effective brushing and flossing. Unlike toothbrushing, flossing up to this point is normally accomplished solely by the parent(s). Parents should be advised to explain to their child what they are doing, allow the child to observe the procedure, and try to floss one or more teeth to get the feel of the technique required. This enables the child to be both familiar and comfortable with the task once he is awarded the responsibility.

Praise and reinforcement by parents and the dental health educator for effective plaque control procedures performed at home encourages learning in the child; much like an insurance policy, these practices will be continued throughout life and passed on to future generartions.

Nutrition

Prior to a child's entrance into school, his diet is greatly influenced by experiences within the family. He is willing to try new foods, and parents have control over the amount and types of foods consumed.[9] The educational environment and social pressures during the day and after school can challenge a child's dietary practices. Many children return home from school at the end of the day to an empty house where they make a snack and wait for their parents to come home from work (latch-key children).

Vending machines at school, convenience stores, and radio and television commercials are constant enticements for the child to eat unhealthfully.[2]

Although eating habits and food preferences are firmly established by late childhood, parents can counterbalance the effects of school activities and the media by purchasing and preparing healthful foods. Foods high in sucrose, sodium, and fat should not be kept in the house. Family meals, particularly breakfast, should not be skipped. Meals should not be eaten on the go, in shifts, in front of the television, or at fast-food establishments despite the fact that a large percentage of American families behave in this manner. Statistics reveal that the average American consumes approximately 123 pounds of sugar and other caloric sweeteners annually. Schools can also modify their nutritional practices by eliminating cariogenic foodstuffs from vending machines and lunch programs.[10] Teaching children about the fat and sugar content of foods, how to read ingredient labels, identify hidden sugars, and prepare foods they enjoy by substituting artificial sweeteners and polyunsaturated fats is also extremely valuable in preparing a child to make sound nutritional choices on his own.[11] Nutritional requirements during this stage of development vary from an initial period of slow growth to rapid physical growth by age 12. An increase in activity and metabolism requires additional high-energy foods incorporated into a well-balanced diet consisting of all four food groups. The two most common nutritional disorders currently affecting children in the United States are obesity and iron deficiency anemia.[8]

Iron deficiency anemia affects significant numbers of children and adolescents, primarily females. This condition can be attributed to the start of menses and self-imposed dieting. Meats are the best source of iron.

Obesity in childhood and subsequent adulthood is associated with excessive caloric intake in infancy through bottle feeding and early weaning. It is believed that by breast feeding, solid foods are introduced much later, therefore reducing the risk of overfeeding. Weight loss for the obese child must be monitored carefully so normal growth is not disturbed. A moderate diet coupled with exercise is recommended to prevent the deposition of fatty tissue while promoting typical body growth and development for a child of this age group.[8] Common practices among parents that are believed to encourage obesity are giving a child large portions, recommending they eat seconds, forcing them to clean their plates, and giving food as a reward for desired behavior.

Fluoride

Dental caries rates among children over the past decade have been plummeting despite the fact that 80% of the sugar in the American diet is derived from simple sugars rather than complex carbohydrates. Fluoride is largely responsible for this phenomenon.

During late childhood, fluoride administration is vital for several reasons: (1) the crowns of numerous permanent teeth are still forming during this developmental period, (2) the permanent molars and premolars are highly susceptible to decay as they erupt, and (3) children are acquiring their independence and are becoming increasingly responsible for their own oral hygiene.[2]

Optimal caries protection can be afforded the child by using all the forms of fluoride available. Water fluoridation is ideal during the pre-eruptive period.[12] A child residing in a fluoride-deficient community should remain on fluoride supplementation until age 13 to guarantee maximum protection to the posterior teeth. Concentrated topical fluoride treatments professionally applied on a semiannual basis are recommended once the permanent teeth begin to erupt. Several lower-dosage home care gels (0.5% APF, 1.1% NaF, or 0.4% stannous fluoride) have been shown to be effective in reducing the risk of caries when used daily in patients with rampant decay or individuals with disabilities (see Chapters 3, 8, and 9). Frequent use of relatively low-concentration fluoride toothpastes and mouthrinses are also believed to be highly effective forms of fluoride therapy. Mouthrinses appear to be most beneficial for children age 10 or older because they bathe the posterior teeth more routinely with fluoride as they erupt into the oral cavity.

Sealants

The prevalence of occlusal caries justifes the need for pit and fissure sealants as a preventive measure. When buccal and lingual pits are included in the statistics for pit and fissure surface decay, this surface area accounts for 80% of the total caries experience in children and adolescents.[13]

Deeper fissures tend to be more susceptible to caries. The cuspal inclines that create the walls of a fissure demineralize first and become weak. The wall lesions join at the base of the fissure to form one lesion, which can then spread laterally to the dentinoenamel junction. Cavitation of the fissure eventually results in a clinically detectable lesion.[2]

Sealants, when applied correctly (see Chapter 3), are highly effective in the prevention of pit and fissure caries. Various manufacturers supply both clear and tinted materials. The tinted materials are usually opaque white or transparent pink or yellow. The opaque white and clear are preferred esthetically, but the colors enable the dental health educator to teach the parent and child how to visually monitor the sealant's retention.

ESTHETIC DENTAL MANAGEMENT

Dental anomalies found in a 5-year-old might be disturbing only to the child's parents. Yet, by approximately 8 years of age, ridicule from peers over tetracycline-stained teeth, for example, might not only be humiliating to the child, but suggest to him that he is different. By age 12, that same child might be withdrawn, self-conscious, and rarely smile due to the verbal abuse he has received from his peers.

Resins, Veneers, and Bleaching

Dental health educators must be aware of this critical emotional stage and provide the parents and child with cosmetic solutions to image problems that are encountered in late childhood and early adolescence. With the advent of bleaching techniques, restorative veneers, and composite resins, the appearance of many broken, chipped, cracked, malformed, widely spaced, discolored, or stained teeth can be significantly improved. (This topic is discussed further in Chapter 6.)

Orthodontics

The irregular alignment of teeth can cause emotional problems as a result of the effect it can have on a child's appearance. Malocclusion can be inherited or caused by harmful habits such as digital sucking, mouthbreathing, pushing the tongue against the teeth, or biting the lips. Aberrations in dental and jaw development can increase a child's susceptibility to dental injury, dental disease, and poor nutrition. Teeth that protrude are traumatized more easily, resulting in fracture, dislocation, or avulsion. Plaque removal tends to be more difficult when the teeth are malaligned, predisposing these teeth to dental caries and periodontal disease. Mastication is also more arduous if the teeth are out of alignment. The foods that are easiest to chew are usually soft, non-nutritious, fermentable carbohydrates, which compound the child's risk of dental decay and periodontal problems due to insufficient stimulation of the periodontium.

The correction of a malocclusion therefore promotes physical, oral, and emotional health. Treatment includes a variety of both removable and fixed appliances according to the child's occlusal analysis and individual needs. Prior to the 1970s, an orthodontic patient was referred to as "metal mouth,"

arousing as much or more mockery from peers as the malocclusion itself. The availability of lingual braces and ceramic brackets changed such a sterotype. Bonding allows brackets to be attached to the lingual surfaces of anterior teeth, rendering them virtually undetectable. When lingual bonding is contraindicated, ceramic brackets that are almost invisible are bonded to the facial surfaces of teeth using conventional resin techniques.[14]

Orthodontic treatment for children usually ranges from 18 to 30 months in duration. With computer-enhanced facial software, the orthodontist can actually show the child what his profile will look like at the conclusion of his treatment. The child is normally required to wear a retainer after the removal of braces to stabilize the teeth in their new position. The retainer is usually worn daily for several months until the teeth become more stationary.[15] Appliances fabricated in a variety of colors and designs have generated a great deal of enthusiasm among orthodontic patients, increasing their compliance in wearing the device (Fig. 5-1). The orthodontic patient's oral hygiene and diet are addressed in Chapter 6, and orthodontics for the adult patient is discussed in Chapter 7.

TRAUMATIC INJURIES

Schoolchildren frequently injure their newly erupted permanent teeth as they engage in play activities. During late childhood and adolescence, organized sports greatly increase the risk of dental injury (see Chapter 6). In contrast to the primary dentition, the crowns of the permanent teeth are more often fractured than dislocated.[2] Annually, over 25,000 school accidents involve injury to the teeth. Many of these incidents, e.g., fractures, dislocations, and avulsions, are serious enough to require professional attention.

The dental health educator should be very solicitous when observing and treating a traumatized permanent incisor because

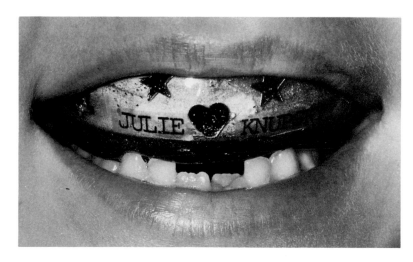

Figure 5-1. Designer orthodontic appliance. Courtesy of C. A. Spear, R.D.H., M.S., and Rajiv Paonaskar, DDS, MS, West Virginia University.

only a slight injury can result in nerve degeneration, loss of vitality, and discoloration of the affected tooth. The extreme can require root canal therapy and bleaching. Minor fractures, on the other hand, are repaired easily and esthetically by the use of bonding or veneers.[16]

At the scene of any accident the oral activity should be examined for evidence of soft tissue lacerations or contusions (Fig. 5-2) and teeth that have been knocked out. If a tooth is missing, it should be located and the following steps should be taken:

1. The tooth should be immediately reimplanted, or
2. If the tooth is dirty, it should be rinsed in water or saline, but not scrubbed and then reimplanted, or
3. If reimplantation is not feasible because of other injuries, or the individual is not able to cooperate, the patient should be transported having him either hold the tooth in the buccal vestibule or in a wet washcloth or cup of cold water or saline.[16]

The dental health educator should assess the patient's medical history after an accident to determine the need for a tetanus injection. Loss of consciousness, disoriented behavior, and nausea are also significant symptoms to address. Positive findings warrant an immediate medical evaluation.[2]

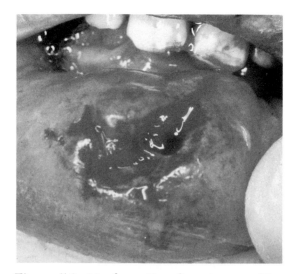

Figure 5-2. Lip laceration from trauma. The maxillary incisor teeth have perforated the soft tissue as a result of a fall.

CHILD ABUSE AND NEGLECT

Precise statistics defining the prevalence of child abuse and neglect do not exist. The National Center on Child Abuse and Neglect estimates a minimum of 2 million cases of child abuse and neglect annually. Only 40% of these incidents are actually reported.[17]

Characteristics of Child Abuse and Neglect

Child abuse and neglect are two different entities. Any deliberate physically, sexually, or emotionally traumatic act inflicted on a child (nonaccidental trauma) is known as child abuse. Child neglect refers to failure to care for a child's physical or emotional needs: omission of food, shelter, supervision, clothing, and health care.[18] Abuse and neglect are widespread. Abusers come from all social, educational, and economic walks of life. Someone who abuses has most likely been abused as a child. Ninety-five percent of abusers are parents.[2]

Almost 30 years ago, Dr. C. Henry Kempe coined the term "battered child syndrome."[19] Today, 10 subtypes of child abuse and neglect can be identified by their characteristics (Table 5-1).[20]

Severe physical injuries are usually directed toward preschoolers; 70% of abuse-related deaths occur during this age period. Physical abuse of males tends to decrease with age. This is not the case for females. Adolescent males more frequently experience emotional and educational abuse, whereas adolescent females are most often victims of sexual abuse.[8] An estimated 25 to 50% of abused children have some form of disability, e.g., sensory, psychological, mental retardation, cerebral palsy.[21] These disabilities may be acquired (physical and psychological problems caused by child abuse and neglect) or congenital (many children who are disabled at birth are perceived by their parents as different, abnormal, or a nuisance). These disabilities act as stimuli to the parents, placing the child at high risk for abuse. Some handicaps are actually exacerbated by abuse.[22]

Table 5-1. Types of Child Abuse and Neglect by Distinguishing Characteristics

Type	Characteristics
Physical abuse	Physical trauma: Mild—a few bruises, cuts, and scratches Moderate—many bruises in atypical areas of body, minor burns, and a single fracture Severe—large burns, CNS or abdominal injury, multiple fractures, or other life threatening injuries
Sexual abuse	Molestation, nonassaultive intercourse, or family-related rape
Failure to thrive	Nutritional neglect caused by parent forgetting to feed child; underweight, malnourished appearance
Intentional drugging or poisoning	The child is given alcohol, drugs to produce intoxication, drug addiction, death
Munchausen syndrome by proxy	Parent fabricates illness for child, e.g., giving child laxatives to induce diarrhea or rubbing the skin to produce a rash so unnecessary medical treatment can be obtained
Medical care neglect	Failure to seek medical care for a child when warranted; parental refusal due to denial or religious beliefs. This results in an increase in the severity of a condition that, if treated early, would have lacked complications
Dental care neglect	Failure to seek treatment for a child with caries, oral infections, or pain; negligence in following through with treatment once informed of the diagnosis and treatment plan
Safety	A gross lack of supervision, particularly of the child under 4 years, leading to burns, poisonings, falls, or other preventable accidents
Emotional abuse and neglect	Failure to stimulate mental growth by rejection of the child; verbal abuse or terrorizing of the child with horrible images and stories
Physical neglect	Poor diet, personal hygiene, or unsanitary home environment
Educational abuse	The child is allowed to be truant; failure to enroll the child in school

Adapted from Schmitt, B. D.: Types of child abuse and neglect. Pediatr. Dent., 8:67–71, 1986.

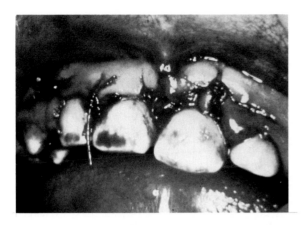

Figure 5-3. Frenum tear. Copyright of the American Society of Dentistry for Children. Child Abuse and Neglect: The Dental Professional Can Help—slide series; slide #6. Reprinted with permission.

Orofacial Trauma

The head and face are often involved in child abuse because they are readily accessible, exposed areas that are significant to a child's whole being.[23] In a 1966 medical study of 29 fatal cases of child abuse, half of the children exhibited injuries to the head and associated areas of the face and oral cavity.[24] Predominant soft-tissue injuries included lacerations of the mucosa of the inner aspect of the upper lip near the frenum, frequently resulting in a tear of the lip from the alveolar margin of the gingiva (Fig. 5-3). Such lacerations can be accomplished by a slap to the mouth or forcing a spoon intraorally when a child is eating too slowly. A toddler learning to walk can injure himself in this manner by falling, but if these intraoral findings are observed on a nonambulatory child or an older child, abuse can be suspected.

Bruises on the face and sides of the head suggest blows with a fist or open hand[25] (Fig. 5-4). Other bruises can be caused by pinching, straps, bites, sticks, boards, hairbrushes, wire, or cord[25] (Fig. 5-5). Bruises vary in color with stage of healing. Red, blue, or purple bruises are up to 3 days old, green to greenish-yellow bruises are between 4 days and 1 week old, and yellow to yellow-brown bruises are 8 to 38 days old.[26]

Burns associated with scalding occur in approximately 10% of abuse cases. Burns can also result from hot objects and toxic chemicals.[25] (Fig. 5-6). Although ocular and auricular trauma can induce severe vision and/or hearing loss, bruising around these areas is more common. Inflicted head injuries include bruises, hematomas, hemorrhage, and alopecia or hair loss from hair-pulling.[23,27] Fractured, discolored, or avulsed teeth can also be indicative of child abuse.[25]

Treatment of Orofacial Injuries. The goal of treatment for the abused or neglected child is the performance of definitive care during the initial visit, if at all possible. Once it is revealed to the parent or the caretaker that child abuse is suspected, follow-up appointments are rarely kept.

If the initial examination exhibits severe trauma beyond the scope of "same day care," emergency treatment should be conducted and appropriate referrals made, e.g., to an oral surgeon, plastic surgeon, or neurologist. Depending on the type of wound inflicted, a tetanus injection might be war-

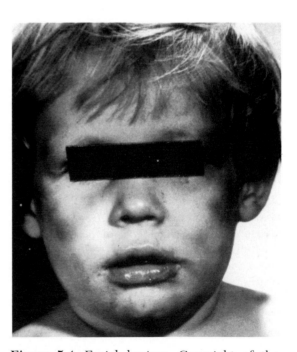

Figure 5-4. Facial bruises. Copyright of the American Society of Dentistry for Children. Child Abuse and Neglect: The Dental Professional Can Help—slide series; slide #45. Reprinted with permission.

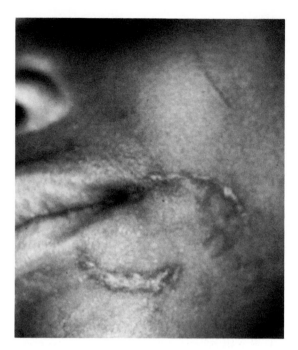

Figure 5-5. Bruising associated with bite marks on the face. Copyright of the American Society of Dentistry for Children. Child Abuse and Neglect: The Dental Professional Can Help—slide series; slide #7. Reprinted with permission.

ranted. Initial treatment and referrals must be conducted prior to discussing with the parents or caregivers the suspicion of child abuse. Intimating that an individual might be a child abuse offender can be threatening and can jeopardize the child's presence at scheduled follow-up visits; therefore, it is imperative that primary care be accomplished that day.

Bruises benefit most from the application of ice during the first 24 hours. A cold compress produces vasoconstriction, which decreases swelling and inflammation.

Frenum lacerations only require sutures and a local anesthetic when the wound is large enough to expose alveolar bone or to separate when the lip is retracted. Abrasions are managed by gently cleansing the wound with warm water and soap to dislodge debris. Irrigation with an antiseptic solution should follow. A sterile dressing, changed daily, is placed over the site to protect it and promote healing. Human bites must also be cleansed and debrided to prevent infection.

A tetanus injection and an antibiotic are recommended to reduce the risk of infection.

Electrical burns can also pose a threat to a patient, often requiring hospitalization and surgical repair if severe (see Chapter 4). Minor electrical burns are treated with topical antibiotics. Antibiotics should be applied to thermal burns and covered with a sterile dressing. If ulcerations form from a thermal injury, topical steroids or topical anesthetics, can be applied to alleviate pain and promote healing. Voluntary or involuntary ingestion of a chemical agent can result in necrotic oral epithelium, excessive salivation, drooling, and dysphasia. These clinical findings manifest from the corrosive action of the caustic substance on the mucosa. Oral mucosal sloughing and esophageal mucosal irritation produce pain. If damage to the mucosal nerve endings results, numbness is exhibited. Flushing the chemical residue with copious amounts of water is recommended.[23]

Child Abuse Intervention

By 1966, all 50 states had passed laws mandating that health science professionals

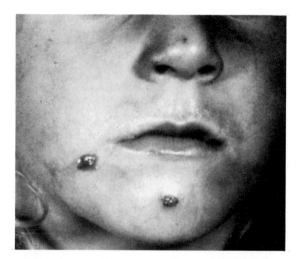

Figure 5-6. Facial cigarette burns. Copyright of the American Society of Dentistry for Children. Child Abuse and Neglect: The Dental Professional Can Help—slide series; slide #3. Reprinted with permission.

report suspected child abuse cases.[2,28] The dental health educator in particular has ample opportunity to identify children he suspects are being abused by conducting a thorough orofacial examination. If suspicious areas are encountered a cursory physical examination should also be performed with a witness present, e.g., a dental assistant. Not all injuries are observable; therefore radiographs can be used to detect more subtle areas of trauma and untreated fractures. A thorough medical history is also necessary.[29] Injuries that are inconsistent with histories obtained from parents, caretakers, or the child himself should be questioned.[30]

The dental health educator should observe the parent-child interaction for hostile, resentful behavior.[29] The younger child might have difficulty verbalizing the abuse and might experience insomnia, anxiety, and recurrent fearful dreams and exhibit withdrawal behavior, e.g., truancy, running away from home, and behavior disorders in the classroom.[31] If abuse is suspected, the child should be interviewed separately from the parents. The dental health educator is not a detective and should interview the parents in a non-threatening style while attempting to alert the parents of his concerns. The dental health educator should avoid being angry or judgmental with these individuals and deal with potential cases objectively.[32] Seeking information is acceptable behavior, and most parents will allow this if it is done tactfully. If the story conveyed by the parent is not congruent with the data gathered concerning the signs, symptoms, and possible causes of the injury, however, further questioning is necessary. If it is concluded that the injury was not an accident, then it is the professional's obligation to notify the proper agency (see Appendix A) so that they can further explore the problem.[33] Prior to filing a child abuse report, the dental health educator should tell the parents that the authorities are being contacted. The dental health educator should also explain his rationale for suspecting child abuse. If the dental health educator has been threatened by parents and is concerned for his own safety as a result of intending to disclose this information,[30] an anonymous report can be made to the authorities that cannot be traced back to the health professional.

The patient's records should be explicit concerning the clinical findings. Photographs or illustrations, and documentation of the interview should be included.[30]

In many schools across the nation children are being taught about child molestation and what they can do to avoid the problem.[34] The dental health educator has a responsibility for being knowledgeable concerning the recognition, treatment, and reporting of this critical health care issue.[35]

Abuse is not confined to children and the disabled. Spouse abuse and abuse of the elderly are also considerable problems in the United States. Approximately 1.8 million women are battered yearly; a violent act occurs every 18 seconds. The United States House Committee on Aging estimated that 4% or 1 million of the nation's elderly are victims of abuse each year.[36] The clinical signs and symptoms described previously are encountered in these adults as well.

SCHOOL DENTAL HEALTH PROGRAMS

School dental health programs encompass a wide variety of activities. Some schools have extensive programs as part of their curriculum, others include dental health as a unit in a health course, and some schools provide isolated dental health presentations to their students, usually centered around Children's Dental Health Month. Large amounts of manpower and financial resources are invested yearly for the promotion and implementation of these programs.

Program Effectiveness

Public schools in the United States have accepted the responsibility for dental health education since the 1940s. Historically schools emphasized learning facts about the teeth and their functions. By the 1960s it became evident that such knowledge had little effect on the child's oral health status. Although the emphasis was changed to include teaching oral health practices, numerous studies concluded that classroom preventive instruction was of limited value in changing behavior.[13,37-43]

Oral hygiene attitudes and behavior can be improved by the inclusion of seven educational strategies into a school dental health program.

1. Preschool-to-secondary-school dental health programs should be developed that include information and experiences that escalate in complexity. Standardization of a K–12 dental health curriculum would be extremely helpful in accomplishing this goal.[44]
2. Parental involvement in dental health program activities on plaque control, fluoride, and diet are necessary to provide continuity from the school to the home.
3. Student participation should be encouraged. Refrain from overwhelming the child with too much information at one time; the more involved children are, the more cooperative they will be.[45]
4. Repetition and reinforcement of oral hygiene skills leads to the improved oral health of children.[46,47]
5. Adequate time and resources for dental health education should be provided. Effectively designed and implemented programs using more innovative curricular materials and media are needed. Health fairs, audio-visuals, puppet shows, etc. can be useful in developing oral hygiene techniques, alleviating the apprehension associated with dental treatment, displaying the relationship between nutrition and dental health, and increasing a child's knowledge and understanding of dental disease and dental procedures.[48,49]
6. A comprehensive school-based program should also include early identification of dental needs through screenings of all children on a yearly basis. Follow-up can be provided by fixed or mobile clinics made available by the county school system or public health department, or a contract can be drawn up between local practitioners and the board of education to volunteer or offer services for predetermined fees.[42]
7. Evaluation is necessary to assist health professionals and school personnel in assessing the effectiveness of a program and establishing guidelines for further program development.

Caries Preventive Programs

Today, in addition to oral hygiene practices, school programs concentrate on the multisystem fluoride approach and the application of dental sealants.[50]

Communal and school water fluoridation continue to be the most effective and least costly methods for preventing dental caries (see Chapter 3). Approximately 500 schools across the nation add fluoride to their water supplies, serving over 170,000 students.[51]

The Preventive Dentistry Demonstration Program[13] suggested fluoride mouthrinses were of limited value. Yet, in a 7-year study assessing a fluoride mouthrinsing program in a New York elementary school, a 50% reduction in caries was found. This and other literature advise that the benefits of rinsing directly relate to the duration of participation in the program.[44] The majority of caries observed in this study were on the pits and fissures of the occlusal surfaces. When the study was supplemented with sealants, the children remained 96% caries-free after 2 years.[52,53] Despite the effectiveness of sealants, their cost might prohibit mass application for schoolchildren.[13] In the 1986–1987 NIDR survey, discussed in Chapter 3, only 7.6% of schoolchildren in the United States had dental sealants placed on one or more teeth. School fluoride rinse programs have been popular since the 1960s. These programs are inexpensive to operate and continue today as a feasible alternative to sealants. In 1989, the NIDR reported that approximately 13 million schoolchildren across the country were participating in fluoride rinse programs.[51]

REFERENCES

1. Lowrey, G. H.: Growth and Development of Children. 6th Ed. Chicago, Year Book, 1973.
2. Watson, E. H., and Lowrey, G. H.: Growth and Development in Children. 5th Ed. Chicago, Year Book, 1967.
3. Piaget, J., and Inhelder, B.: The Psychology of the Child. New York, Basic Books, 1969.
4. Finn, S. B.: Clinical Pedodontics. 4th Ed. Philadelphia, W. B. Saunders, 1973.
5. Stone, L. J., and Church, J.: Childhood and Adolescence. 3rd Ed. New York, Random House, 1975.
6. Suomi, J. D., et al.: Oral calculus in children. J. Periodontol., 42:341-345, 1971.
7. Murray, J. J.: The prevalence of gingivitis in children continuously resident in a high fluoride area. J. Dent. Child., 41:133-139, 1974.
8. McDonald, R. E., and Avery, D. R.: Dentistry for the Child and Adolescent. 5th Ed. St. Louis, C. V. Mosby, 1987.
9. Anderson, T. A., Wei, S. H. Y., and Fomon, S. J.: Nutritional counseling and the development of eating habits. In The Food That Stays: An Update on Nutrition, Diet, Sugar and Caries. Edited by E. A. Sweeney, New York, Medcom, 1977.
10. Guthrie, H. A., and Sheehe, M. P.: Nutrition messages in elementary school textbooks. J. Sch. Health, 54:126-127, 1984.
11. Weinstein, L. B., Abrams, R. A., and Ayers, C. S.: Increasing awareness of sugar ingestion among children. Pediatr. Nurs., 14:277-279, 1988.
12. Van Eck, A. A. M. J., Groenveld, A., and Backer Dirks, O.: Pre and post-eruptive caries reduction by water fluoridation. Caries Res., 19:163, 1985.
13. Bohannan, H. M., et al.: A summary of the results of the National Preventive Dentistry Demonstration Program. J. Can. Dent. Assoc., 6:435-441, 1985.
14. Martin, F. J.: New age dentistry for children. Dent. Tmwk., 1:220-223, 1988.
15. Maloney, L. R. (Ed.): Guide to Dental Health. J. Am. Dent. Assoc., Special Issue, 1987.
16. Wei, S. H. Y. (Ed.): Pediatric Dental Care: An Update for the Dentist and for the Pediatrician. New York, Medcom, 1978.
17. National Center on Child Abuse and Neglect: Child Abuse and Developmental Disabilities: Essays. Washington, DC, U. S. Department of Health and Human Services. publication No. 79-30226, 1980.
18. Davis, G. R., et al.: The dentist's role in child abuse and neglect. J. Dent. Child., 46:185, 1979.
19. Kempe, C. H., et al.: The battered child syndrome. J. Am. Med. Assoc., 181:17, 1962.
20. Schmitt, B. D.: Types of child abuse and neglect. Pediatr. Dent., 8:67-71, 1986.
21. A report on the first national conference on the implications of child abuse and neglect for dental education and dental health care. J. Dent. Child., 48:311-312, 1981.
22. Mullins, J. B.: The relationship between child abuse and handicapping conditions. J. Sch. Health, 56:134-136, 1986.
23. Needleman, H. L.: Orofacial trauma in child abuse: Types, prevalence, management, and the dental profession's involvement. Pediatr. Dent., 8:71-79, 1986.
24. Cameron, J. M., Johnson, H. R., and Camps, F. E.: The battered child syndrome. Med. Sci. Law, 6:2-21, 1966.
25. Sanger, R. G., and Bross, D. C.: Clinical Management of Child Abuse and Neglect. Chicago, Quintessence, 1984.
26. Wilson, E. F.: Estimation of the age of cutaneous contusions in child abuse. Pediatrics, 60:750, 1977.
27. Schmitt, B. D.: Physical abuse: Specifics of clinical diagnosis. Pediatr. Dent., 8:83-87, 1986.
28. Regis, J. S.: Early detection of child maltreatment. Dent. Hyg., 59:62-64, 1985.
29. Child abuse recognition and reporting. Sp. Care Dent., 6:62-67, 1986.
30. Symons, A. L., Rowe, P. V., and Romaniuk, K.: Dental aspects of child abuse: Review and case reports. Aust. Dent. J., 32:42-47, 1987.
31. Kempe, C. H.: Sexual abuse, another hidden pediatric problem: The 1977 C. Anderson Aldrich lecture. Pediatrics, 62:382-389, 1978.
32. Luther, S. L., and Price, J. H.: Child sexual abuse: A review. J. Sch. Health, 50:161-165, 1980.
33. Goldson, E.: Child abuse: A social-psychological-medical-disorder. In Psychological Aspects of Pediatric Care. Edited by E. Gellert. New York, Grune and Stratton, 1978.
34. McNab, W. L.: Staying alive: A mini-unit on child molestation prevention for elementary schoolchildren. J. Sch. Health, 55:226-229, 1985.
35. Carlin, S. A., and Polk, K. K.: Teaching the detection of child abuse in dental schools. J. Dent. Educ., 49:651-652, 1985.
36. King, N. R.: Exploitation and abuse of older family members: An overview of the problem. In Abuse of the Elderly. Edited by J. Costa. Lexington, MA, Lexington Books, 1984, pp. 3-6.
37. Smith, L. W., et al.: Teachers as models in programs for school dental health: An evaluation of the "Toothkeeper." J. Pub. Health Dent., 35:75-80, 1975.
38. Croft, L. K.: The effectiveness of the Toothkeeper program after six years. Tex. Dent. J., 98:4, 1980.
39. Graves, R. C., et al.: A comparison of the effectiveness of the "Toothkeeper" and a traditional dental health education program. J. Pub. Health Dent., 35:85-90, 1975.
40. Kleinman, P. R., et al.: An assessment of the Alabama Smile Keeper school dental health education program. J. Am. Dent. Assoc., 98:51-54, 1979.
41. Melson, B., and Agerback, N.: Effect of an instructional motivation program on oral health in Danish adolescents after 1 and 2 years. Comm. Dent. Oral Epidemiol., 8:72-78, 1980.
42. Horowitz, A. M., et al.: Effects of supervised daily dental plaque removal by children: 24-month results. J. Pub. Health Dent., 37:180-188, 1977.
43. Horowitz, A. M.: A comparison of available strategies to affect children's dental health: Primary preventive procedures for use in school based dental programs. J. Pub. Health Dent., 39:268-274, 1979.
44. Harris, N. O., and Christen, A. G.: Primary Preventive Dentistry. 2nd Ed., East Norwalk, CT, Appleton & Lange, 1987.
45. Logan, H. L., Shepardson, R., and Hayden, H.: Oral care instruction in the public classroom: Some tips. Dent. Hyg., 53:459-461, 1979.
46. Emler, B., et al.: The value of repetition and reinforcement in improving oral hygiene performance. J. Periodontol., 51:4, 1980.

47. Lee, A. J.: Daily, dry toothbrushing in kindergarten. J. Sch. Health, *50*:506-508, 1980.

48. Levy, G. F.: A survey of preschool oral health education programs. J. Pub. Health Dent., *44*:10-18, 1984.

49. Hawkins, C.: The Newport News, Virginia dental health fair. J. Sch. Health, *56*:292-293, 1986.

50. Flanders, R. A.: Effectiveness of dental health educational programs in schools. J. Am. Dent. Assoc., *114*:239-242, 1987.

51. McCann, D. (Ed.): Fluoride and oral health: A story of achievements and challenges. J. Am. Dent. Assoc., *118*:529-540, 1989.

52. Ripa, L. W.: The surface-specific caries pattern of participants in a school based fluoride mouthrinsing program with implications for the use of sealants. J. Pub. Health Dent., *45*:90, 1985.

53. Ripa, L. W.: Caries prevention in children: The use of fluoride mouthrinses and pit and fissure sealants. N. Y. St. Dent. J., *53*:16, 1987.

Chapter 6

THE ADOLESCENT

*Fifteen is really medieval and pioneer and
nothing is clear and nothing is sure, and nothing
is safe and nothing is come and nothing is gone
but it all might be.*

Gertrude Stein
Gertrude Stein: Her Life and Her Work
by Elizabeth Sprigge

PHYSICAL, INTELLECTUAL, AND PSYCHOSOCIAL CHANGES

The period of growth and development that occurs in an individual as he moves from childhood to adulthood is known as adolescence.[1] In U.S. society the term teenager has become synonymous with adolescent, characterizing the individual between 13 and 20 years of age.[2] With emphasis on the physical activity of the individual rather than chronological age, adolescence is often described as beginning with the onset of puberty and ending when morphologic and physiologic growth and development are largely completed.[1] Development of the secondary sexual characteristics associated with puberty occurs approximately 2 years earlier in females (12 to 13½ years) than males (13 to 15½ years).[3] During this growth spurt, an increase in muscle mass, body fat redistribution, and skeletal growth can also be observed.[4] Menarche usually signals the end of a female's growth spurt, whereas males have no such indicator and usually continue to grow over a longer period of time. The average child can expect a 20 to 25% increase in height and a 100% gain in weight during adolescence.[5]

Intellectual capacity also increases consistent with physical growth. Piaget refers to this period of intellectual development as the formal operational stage.[6] The adolescent becomes capable of thinking more abstractly and understanding logic and deductive reasoning.

Psychosocial development is greatly influenced by a teenager's experiences with his environment. Successes or failures encountered during the previous physical and intellectual developmental stages will determine an individual's sense of identity and level of self-confidence. For instance, the young adolescent who appears more advanced in height, weight, or sexual maturity will often be shunned or ridiculed by the "normal" adolescent group and will have great difficulty coping with his own body image until that time when the norm group catches up to him. Often the damage to this individual's self-worth cannot be erased, affecting his capacity for intimacy and trust in future relationships.

By mid-adolescence, emotional independence from parents and more mature relations with peers emerge, furthering gender differentiation and sexual identity.[3] It is because teens seem to profit from interaction with secure, satisfied adults outside the family that role models are extremely important in guiding an adolescent's thinking and behavior. Teenagers live in a confusing world with an ever-changing social value system (drugs, promiscuity, and communicable disease constitute particularly problematic issues). This situation creates a great deal of anxiety in the adolescent, who, as he approaches adulthood, looks to his role model(s) for answers to what is considered okay to do versus what is considered to be undesirable behavior. Overly strict or ineffective parents or significant others can lead to defiance and resentment.

Delinquency, attempted or successful suicide, smoking, eating disorders, alcohol and drug abuse, and irresponsible sex practices are just a few of the typical behaviors of a maladjusted adolescent. The patterns of behavior and attitudes acquired during this transition period known as adolescence determine an individual's present and future health, degree of psychosocial "belonging," and future economic productivity.[1]

Late adolescence or young adulthood offers continued separation from parents and individualization. The teenager begins to develop a concern for those beyond himself. Feelings about long-term commitment, e.g., marriage, family, and career, are being formulated. If conflicts with parents exist they are usually resolved, accepting parents for the people they are.[3]

Orofacial Growth and Development. The anatomy of the face and head is finalized during adolescence. The nose and chin become more pronounced, and the ramus of the mandible increases in vertical dimension to accommodate the expansion of the nasal region and the remaining erupting permanent teeth. By ages 12 to 13 the second molars erupt; they are followed by the third molars, which usually erupt between 17 and 21 years of age.

By the close of adolescence the 27 bones that once comprised the skull of a newborn have now joined to form 22 bones.[4]

DEMOGRAPHICS

There are over 33 million adolescents in the United States. In recent decades, the adolescent/young adult population in America has considerably increased relative to other age groups.[1] These statistics are influenced by the "baby boom" phenomenon of 1945–1965. The large numbers of individuals born during this 20-year period now have adolescent offspring of their own. Currently there are 20 persons 65 and over and 42 children under 18 for every 100 persons of working age (18–64 years). However, these relationships are changing; by 2030, when the last of the baby boom generation will have reached 65, the ratio of elderly to working-age persons will be greater than the ratio of children to working-age persons (Table 6-1).[7]

Today, many adolescents reside in one-parent families. The U.S. Census Bureau notes that 19% of children under 18 years of age live with a single parent. This figure is considerably higher for blacks.[8] Generally, youths from these homes are discipline problems. They are frequently truant, drop out of school, display poor academic perfor-

Table 6-1. Middle Series Population Projections (In Thousands)

Age	Year			
	1987	2000	2030	2050
Under 17	63,542	65,713	62,161	59,764
18 to 64	150,536	167,672	172,864	171,552
65 and over	29,835	34,882	65,604	68,532
Total	243,913	268,267	300,629	299,848

From U.S. Bureau of the Census, Current Population Reports: Population Estimates and Projections. Series P-25, No. 1018, Washington, DC, U.S. Government Printing Office, 1989.

mance, and often have difficulty coping socially and emotionally. The statistics are alarming:[5]

1:2   adolescents (15–19 years) is sexually active.

1:4   adolescents (11 years and older) drops out of school prior to graduation.

1:8   high school students (17 years) is functionally illiterate.

1:10 adolescent females (15–19 years) becomes pregnant annually.

1:30 adolescents (10–19 years) runs away from home.

THE ADOLESCENT DENTAL PATIENT

Dentistry for the adolescent usually begins after the eruption of the permanent premolars and canines. Orthodontic intervention initiated during late childhood is a common form of dental therapy for this age group. Other dental concerns such as caries and periodontal disease seem to be most severe during the teen years. Hormonal changes, rapid growth, and the quest for independence as exemplified by poor oral hygiene and erratic eating patterns have been implicated as plausible causes.[9]

Esthetic dental procedures and protection of the teeth during athletic competition are of great interest to the adolescent during a period when appearance and popularity are extremely pertinent to a successful lifestyle.

Communication

An open line of communication is essential with all persons if behavioral change is expected. Young adolescents present a challenge for communication because they are often moody and sensitive, particularly during pubescence.[10] In an effort to gain independence the adolescent will frequently resist advice from an authority figure and refute any rules or regulations handed down

from a parent or teacher. Successful dialogue with teens lies in determining what motivates existing habits, so the dental health educator can relate more desirable behavior to what currently serves as an incentive to the individual. The adolescent is often motivated by appearance, popularity, and sports.

The dental health educator can be more effective if he works with the teenager alone, rather than in the presence of parents or peers. This interpersonal setting ensures that the adolescent will receive the educator's complete attention and no disruptive interaction will occur. Many teens cannot be truthful in front of their parents or peers; in the presence of such persons they will try to act in the manner expected of them by each, which is often contradictory. For instance, in a dental health counseling session, a teenager will rarely admit to smoking or eating junk foods with a parent present for fear he will be scolded. Having a judgmental parent in the room places the teenager in the child's role, and he becomes embarrassed. He retreats into silence or one-word responses as his parent begins talking for him. Parents also do not like to be embarrassed, and they will answer for their child in a style that they believe to be appropriate.

Teenagers need to be treated as adults. Although it is often difficult for the dental health educator, he should never pass judgment on the adolescent's lifestyle or attitudes even when they conflict with his own. A nonjudgmental approach leads to open and honest communication and a more trusting relationship. The wonder of health education lies in allowing the patient to draw his own conclusions and make his own decisions on the basis of a sound, clear explanation of the problem by the educator.[9]

Dental Caries

Despite the decline in caries nationally among children, the caries activity of adolescents remains significantly high for many individuals. Rampant caries is more common in the female adolescent. Recall from

Chapter 3 that decayed, missing, and filled permanent tooth surfaces increased from 2.7 surfaces in the 12-year-old to 8 surfaces for the average 17-year-old.[11]

Emotional disturbances have been suggested as a possible cause in some cases of rampant caries. Certainly this theory supports a higher prevalence of caries among adolescents who routinely experience feelings of tension and anxiety related to school, home, and appearance. Depression or frustration often leads to overindulging in sweets or snack foods. These foods are high in fermentable carbohydrates and promote tooth decay. The emotionally disturbed teenager also sustains a noticeable reduction in salivary flow, or xerostomia. Antidepressant or antipsychotic drugs prescribed for the nervous or anxious patient further depress salivary function, resulting in an increase in caries susceptibility due to impaired remineralization.[12]

Periodontal Disease

Evidence of periodontal disease in adolescents exists at a level higher than one might suspect. Loss of periodontal attachment and supporting bone in one or more locations occurs in 5 to 46% of teenagers depending on the method of diagnosis and the population surveyed. Generalized and localized forms of gingivitis affect a much larger percentage of this age group. Adolescent gingiva appears to be more sensitive to local irritants, e.g., plaque and trauma, than the gingiva of a child. Histologically, gingivitis in adolescents also mimics that of an adult rather than that of a child, with plasma cells predominating at the affected site. Unlike gingivitis in the child, gingivitis in the adolescent can and will progress to periodontitis if untreated. These factors suggest that periodontal involvement during adolescence is the result of a transition period in the body's immune response as well.[4]

PUBERTY GINGIVITIS

Gingival inflammation exaggerated by the hormonal fluctuations experienced during

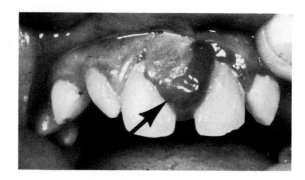

Figure 6-1. Puberty gingivitis. Courtesy of J.E. Bouquot, DDS, MS, West Virginia University.

puberty is a common phenomenon in adolescents. As in gingivitis induced by pregnancy or oral contraceptives (see Chapter 7), the interproximal gingiva, particularly in the anterior segment, becomes edematous and bleeds spontaneously (Fig. 6-1). Overall, the gingival response is far greater than normally expected from the presence of plaque and calculus on the teeth. By age 18, the hormonal influence on the gingiva usually diminishes. In a study conducted by Sutcliffe of children between the ages of 11 and 17, both sexes displayed a high prevalence of gingivitis. Although 90% of 11- and 12-year-olds were affected, the prevalence tended to decline with age.[13]

Other local factors that aggravate the gingivae in this age group are orthodontic appliances, restorations with overhangs, and carious teeth.

The dental health educator must warn parents and children in the late childhood years of this hormonal condition and the extreme importance of proper oral hygiene in reducing its sequelae. Treatment should begin with an oral prophylaxis and oral hygiene instruction relative to the patient's needs to ensure thorough and routine removal of bacterial irritants. Often the adolescent's diet is poor and dietary counseling is indicated. Overhanging margins on fillings must be removed, and carious teeth must be restored. If orthodontic appliances harbor plaque, the gingiva will respond adversely. Meticulous oral hygiene and the relatively smooth surface created by orthodontic bonding can reduce the risk of gingival disturbances among adolescents.

JUVENILE PERIODONTITIS

Juvenile periodontitis is an aggressive form of periodontal disease that causes a rapid loss of the alveolar bone and periodontal ligament supporting the permanent teeth.

If it is the localized type of juvenile periodontitis (LJP), the first molars and incisor teeth are commonly involved. Some believe that localized juvenile periodontitis is a hereditary neutrophil disorder of function, transmitted by an autosomal recessive or an x-linked dominant gene.[14] Pubescent and adolescent youths (10 to 15 years of age) tend to be at greatest risk for developing LJP. Estimates of the prevalence of LJP range from 0.1% to 15% in this age group.

On clinical examination the gingiva appears normal. The condition is virtually undetectable until periodontal probing is conducted and bleeding from the infected gingival sulci occurs. Actinobacillus actinomycetemcomitans is the organism believed to penetrate the crevicular epithelium. If LJP is diagnosed and treated early, severe bone loss, tooth mobility, and eventual tooth loss can be prevented in these young individuals. Figure 6-2 illustrates bone loss in a more advanced case of LJP.

Generalized juvenile periodontitis is similar to LJP except that more than half or all of the permanent dentition is affected, and heavy accumulations of plaque with observable gingival inflammation are present.

Treatment for both the generalized and localized forms of juvenile periodontitis consists of scaling, root planing, and curettage of infected tissue; periodontal surgery if hard and soft tissue deformities exist, and a 2-week or longer regimen of tetracycline antibiotic therapy.[4,12]

The dental health educator must work closely with the adolescent suffering from juvenile periodontitis. Frequent intervals of preventive maintenance, beginning with weekly appointments and progressing to

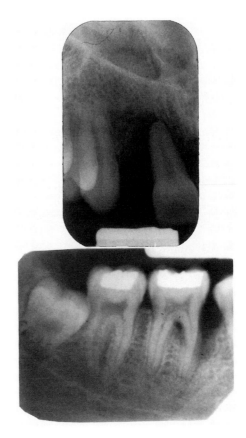

Figure 6-2. Periapical radiographs illustrating alveolar bone loss associated with juvenile periodontitis. Courtesy of R. J. Crout, DMD, PhD, West Virginia University.

monthly sessions, are necessary to avoid recurrence.

ACUTE NECROTIZING ULCERATIVE GINGIVITIS

A noncontagious infection common in young adults is known as acute necrotizing ulcerative gingivitis (ANUG), Vincent's infection, or trench mouth. Spirochetes and fusiform bacilli are responsible for this infection; they usually attack when the individual's resistance is low during periods of stress or illness. Adolescents frequently experience ANUG during examination week, when rest, and good dietary and oral hygiene practices are often ignored.

The clinical manifestations include blunt-

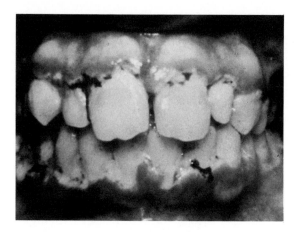

Figure 6-3. Acute necrotizing ulcerative gingivitis.

ing or cratering of the interdental gingival papillae, gingival inflammation and bleeding, a grayish pseudomembrane covering the gingival margin, oral pain, a fetid mouth odor from bacterial accumulation and tissue necrosis, poor appetite, fever, lymphadenopathy, and a feeling of general malaise (Fig. 6-3).

A remarkable change in the gingival tissue can occur within 1 to 2 days following treatment. Depending on the severity of the condition, a series of appointments should be scheduled until the patient's acute symptoms have subsided. The first meeting should consist of thoroughly explaining the following to the patient: (1) the nature of the condition; (2) oral hygiene care recommendations,which include a rinse consisting of equal parts of 3% hydrogen peroxide and water hourly for the first 2 to 3 days, followed by saline rinses every 2 hours thereafter; (3) the importance of avoiding alcoholic beverages and smoking products; and (4) the need for a well-balanced diet: bland liquids and soft foods should be consumed for the first 2 days following initial treatment. Rinsing with an anesthetic solution, e.g., viscous lidocaine (Xylocaine) or dyclonine (Dyclone), might be necessary to alleviate the discomfort associated with eating. Foods should be served at a temperature soothing to the oral tissues. Therapeutic doses of vitamins B and C are also recommended.[15] Subgingival scaling started at the

first visit should be continued until healing is complete in all gingival areas. If one or more areas do not respond, gingivoplasty might be needed to correct a soft tissue defect. When bony cratering is present, flap surgery with osseous recontouring is indicated. Therapeutic antibiotics can be administered to eliminate systemic symptoms.[4,12,16]

RECURRENT APHTHOUS ULCER

The recurrent aphthous ulcer (RAU) is also called a canker sore. These ulcerations are most prevalent in adolescents and are experienced by females twice as often as males. Although aphthae are believed to be caused by bacteria,[17] some conjecture RAU is the result of a cell-mediated immunity.[18] Nonetheless, the susceptibility of certain individuals to aphthae appears to be related to (1) localized trauma, e.g., cheekbiting and impingement of dental films on the oral soft tissue; (2) stress; (3) nutritional deficiencies particularly, iron, B_{12}, and folic acid; and (4) gastrointestinal disorders.[19]

RAU typically develops on nonkeratinized oral mucosa (Fig. 6-4). The ulcers ap-

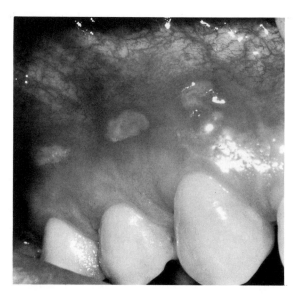

Figure 6-4. Recurrent aphthous ulcers (RAU), or canker sores. Courtesy of C.A. Spear, BSDH, MS, West Virginia University.

pear as white, round, or oval crater-like centers bound by an erythematous margin. Sometimes they erupt singularly or in clusters to form a lesion of approximately 1 to 3 mm in diameter. They are painful and have a duration of 4 to 12 days.

Numerous over-the-counter (OTC) preparations are available to soothe the pain and promote eating without discomfort. Some of the antibacterial mouthwashes with low alcohol content have been reported as helpful. A list of these agents can be found in Table 6-2.[20]

PERICORONITIS

The adolescent might also experience pericoronitis as the third molars (wisdom teeth) begin to erupt. This condition arises when an operculum or a flap of tissue from the retromolar pad extends over the crown of the erupting tooth (Fig. 6-5). Food can become impacted under this tissue covering, producing an acute infection. Trauma to the operculum from an opposing tooth is also a common cause. Symptoms include halitosis from the collection of debris beneath the operculum, pain associated with the edema and sensitivity of the area, and an inability to obtain complete jaw closure due to tissue thickness and irritation.[4] Treatment ranges from tooth extraction to excision of the tissue tag to simple debridement of the area with saline. Antibiotics might be required for extensive inflammation. The patient can be instructed to irrigate the site at home.

Radiographic Assessment

Radiographic examination is essential to the proper detection of dental caries and periodontal disease in the adolescent. If the teenager's oral cavity is large enough, an adult radiographic survey can be taken with size 2 intraoral films to ensure tissue coverage. The type of radiographs (panoramic, bitewings, periapicals) should be dictated by the number of teeth present and the reason for the radiographic appraisal. Assessing

an adolescent's growth and development is primarily an inquiry into the status of canines, premolars, and third molars.

For the adolescent with rampant caries and possible periapical pathosis, periapical films are necessary. To assess areas of interproximal decay or alveolar bone height, particularly in a teenager with LJP, bitewing radiographs are indicated. The panogram is ideal for a new patient with minimal or no treatment needs. This film gives the dental health educator the full scope of the patient's development from the presence or absence of certain teeth to a gross display of the sinus and temporomandibular joint.[4] In addition to their function as diagnostic tools, dental radiographs serve as outstanding patient education devices.

PREVENTION OF DENTAL DISEASE

The health of the teeth and periodontium becomes critical during adolescence. Although gingivitis in the child appears to have no long-term consequences on the periodontal status of the adult, gingival inflammation around an adolescent's permanent teeth can lead to fibrotic tissue, recession, and crestal bone loss.[4] Similarly, rampant or single advanced carious lesions in the permanent dentition can result in a loss of teeth with no natural replacements. This loss can cause periodontal, esthetic, and masticatory problems, and restoring function can be costly. Daily, thorough oral hygiene is the mainstay for preventing irreversible damage associated with caries and periodontal disease. When dental health is meaningful to the adolescent, he is likely to practice routine oral hygiene, a healthful habit he will retain through adulthood. Unfortunately, although most adolescents possess the dexterity to brush and floss adequately, they lack the motivation to perform these procedures on a regular basis.

Table 6-2. OTC Preparations for the Treatment of Oral Ulcerations
(Cold Sore/Canker Sore Preparations)

Product (Manufacturer)	Ingredients
Anbesol (Whitehall)	Benzocaine 6.3%, phenol 0.5%; povidone iodine (0.04% available iodine), alcohol 70%
Anbesol Gel (Whitehall)	Benzocaine 6.3%, phenol 0.5%, alcohol 70%; viscous water-soluble base
Baby Anbesol (Whitehall)	Benzocaine 7.5%; viscous water-soluble base without alcohol
Baby Orajel (Commerce)	Benzocaine 7.5%; viscous water-soluble base
Benzodent (Vicks)	Benzocaine 20%, eugenol 0.4%, hydroxy-quinoline sulfate 0.1%; denture-adhesive-like base
Blistex Lip Ointment (Blistex)	Camphor 1%, phenol 0.45%
Butyn Dental Ointment (Abbott)	Butacaine 4%
Campho-Phenique Liquid and Gel (Winthrop)	Phenol 4.7, camphor 10.8%
Cankaid (Becton Dickinson)	Carbamide peroxide 10%, anhydrous glycerol; flavor
Cold Sore Lotion (Pfeiffer)	Gum benzoin 7.0%, alcohol 85%
Gly-Oxide (Marion)	Carbamide peroxide 10%, anhydrous glycerol
Herpecin (Campbell)	Pyridoxine hydrochloride, Padimate O
Herpes Simplex Relief Formula (DeWitt)	Gum benzoin 1.2%, alcohol 90%; menthol 0.3%, camphor 3.7%, phenol 0.3%
Kank-A Liquid (Blistex)	Benzocaine 20%, cetyl pyridinium chloride 0.5%
Lysine (amino acid supplement)	
Orabase with Benzocaine (Colgate-Hoyt)	Benzocaine 20%, pectin, gelatin, carboxymethyl cellulose sodium, polyethylene, mineral oil
Orajel (Commerce)	Benzocaine 10.0%, polyethylene-glycol-like base 62.7%
Ora-5 (Premier)	Copper sulfate, iodine, alcohol 1.5%
Ora-jel Extra-Strength (Commerce)	Benzocaine 20%
Proxigel (Reed & Carnrick)	Carbamide peroxide 10%; water-free gel base
Rexall Cold Sore Lotion (Rexall)	Phenol, menthol, benzoin, camphor; alcohol 90%
Rexall Cold Sore Ointment (Rexall)	Phenol, menthol, benzoin, camphor, alcohol 30%; viscous base
Ulcerease (Med-Derm)	Phenol, 0.6%, glycerine, water, sodium bicarbonate, sodium borate
Zilactin (Zila)	Hydroxypropylcellulose, tannic acid 7%, alcohol 80%

Adapted from Baker, K.A., and Helling, D.K.: Oral Health Products. In Handbook of Nonprescription Drugs. 8th Ed. Washington, DC, American Pharmaceutical Association, 1986, pp. 477–505.

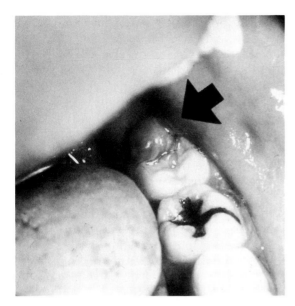

Figure 6-5. Pericoronitis. Courtesy of D. Terrill, DDS, MS, Fredericksburg, VA.

Oral Hygiene

The parents' role in an adolescent's dental home care is relatively minimal. The teenager has a strong desire to control his own life, voicing his independence by his ability to take care of himself. Therefore, the adolescent accepts oral home care as his own responsibility. Some adolescents take the job seriously, but others lack the motivation to practice routine oral hygiene. The dental health educator functions by both educating and motivating teens to proper oral health, reducing the risk of caries and periodontal disease.

The dental health educator's first encounter with a patient involves communication through a medical and dental history and an oral inspection. The educator's mind should be constantly working, developing a mental list of oral problems and solutions before doing any teaching.

Determining what motivates the adolescent is the first step to successful dental health education. Perhaps appearance, e.g., having a pretty smile, is the teenager's primary concern in the area of oral health. The dental health educator must encourage good oral hygiene as a "smile enhancer," addressing the role of plaque in inflammation and disease and how its presence detracts from one's appearance. The second step requires an investigation of the adolescent's present oral hygiene practices. The teenager might report that he brushes only in the morning before school. While conducting the examination the educator remembers plaque on the cervical thirds of virtually all of the adolescent's teeth and generalized mild to moderate gingivitis. The third and most important step in the education process involves giving a mirror to the patient and asking him what looks unpleasing to him in his own mouth, e.g., red, puffy gums and an accumulation of yellow plaque. Instead of suggesting he brush better and floss, the educator might inquire as to what he thinks he should do to improve his oral appearance. The teen might answer that he thinks he needs to brush closer to his gums. A patient who draws his own conclusions is essentially giving the educator a verbal commitment that he will do so. Praising the patient for his astute deduction is important, even if the educator does not find it to be the ideal or total solution to the problem. Although flossing is also crucial, the educator should not bombard the patient with new information; instead he should take the passive role and review the Bass method of brushing. The patient is more apt to improve his toothbrushing if he has decided what change is needed in his own mouth to enhance his appearance. Flossing can be introduced at a subsequent appointment after effective toothbrushing has been mastered.

The ultimate regimen of adolescent oral hygiene involves at least one thorough toothbrushing and flossing session daily, preferably at bedtime, with vigorous oral rinsing[4] or gum-chewing after meals (see Chapter 3). In a 1976 study of high school students in their sophomore year, only 10% were found to floss their teeth daily.[21] Another study found adolescents brushed their teeth for an average of only 90 seconds, frequently missing the lingual surfaces.[22] Consequently, proper angulation of the toothbrush, time spent brushing, and flossing technique are important lessons when teaching oral hygiene to an adolescent patient.

The Orthodontic Patient. Oral hygiene measures for the orthodontic patient present new challenges for instruction. If orthodontic appliances are being worn by the patient, oral hygiene modifications, which include a group of specialized toothbrushes, floss threaders, and an oral irrigator, can be extremely helpful. Digital massage of the marginal gingiva to enhance circulation can also be beneficial.

Tooth movement in the presence of gingivitis can cause rapid and irreversible periodontal destruction. The gingival margins and papillae between brackets are the first areas to respond to plaque accumulation. Plaque removal with a two-row sulcus brush placed above the brackets and angled gingivally is excellent for orthodontic patients. The drawback of using the sulcus brush relates to the additional placement of the brush below the brackets to cleanse the incisal one-third of the tooth. Orthodontic brushes designed to reach above and below the brackets, while additionally cleaning the bracket with an indented middle row of bristles, have become quite popular. End-tufted brushes can also be helpful for removing plaque around brackets and archwires (Fig. 6-6). The Interplak automatic toothbrush described in Chapter 3 can provide the orthodontic patient with an effective alternative to manual brushing. Although time-consuming, the use of Super Floss or floss threaders makes flossing possible for the orthodontic patient. Deliberate yet gentle flossing strokes are necessary to avoid dislocating bands or bending archwires. The floss is removed from the interproximal area by pulling the floss through the embrasure from the facial aspect.[12]

Oral irrigation devices are recommended as useful adjuncts to toothbrushing for the removal of debris around orthodontic appliances. Care should be taken to use a low-pressure, horizontal stream of water, aimed interproximally and perpendicular to the long axis of the tooth. The tip should not be directed into a sulcus.[16]

Fluoride

Most or all of the permanent teeth, with the exception of the third molars, have erupted by early adolescence. Reducing the susceptibility of these teeth to decay is paramount. Because oral hygiene and dietary practices among adolescents are often capricious, fluoride continues to play an integral part in the preventive dental program plan. Daily OTC rinses are highly recommended for the individual experiencing rampant caries or wearing orthodontic appliances. Because fluoride rinsing requires the adolescent's compliance, appealing to the teenager's personal appearance can serve as a powerful motivator for establishing a daily fluoride rinse regimen because dental caries are both noticeable and unattractive. The adolescent's desire to be autonomous is also respected because he is capable of purchasing and administering his own fluoride therapy.

Nutrition

The growth spurt experienced during adolescence is second only to that of infancy. Rapid growth and development require nutrients and energy beyond that needed for adulthood. A teenager's particular growth

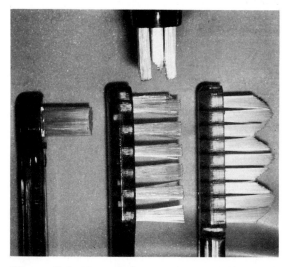

Figure 6-6. From *left to right*: end-tufted, orthodontic (side and front view), and sulcular toothbrushes. Courtesy of C.A. Spear, BSDH, MS, West Virginia University.

pattern, heredity, and activity level dictate his nutritional requirements.

A balanced diet high in protein, vitamins, and minerals is recommended. From mid-childhood on, approximately one-fifth of an individual's total body weight is comprised of protein. During adolescence, protein intake must increase to accommodate the deposition of new tissue, chiefly associated with the development of the sex characteristics.

Vitamin requirements for adolescents have not been standardized and to a large extent have been extrapolated from infant and adult allowances.[1] Meeting these requirements through the diet is preferable to supplementation. Teenagers have been shown to consume diets deficient in vitamin A. Several compounds possess vitamin A activity, but most diets contain beta carotene as the primary source of the vitamin.

Calcium intake is related to the formation and maintenance of skeletal length and mass. Endochondral growth associated with puberty places an increased demand for calcium on the adolescent's diet. The National Research Council recommends a calcium intake of 1200 mg/day for the adolescent.

The teenage male increases his red cell mass by one-third during puberty. A resultant loss of iron ensues, as with menstruating females of the same age group. The recommended allowance for iron is 18 mg/day.

Snacking

In 1977, Congress enacted the National School Lunch Act and Child Nutrition Amendment, which appropriated state funds to advance nutrition programs in public schools, day care centers, and family care centers. Unfortunately, in many schools nutrition education activities are virtually nonexistent. Vending machines and high-carbohydrate foods are often the student's only alternatives. Even if the choice for more nutritious foods is available, the search for social independence and peer approval and the disregard for parental rules and regulations increase the popularity of nonnutritious snacking behavior. Over 60% of the American population snacks between meals; this percentage is higher for teens.[23] Moreover, teenagers consume approximately half of their daily calories from snacks.

Foods eaten between meals are usually "empty" calories, high in fat, sodium, and sugar. Suggesting to teens that they avoid snacks is unrealistic. Instead, the dental health educator should offer the adolescent alternative snack foods that are nutritious and non-cariogenic. A teenager who passes a convenience store daily with his friends on his way home from school should not be told to wait outside while his peers consume mass quantities of junk food. He might decide though, to buy a bag of peanuts instead of candy.

A 5- or 7-day diet diary aids the dental health educator in determining existing habits and daily routine. The educator should fill out the form for the first day's intake as the patient recalls what he has eaten over the past 24 hours (Fig. 6-7).[15] All liquid and solid foods consumed during mealtime and snacking should be included. Amounts and food preparation, e.g., baked, fried, or boiled, are also significant. On receipt of the completed food dairy, the dental health educator needs to review the form, identifying fermentable carbohydrates and foods that are retentive by circling them in red. The degree of parental or adolescent control over food preparation might also be pertinent. Most importantly, the dental health educator needs to evaluate the diet for balance by determining the extent to which the four food groups are incorporated into the diet. Unusual foods or dietary patterns should be listed.[4]

Effective, nonjudgmental communication with the adolescent now becomes the key focus. Following a basic description of how the foods were categorized and what was meant by the red circles, the dental health educator should record a list of the individual's dietary adequacies and inadequacies from the patient's viewpoint. The patient should then be asked to prioritize his problem areas and devise some solutions for change. If the teenager makes these decisions himself, he is more apt to alter his behavior. This dietary plan of action can be

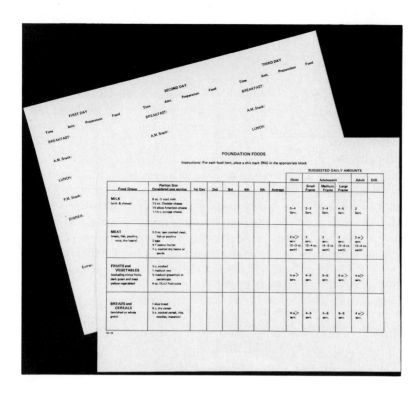

Figure 6-7. Five-day food dairy and foundation food (four food groups) worksheets.

reviewed by the dental health educator at periodic recalls and evaluated for both successes and failures.

Parental involvement is not required unless typical problems exist relative to food preparation by a parent. Adolescents can find nutrition fascinating, and their eating practices can improve if they become involved in shopping and cooking early in life; home economics in a junior high curriculum can help in the attainment of this goal. Teenagers should not be taught that their favorite foods are forbidden; rather they should be taught what nutrients these foods contain and how they can be varied and incorporated into a balanced, healthy diet.

Nutritional Trends

Several trends in food consumption and vitamin supplementation have flourished in response to an increased public awareness of the relationship of nutrition to health. These trends include health foods, organi-

cally grown foods, natural foods, vegetarianism, and megavitamin therapy.

Health foods are professed to have health-giving curative properties beyond their proven nutritional value. *Organically grown foods* are cultivated without the use of chemicals and fertilizers. Chemical processing using food additives and preservatives is also prohibited. Only fertilizers and pesticides that have originated from animals or vegetables can be used to enhance growth. *Natural foods* are in their original state and involve little or no processing. *Vegetarianism* constitutes abstinence from the consumption of meat, fowl, and fish with or without eggs or dairy products. Ovolacto-vegetarians eat vegetables, milk, cheese, and eggs; lactovegetarians eat vegetables, milk, and cheese, and strict vegetarians eat a pure vegetable diet. A vegan diet, if balanced and supplemented with vitamin B_{12}, can offer many health benefits such as a lower incidence of hypertension, atherosclerosis, and several forms of cancer, such as breast, lung, intestinal, and oral. *Megavitamin therapy*, which involves the intake of fat-soluble vitamins over a period of time, can be toxic when high levels accumulate in the body. Megadoses of vitamin C can cause acidic urine and burning on urination; kidney stones can also result.[15,24]

The individual credited as being the first *food faddist* was a Roman named Cato, who lived during the second century A.D. Cato believed that cabbage was the perfect food, capable of curing all ailments. Food fads comprise a billion dollar market annually in the United States. Effective marketing of diet foods and drinks persuades the consumer to patronize certain brands and special stores where these products are sold. Hundreds of diet books are circulated in retail establishments across the country. A 1972 study conducted by the Food and Drug Administration reported that 26% of the population used nutritional supplements without a physician's advice and nearly one-tenth of the sample had eaten organic or natural foods.[25] Teens are often the first to try a new diet craze when weight loss is desired quickly.

Much of the phenomenon of food faddism is a result of the notion that certain foods will produce health benefits. On the contrary, addiction to fad diets can (1) cause an unnecessary strain on the budget, (2) result in malnutrition due to the consumption of an unbalanced diet, and (3) be a symptom of a psychologic disorder.[26] According to Jalso et al., rigid personal traits were positively correlated with faddist beliefs and practices, including the consumption of health foods and nutritional supplements.[27] Obsession with some fads, such as the liquid-protein diets, has actually been directly linked to fatalities. Ice cream diets and grapefruit diets have also become popular food fads. The *Zen macrobiotic diet* is a 10-stage diet that culminates in the sole consumption of wholegrain cereals. Fluids and sugars are eliminated.[24] Needless to say, this diet is extremely dangerous. Patients must be taught how to modify their eating behavior to establish good habits. The ingestion of well-balanced meals and nutritious snacks coupled with regular exercise promotes health and weight regulation throughout life.

ADOLESCENT HEALTH CONCERNS

Eating Disorders

Although anorexia and bulimia are two distinct eating disorders, their associated behaviors can overlap. Both entail a set of abnormal behaviors associated with food and weight. A preoccupation with slimness in American society has been responsible for an increase in these conditions. In general, these eating disorders are most common in Caucasian female adolescents and young adults of upper socioeconomic status.[28]

ANOREXIA NERVOSA

Individuals suffering from anorexia attempt to control their body weight by severely restricting the amount of food they consume and exercising to extremes. Although 5 to 10% of persons who have this condition are males, most are females who first display signs of the disorder between the ages of 12 and 18 years.[29,30] The prevalence among adolescent white females has been estimated to be as high as 0.5 to 1%, with a mortality rate that ranges between 7 and 21%.[30] Anorectics who die as a result of their disease typically die from malnutrition, infection, and suicide.

Anorectics are frequently described as obedient, cooperative overachievers striving to be the perfect child. They usually possess above-average intelligence and lack interest in their own sexuality. They express a sense of insecurity or inadequacy; they are never able to feel that they have satisfied their parents' expectations or their own perceptions of what is required to become fulfilled. Consequently, they derive satisfaction from their heightened sense of power over what and how much they consume. Anorectics have a distorted view of their own emaciated appearance, believing that they are still overweight. It is not uncommon for anorectics to lose up to 25% of their original body weight.[31] In addition to a reduction in weight from starvation, anorectics display several other clinical signs. They include amenorrhea (absence of menstrual periods); lanugo (fine, silky body hair); dry, flaky skin; constipation; and a lowered body temperature, pulse, and blood pressure.[32] Approximately 50 to 75% of anorectics refuse to eat, fasting continuously. The remaining individuals experience episodes of binging followed by guilt-induced purging or vomiting.[30]

Food is consumed in private so portions can remain minute without criticism from family or peers. Many anorectics practice strange eating rituals such as cutting food in small pieces, rearranging food on their plates, counting the number of times they chew their food, and preventing food from touching their lips.[33]

BULIMIA

Bulimia means "voracious appetite" or "ox hunger."[34] Bulimics secretly consume large amounts of food in a short period of time (binging) followed by self-induced vomiting (purging) and use of laxatives, diuretics, or enemas to prevent weight gain.[35] Bulimic episodes can occur between one and 18 times per week. The average bulimic will binge for 1½ to 2 hours, consuming as much as 4000 calories,[36] and then vomit for 5 to 30 minutes.[37] Ingesting two times the daily dosage to handfuls of laxatives to rid their bodies of the food just eaten is also characteristic of bulimics, but it is practiced less frequently than vomiting. Initially bulimics induce vomiting by inserting their fingers, a toothbrush, or a spoon against the soft palate to stimulate the gag reflex.[35] With time, the bulimic can vomit at will by merely contracting the abdominal and throat muscles. Ipecac syrup is also commonly employed to induce vomiting.[38] Chronic vomiting and laxative abuse can result in serious systemic consequences such as dehydration, an imbalance of electrolytes, esophageal rupture, and gastrointestinal disturbances.[32] Addictive use of syrup of ipecac can lead to muscle tissue damage or myopathy.[16] Hypokalemia, or a depletion of potassium, can result in cardiovascular or renal failure.[39]

Although the prevalence of bulimia is difficult to ascertain due to the extreme secrecy maintained by bulimic patients, the disorder is believed to occur more frequently than anorexia.[38] The majority of known bulimics are Caucasians between 12 and 35 years of age, with 18 as the mean age of onset.[40] In contrast to anorectics, bulimics are generally of normal weight, socially outgoing, and sexually active (Table 6-3).[28] The problem often manifests after numerous attempts to diet have been unsuccessful. The dieter loses control when eating and begins binging. Weight gain and frustration cause the individual to turn to purging as a method of weight control.

ORAL MANIFESTATIONS

A patient suffering from either eating disorder might exhibit one or more of the following: perimylolysis, an increase in pit and fissure and smooth surface caries, oral mucosal irritation, cheilosis, xerostomia, and chronic swelling of the parotid glands.[28,41]

Perimylolysis is the erosion of enamel on the lingual, occlusal, or incisal surfaces of the teeth, primarily the maxillary incisors (Fig. 6-8). This occurs from the chronic regurgitation of low-pH gastric contents. Particularly in prolonged cases of bulimia, the teeth appear stained from exposed dentin and the incisal edges of anterior teeth have a "moth eaten" appearance (Fig. 6-9). The loss of enamel from the occlusal surfaces of restored teeth gives the filling material the appearance of being elevated, i.e., amalgam islands (Fig. 6-10).[42] Teeth with erosion also experience thermal sensitivity due to dentinal exposure.

Dental caries activity can increase due to an increase in carbohydrate consumption during binging, a decrease in the salivary

Table 6-3. Characteristics of Patients with Eating Disorders

Anorexia	Bulimia
Abnormal fear of weight gain	Excessive fear of being overweight
Distorted body image	Usually within normal weight range
Loss of up to 25% of normal body weight	
Self-induced starvation	Compulsive binge eating
	Inconspicuous eating
	Vomiting or purging
Dry skin	Dry lips
Fine, generalized body hair (lanugo)	Blotched, dry skin from dehydration
Loss of hair (alopecia)	
Brittle fingernails	
Hypothermia	
Amenorrhea	
Shy and introverted	Gregarious and socially outgoing
High achiever, rigid compliance	Alternates between self-control and impulsiveness
Feelings of inadequacy and unworthiness	Low self-esteem, depression
	Guilt-ridden following purging
Referred for treatment by concerned individual; rarely looks for help	Often seeks out assistance in gaining control over behavior

From Gross, K.B.W., Brough, K.M., and Randolph, P.M.: Eating disorders: Anorexia and bulimia nervosas. J. Dent. Child., 53:379, 1986.

pH, a decrease in the quantity and buffering capacity of the saliva, and poor oral hygiene. The perioral area, intraoral mucous membranes, and the periodontal tissues can be inflamed and dry from existing vitamin deficiencies and from xerostomia, which serves to dehydrate the oral mucosa. An iron deficiency will produce atrophy of the filiform papillae of the tongue and pallor of the lips, tongue, and mucous membranes. A B-complex deficiency causes glossitis, papillary hypertrophy of the tongue, and angular cheilosis. Bleeding gingivae are often observed in individuals with a vitamin C deficiency. Sore throat, burning tongue, and cheilosis can also be caused directly by the eating disorder if the oral environment remains acidic from frequent vomiting. Furthermore, the throat can be sore due to abrasions on the pharyngeal wall from using fingers or other objects to induce vomiting.[38]

Enlargement of the salivary glands, although not fully understood, appears to be related to nutritional deficiencies and atypical eating behaviors.[43] The cheeks look puffy, and pain can be present (Fig. 6-11). The parotid gland in particular undergoes work hypertrophy because it is taxed from repeated abrupt binging episodes and irritated by gastric juices flowing through the

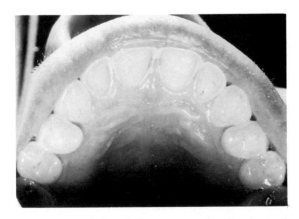

Figure 6-8. Perimylolysis. Note the flat lingual surface created by the enamel erosion. Courtesy of J.E. Bouquot, DDS, MS, West Virginia University.

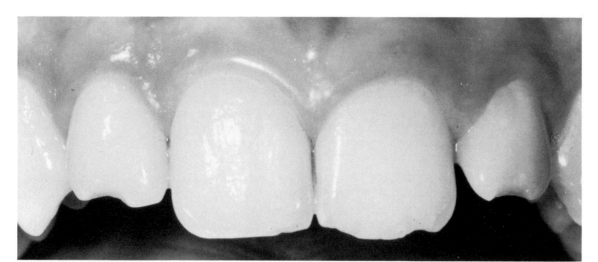

Figure 6-9. "Moth-eaten" appearance of incisal edges due to enamel erosion. Courtesy of C.A. Spear, BSDH, MS, West Virginia University.

opening and lining of the ducts.[44] Xerostomia might be associated with parotid swelling, but it is directly related to the loss of body fluids from vomiting and diuretic abuse. Depression and anxiety can also decrease salivary output.

INTERVENTION

The dental health educator can be an integral part of the team approach used to treat patients with eating disorders. Frequently the dental health educator is the first professional person to recognize the disorder by the existence of certain visual signs descriptive of the malady e.g.,. enamel erosion, tooth abrasion, or calluses across the knuckles of the dominant hand used to initiate the gag reflex (Fig. 6-12).

Counseling the patient not only requires knowledge of the signs and symptoms of an eating disorder, but more important, it demands communication, which reflects support, respect, and empathy for the individual's predicament.[45] Many individuals become extremely relieved when they can share the burden of their problem with someone who will not pass judgment on them. People with eating disorders cannot

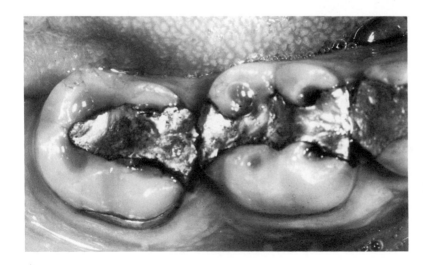

Figure 6-10. "Amalgam islands" resulting from occlusal erosion. Courtesy of C.A. Spear, BSDH, MS, West Virginia University.

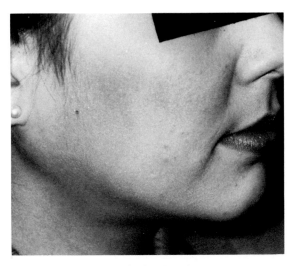

Figure 6-11. Parotid gland enlargement. Courtesy of J.E. Bouquot, DDS, MS, West Virginia University.

resolve their condition until they admit its presence and willingly accept and remain in treatment.[46] The dental health educator must emphasize to the adolescent or young adult the significance of parental communication and therapy that involves the family unit. If an eating disorder is strongly suspected, it is the educator's responsibility to notify the parents or guardians of a minor and make the proper medical and psychiatric referrals. Accusations without sufficient evidence are not recommended.[45]

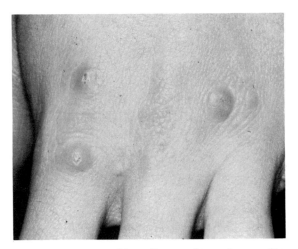

Figure 6-12. Knuckle callouses from chronically inducing vomiting. Courtesy of J.E. Bouquot, DDS, MS, West Virginia University.

Resource groups for individuals with eating disorders are listed in Appendix B at the end of the text. Educational programs at the junior high and high school levels to assist in the prevention of anorexia and bulimia related behaviors, particularly among adolescent females, are suggested.

Dental intervention procedures begin with a complete dental evaluation to assess a patient's orodental involvement. These baseline data provide the dental health educator with information for comparison during subsequent dental visits (Fig. 6-13). Patients exhibiting eating disorders also need nutritional guidance for making alternative noncariogenic food choices. Although meticulous oral hygiene is paramount, toothbrushing after emesis is contraindicated. The acids from the vomitus will demineralize the tooth, and immediate toothbrushing can abrade the weakened outer enamel surfaces, expediting erosion. Rinsing with a sodium bicarbonate solution or allowing antacid tablets to dissolve in the mouth immediately after vomiting will neutralize residual gastric acids in the oral cavity. A daily neutral sodium fluoride rinse in a 0.05% concentration or a fluoride gel (0.4% stannous fluoride or 2.0% neutral sodium fluoride) applied daily with a toothbrush or a custom tray in conjunction with a fluoride dentifrice are advised to prevent decay and minimize enamel erosion and subsequent tooth sensitivity.[28,29,38,44] Therapeutic fabrication of a dental prosthesis to prevent the progression of enamel erosion from routine vomiting can also be employed (Fig. 6-14).[47]

Extensive restorative dental treatment to stabilize the condition of the oral cavity should not commence until the eating disorder is controlled. The preventive approach, which includes the application of sealants, is usually adequate for the patient with minimal erosion, whereas moderate enamel loss can require a bonded composite resin. Composites are esthetic and also serve to improve the patient's self-image. Permanent crowns become necessary when the patient has experienced severe erosion. The teeth and restorations should be examined for new caries, recurrences, and defects that harbor plaque, on an average of 1

Analysis of Eating Disorders
I. History and Habits

Name _____ Date _____

Gender _____ Birthdate _____

Impression of self _____

_____

Impression of teeth _____

_____

Number of teeth _____

Previous extractions _____

Reasons for tooth loss _____

Frequency of oral prophylaxes _____

Hereditary dental factors _____

Appliances worn _____

Unusual dental experiences _____

Grind or clench teeth _____

Frequency of toothbrushing _____ Brand _____

Frequency of flossing _____ Brand _____

Frequency of mouthrinsing _____ Brand _____

Brand of toothpaste _____

Is community water supply fluoridated? _____

Type, amount, and preparation of foods consumed over a 24-hour period:

Frequently thirsty _____

Frequency of binging _____

Frequency of purging _____

Pre-vomiting habits _____

Post-vomiting habits _____

Alcohol _____

Smoking _____

Medications _____

Regularity of menstrual periods _____

Figure 6-13. A two-part dental evaluation for patients with eating disorders. I. History and habits and II. Clinical signs and symptoms.

Analysis of Eating Disorders
II. Clinical Signs and Symptoms

Name _____

Date _____

DENTAL FINDINGS	Negative (−) or Normal (√)	If positive (+) or abnormal note: (location, severity, extent)
Amalgam islands		
Enamel erosion		
Carious lesions		
Decalcification		
Abrasion		
Staining		
Sensitivity		
Other		

ORAL FINDINGS

Gingivitis		
Periodontitis		
Gingival recession		
Ulcerations		
Frictional abrasion		
Hematomas		
Erythema		
Edema		
Tenderness		
Fibrous hyperplasia		
Sore throat		
Inflamed throat		

Analysis of Eating Disorders
II. Clinical Signs and Symptoms
(*continued*)

	Negative (−) or Normal (√)	If positive (+) or abnormal note: (location, severity, extent)
Salivary gland enlargement		
Salivary gland tenderness		
Facial muscle tenderness		
Xerostomia		
Cheilosis		
Halitosis		
TMJ pain		
TMJ crepitation		
Other		

GENERAL APPRAISAL

Skin texture		
Body hair		
Knuckle abrasion		

Reading (#)

Height	
Weight	
Blood pressure	
Temperature	
Pulse	

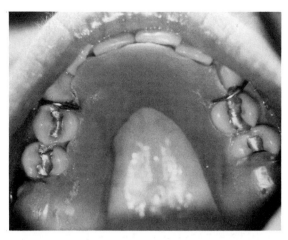

Figure 6-14. Preventive appliance to be worn during vomiting episodes to cover and protect those surfaces most affected by erosion. Courtesy of J.C. Ruff, DDS, and R.A. Abrams, DDS, MPH, MEd, Marquette University. From Ruff, J. C., and Abrams, R .A.: Preventive dental prosthesis for the patient with bulimia. Sp. Care Dent., 7:218–220, 1987.

to 3 months depending on the patient's needs. Fluoride therapy should also be monitored.[29,42]

Suicide

Suicide is the second leading cause of death among adolescents; it is surpassed only by accidents and closely followed by homicide (Table 6-4).[48] Homicide is the leading cause of death among black males ages 15 to 44 years.[49] Although the nation's overall suicide rate has not varied significantly over the past 30 years, the rate for

Table 6-4. Death Rates for Adolescents, Ages 15–25, U.S., 1984 (Rate per 100,000 Population)

Accidents	50.5
Suicide	12.2
Homicide	11.8
Cancer	5.5
Heart disease	2.5
Cerebrovascular disease	0.7

Adapted from U.S. Dept. of Health and Human Services: Disease Prevention and Health Promotion: The Facts. Palo Alto, Bull Publishing, 1988.

adolescents has tripled. White males account for 70% of all suicides.[49] For every successful adolescent suicide, there are as many as 50 to 150 attempts.[50,51] Over half of suicidal behavior in the adolescent population is not reported as such because of religious taboos, insurance policy stipulations, and the social stigma associated with suicide.[52]

Internal pressures felt by the adolescent are common causes of suicidal behavior. Such inner struggles can include (1) competition or a self-imposed need to be successful; (2) personal feelings of inadequacy when faced with social or environmental pressures, e.g., making new friends in a new city, having to deal with the pressures of premarital sex or pregnancy; (3) an inability to cope with independence granted at a young age; and (4) a lack of love or security from boyfriend-girlfriend relationships, or institutions significant in the adolescent's life.[53]

Although suicidal behavior is the culmination of several causative influences, family problems probably pose the greatest threat to an adolescent's emotional stability. A lack of communication between parent and adolescent can leave the adolescent feeling isolated, not understood, and unloved.[52] Many suicidal adolescents are not living at home, indicating a family disruption caused by abuse, divorce, separation, or the death of a parent.[54,55]

Depression in the adolescent has also been associated with suicidal tendencies. Prolonged sleeping, significant gains or losses of weight, an unusual neglect of personal appearance, violent or rebellious behavior, alcohol or drug abuse, a melancholy, hopeless, empty feeling, and a loss of interest in school and peers are characteristic of depression.[53,54]

WARNING SIGNS

Unless the dental health educator knows the adolescent fairly well, he might have difficulty recognizing the etiologic factors described above. Nonetheless, the educator should be aware of one or more of the signals an adolescent might exhibit that indicate an intention to commit suicide.

Previous Suicidal Attempts. Eighty percent of suicide victims have made at least one previous attempt.[56] Teenagers who attempt suicide are not just searching for attention. If their problems are not resolved, there is a good chance they will try again.

Suicidal Threats. Statements regarding an individual's desire to take his own life should be taken seriously. Less direct presuicidal comments might include "Who cares if I die" and "They would be better off without me."

Prolonged Depression with a Sudden Unexplained Improvement. An adolescent who has decided to commit suicide might experience sudden relief from his decision. Suicide can provide an answer for eliminating the individual's feelings of confusion and rejection.

Final Arrangements. Inner feelings are expressed and personal possessions are distributed in the form of a last will and testament.[57]

INTERVENTION

When observation and questioning of an adolescent patient lead the educator to suspect suicidal tendencies, immediate intervention is necessary. Patients are generally willing to discuss their feelings with a health professional who is direct, supportive, and caring. To maintain rapport with the adolescent, the dental health educator should not be judgmental or act shocked. Trite comments, e.g., "Things aren't as bad as they seem" and "It could be worse" can increase the adolescent's sense of guilt and worthlessness. Instead, open communication is advised, along with a recommendation for the adolescent and his parent(s) to seek professional counseling. Private practice psychiatrists, psychologists, and approximately 24 hotlines and 200 suicide prevention centers are available throughout the United States.[58] Arranging the actual appointment might also be necessary to ensure that it is made. If the adolescent refuses to seek help (such refusal might actually be the

decision of his parents), the dental health educator is obligated to take the appropriate action to secure adequate medical or social intervention before it is too late.[57]

Drug and Alcohol Use and Abuse

It might seem that children in elementary schools and junior high are too young to have a problem with drugs, but, sadly, that is not the case. Although drug and alcohol use among adolescents is declining across the country, the statistics remain alarming. In 1988, 50% of 12- to 17-year olds stated that they had tried alcohol at least once and 6% had consumed it within the past week.[59] The three main reasons for this early use are that alcohol is readily available in most homes, alcohol is inexpensive and easy to obtain from peers, adult friends or store personnel, and parents can use or abuse alcohol without the criticism or scrutiny that accompanies use of other substances. For youngsters, physical addiction to alcohol can occur in less than 1 month with daily use.[60] Binge drinking, the consumption of five or more drinks in one evening, remains popular among 39% of high school seniors, particularly on weekends.[61] Among 1987 high school seniors, 5% reported daily alcohol use.[61]

Marijuana is second to alcohol in popularity among adolescents and is considered the most widely abused illicit drug among this age group. In 1988, nearly 4 million teenagers (17%) revealed having tried marijuana.[59] Three percent of 1987 high school seniors reported daily use.[61] Small amounts of marijuana can produce distorted perception and apathy. Because the chemicals in marijuana are only slowly removed from the brain, a residue remains in the fatty cells that results in synaptic gaps that impair or delay electrical brain waves and the storage of thought. The adolescent displays memory loss, sluggish thinking, and little or no motivation for logical, analytical thought. As with any form of substance abuse, relationships with parents and teachers deteriorate because of abrupt changes in behavior. Marijuana can also produce respiratory complications. Emphysema, which takes 10 to 20 years to manifest in a chronic cigarette smoker, can occur in only 1 year from marijuana smoking.[62]

The third most widely used drug among adolescents is cocaine. In 1988, over one-half million 12- to 17-year-olds (3%) divulged having used cocaine. Fifteen percent of high school seniors reported having tried cocaine, more than 3% admitting current use.[59] The use of cocaine has continued to spread since the advent of "crack," the base or sediment of cocaine. Crack is smoked and can produce an addiction in approximately 90 days. Use of the cocaine base only allows the price to drop and makes it more affordable to youths and much more lethal. Cocaine can also be taken orally, intravenously, or most commonly through the nostrils by snorting. Chronic use damages nasal mucous membranes and produces hypertension and tachycardia.[63]

The use of amphetamines also available in a smokable form referred to as "ice" is becoming prevalent among adolescents in the United States. Prolonged use leads to compulsive, repetitious, or stereotypic behavior, and a form of psychosis characterized by delusionary, hallucinatory, hyperactive, and aggressive violent outbursts.[63] Sleep disturbances and elevations in blood pressure also result.[60]

WARNING SIGNS

Adolescents who begin smoking cigarettes frequently graduate to marijuana use within a 2-year period. The patient who appears to have a lack of self-esteem or describes his parents as excessively permissive or demanding might be a substance abuser.[64] The adolescent's performance in school might be suffering, and he might have had an incident with law enforcement personnel. A teen who begins to break dental appointments or displays unusual alterations in his behavior can also be suspected. Watch for changes in a patient's gait, breath odor, eyes, and teeth (poor oral hygiene and green stain can indicate marijuana use); scars along veins can indicate drug abuse.

The wearing of sunglasses or long sleeves at inappropriate times should also alert the dental health educator that he could be dealing with a substance abuser.

INTERVENTION

Once the dental health educator suspects an adolescent's involvement in substance abuse, he must initiate intervention strategies. The dental health educator should share this responsibility with the teenager's physician, parents, teachers, school, and peers. Successful intervention includes giving the adolescent (1) parental support; (2) accurate information about drugs as requested; (3) opportunities for health-promoting activities to replace drug-related behaviors; (4) opportunities to contribute to school and family in a meaningful way; (5) counseling sessions with an adult he respects and who serves as a role model for socially acceptable behavior; and (6) opportunities for continued support so he can develop into a capable, healthy, functioning adult.[60]

Individualized school drug education programs developed with the goal of preventing substance abuse should (1) contain clearly defined objectives that are realistic for the students; (2) include an honest exposition of the costs and the pros and cons of drug use; (3) link the principles and skills required in the classroom with the reality of drugs outside the classroom; (4) possess a sound, theoretical basis for expected social and behavioral outcomes; and (5) devote as much time to the implementation and evaluation of the program as is spent in the design process.[65]

In 1986, Congress passed Public Law 99-570 (Anti-Drug Abuse Bill of 1986). This piece of drug-control legislation authorized expanded programs of law enforcement, prevention, and treatment. The "Just say no" media campaign developed by the Reagan administration[66] and contributions from the Kaiser Family Foundation and the Pew Charitable Trust, which sponsored the "Conference on Community-Based Health Promotion and Drug Abuse Prevention for

Youth," are examples of philanthropic foundations and government programs that have an interest in the prevention and control of substance abuse.[67]

Cigarette Smoking

Although cigarette smoking has declined markedly among adults on the national level, it continues to be a major health issue for adolescents, particularly females (Table 6-5).[68] More than 8.5 million adolescents between the ages of 12 and 17 (42%) have smoked cigarettes.[59] The critical time for cigarette smoking appears to begin during the seventh grade.[69]

A combination of forces, such as the signals sent by parents, peers, and the media, seems to be responsible for encouraging smoking behavior among adolescents.[70] Messages conveyed by parents and the media present cues to adolescents relative to acceptable adult behavior. Many teenagers admit that one of the pressures to smoke was derived from the need to appear grownup. Schools encourage adolescents to "behave like adults," parents desire mature,

responsible offspring, and adolescents want to be older so they can obtain adult privileges. Amidst the numerous pressures to act in an adult manner, the alternatives for becoming an adult overnight are few; smoking is one of the few. Pressure from peers might not be as strong a force as adults believe. Peers often encourage smoking to be recognized, feel independent and mature, and just to have fun.[71]

A number of studies also suggest that an individual's psychologic make-up plays a significant role in determining smoking behavior. Smokers tend to be more anxious,[72,73] more peer-oriented,[74] less socially confident,[75] more extroverted,[73,76] and more impulsive.[74,77] Teenage smokers appear to lack self-esteem.[78]

Smoking Cessation. If a patient asks "Why should I quit smoking?" the dental health educator should be armed to explain the numerous ramifications of continuing the behavior. The risk factors associated with smoking are well known. Cigarette smoking increases the risk of coronary heart disease, lung cancer, chronic bronchitis, emphysema, and gastric ulcers. Tobacco is also linked to oral, laryngeal, esophageal, bladder, kidney, and pancreatic carcinomas, particularly when coupled with alcohol use.[79,80] For women who smoke during pregnancy, the risks of premature birth and spontaneous abortion are high.[81] Other complications and side effects associated with smoking include halitosis, calculus deposition, dental stains, abrasion, hairy tongue, leukoplakia, delayed wound healing, a predisposition to destructive periodontal disease, drying of the skin, sinusitis, and diminished acuity of taste and smell.[80,82]

Because of the magnitude of oral manifestations of smoking, the dental health educator is in an ideal position not only to make the patient aware of the changes occurring in his own body, but also to introduce him to an effective smoking-cessation program. First of all, a patient has to be ready to quit. Once the dental health educator has discussed the risk factors with the patient and taken a history of his smoking patterns, it is up to the patient to make an informed decision to quit or continue the

Table 6-5. Percentage of High School Students Reporting Daily Use of Cigarettes in the Previous 30 Days According to Gender: 1975–1984

Class of	Total	Males	Females
1975	26.8	26.9	26.4
1976	28.8	28.0	28.8
1977	28.8	27.1	30.0
1978	27.5	26.0	28.3
1979	25.4	22.3	27.8
1980	21.3	18.5	23.5
1981	20.3	18.1	21.7
1982	21.1	19.2	22.2
1983	21.2	19.2	22.2
1984	18.7	16.0	20.5

Reprinted with permission from Koop, C.E.: The quest for a smoke-free young America by the year 2000. J. Sch. Health, 56:8, 1986, which listed the following reference: U.S. Dept. of Health and Human Services: Use of Licit and Illicit Drugs by America's High School Students 1975–1984. U.S. Department of Health and Human Services. Publication #ADM 85-1394, Washington, DC, U.S. Government Printing Office, 1985.

habit. Many times individuals are aware that smoking poses a significant health hazard, but other factors in their lives, e.g., job stress, motivate the continuance of the behavior. Don't press the issue with this type of patient. Additional pamphlets and encouraging words to offer future help when he is ready are sufficient at this time. Low-key messages and gentle persuasion are the most effective. A supportive waiting room with "No Smoking" posters and no ashtrays emphasizes the office's serious commitment to quit-smoking efforts for its patients.[79,80]

When the patient selects a date to quit smoking, it should be one that is projected several weeks into the future, to enable him to prepare mentally for this major task. The patient is expected to cease smoking all cigarettes on the date chosen, fully committing himself to this specific personal goal. A light smoker (less than a pack a day) might only require the dental health educator's moral support and referral to enroll in a smoking-cessation course such as those conducted by the American Cancer Society (see Appendix C). The cigarette-smoking addict (a pack or more a day) requires a multifaceted approach. This individual is addicted to nicotine and will benefit most significantly from referral to a quit-smoking clinic and prescription of nicotine-containing chewing gum. Nicorette gum (Lakeside Pharmaceuticals, Merrell Dow, Inc.) helps the cigarette-free patient concentrate on overcoming his psychologic and social needs for smoking by releasing enough nicotine to satiate the individual. The gum should be chewed slowly, and a maximum of 30 pieces are allowed per day. The patient is advised to carry the gum with him at all times to alleviate withdrawal symptoms when the sudden desire to smoke occurs.[83,84] After 3 months of Nicorette gum use, the patient's chewing behavior should begin tapering off. Within 6 months, the patient learns to substitute positive behaviors for smoking and should be gum-free.

Weekly during the entire cessation process, the dental health educator should remain in contact with the patient to offer support and evaluate the individual's progress. Reinforcing the technique for gum therapy and discussing its potential side effects e.g., nausea, hiccups, and belching, are also helpful. This gum is contraindicated during pregnancy and for those with certain cardiovascular disorders.

Smokeless Tobacco

Smokeless tobacco refers to any tobacco that is placed in the mouth or nose without being ignited. It can be found in the United States as finely powdered tobacco known as snuff for dipping and in leaf form for chewing.

Smokeless tobacco has been used by mankind since as early as 3500 B.C. American Indians used tobacco in a variety of forms, and by the eighteenth century many Europeans, particularly royalty, were addicted to snuff. Smokeless tobacco became popular in the United States during the nineteenth century but was replaced by Camel cigarettes in 1913, at which time it was learned that tuberculosis was spread through expectoration. Therefore public spitting was made illegal and deemed socially unacceptable.[85] Only a small percentage of the population, located mainly in the South, continued its use. In the 1970s the interest in smokeless tobacco reemerged. Smokeless tobacco sales have increased 52% since 1978.[86] It is estimated that there are as many as 22 million smokeless tobacco users in the United States, over 3 million of whom are adolescents,[59,87] particularly males.[88-97]

Many users mistakenly believe smokeless tobacco is a safe alternative to cigarette smoking. Sixty percent of students in junior high using smokeless tobacco and 40% of senior high users thought there were no risks associated with "dipping and chewing."[92] Skillful advertising by tobacco manufacturers, featuring entertainers and sports personalities promoting its use as creating a macho image, have transformed an unhealthful, unsightly habit into one that is viewed as attractive, healthful, and highly appealing to youths.[98,99]

HARMFUL EFFECTS

When chewing-tobacco products combine with saliva, nicotine is released and ab-

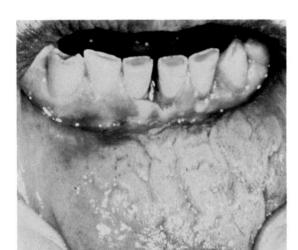

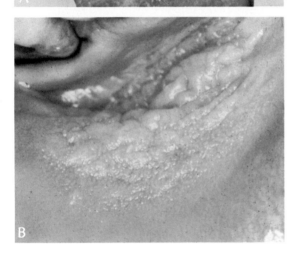

Figure 6-15. Vestibular keratosis or "snuff pouch"—anterior (A) and posterior (B) lesions. Courtesy of J.E. Bouquot, DDS, MS, West Virginia University, and R. Marshall, DDS, Lewisburg, West Virginia.

sorbed by the oral mucosa. Consequently, smokeless-tobacco users have a fourfold greater risk for developing an oral-pharyngeal carcinoma than do nonusers; the risk increases 50-fold for cancers of the gingivae and buccal mucosa.[100] The two types of cancer associated with smokeless tobacco use are the verrucous and squamous cell carcinomas. Verrucous carcinomas rarely metastasize, but the local invasion that they initiate can be severe enough to cause a loss of tissue and function, which in some cases could be fatal.

Clinically, pinches of snuff between the lower lip and gingivae or quids, chaws, or plugs of chewing tobacco placed in the buccal or labial vestibule, cause continuous mucosal irritation. Chronic irritation produces a white to yellowish wrinkled lesion that thickens and furrows with increased duration of the habit, age of the patient, and length and amount of daily exposure[101] (Fig. 6-15). This lesion has been described clinically as leukoplakia or snuff dipper's pouch, but histologically the changes in the epithelium include hyperorthokeratosis or hyperparakeratosis, acanthosis, and dysplasia.[98]

Additional side effects include the following:

1. An increase in heart rate and blood pressure,[102,103] and a greater risk for developing nicotine addiction; coronary and peripheral vascular disease; peptic ulcer (from swallowing nicotine); reproductive disorders; and neuromuscular disease are all possible systemic complications.[92]
2. Gingival recession at the site where the tobacco is placed is common and can give rise to root sensitivity.[90,97]
3. The role of smokeless tobacco in caries formation remains controversial. Exposed root surfaces, bathed in the sucrose contained in these tobacco products, appear to be more susceptible to decay. Greer and Poulson however, found no "tobacco-associated dental caries" in their sample of 1119 adolescent users and nonusers in Colorado.[90] Perhaps the fluoride content of some products and the increase in salivary flow from chewing are capable of preventing caries formation.
4. Tooth abrasion appears to be linked to the high content of abrasive grit found in leaf and plug chewing tobacco, although significant abrasion from a tobacco habit would take several years to occur.
5. Other oral entities observed across the country, which lack substantiated research at this time, are sialadenitis (inflammation of the salivary glands), periodontitis, halitosis, discoloration and staining of the teeth, and a decreased

ability to taste and smell bitter, salty, and sweet foods.[101,104] Oral ulcerations or sores might heal more slowly as a result of smokeless tobacco use.[105]

PATIENT EDUCATION

Public Law 99-252 banned smokeless tobacco television advertising on August 27, 1986 and mandated that warning labels be placed on all smokeless tobacco products as of February 27, 1987. Despite these efforts few users have abandoned the habit. It seems there are two origins of users: (1) the young initiator is primarily from a rural area, and his parents or family influenced him to begin the chewing tobacco habit; and (2) the older initiator is a high school teenager or young adult, from an urban area, where the adoption of snuff was influenced most significantly by his peers.[106] The dental health educator must consider the demographic characteristics of the smokeless tobacco user when attempting to motivate a patient to cease such a habit. The dental health educator must be very skillful when attempting to reverse a behavior that has been passed on from generation to generation. Similarly, the dental health educator's creative talents are required when a new angle must be found to motivate an adolescent to stop using smokeless tobacco, even when the baseball player he worships does.

The dental health educator might find the following procedures helpful when trying to encourage patients to stop using smokeless tobacco:

1. Take a thorough health history. The sucrose, nicotine, and sodium content of smokeless tobacco might aggravate an existing condition such as diabetes or cause an elevation in blood pressure. It is important to make the patient aware of these ingredients and the effects they have on the body as their levels in the blood increase. Personality fluctuations experienced when trying to quit the habit are related to the withdrawal of nicotine from the bloodstream. Routine monitoring of the patient's blood pressure is advisable. A dental history should also be recorded that includes information concerning the type and location of the tobacco used, the frequency and duration of the smokeless tobacco behavior, and attempts by the individual to quit.

2. Oral hygiene instructions should be given to prevent the sequelae of gingivitis. Gingival inflammation is enhanced by the combination of plaque and the irritating chemicals in smokeless tobacco products. For users with an increased risk of dental caries, combined fluoride therapy is recommended.

3. Educate the parents and other significant role models such as teachers, coaches, and sports figures. Athletes who "endorse" smokeless tobacco use by example need to be aware and make impressionable youths aware that it causes vasoconstriction and actually decreases athletic performance.[107]

4. Perform a thorough oral examination and point out to the patient any oral changes that currently exist.

5. Teach the patient how to perform his own periodic oral self-examination.

6. Advise the patient to keep a chart of his tobacco behavior by recording each time he places snuff or chewing tobacco in his mouth and how long he retains it there. This type of recording effort might serve to reduce the habit through behavior modification.

7. Counsel the patient regarding other alternatives for reducing or eliminating the behavior, e.g., changing to a disliked brand, chewing gum, using half the amount of tobacco, moving the quid to a less comfortable area of the mouth, and setting a quitting date.

8. Refer the patient to a community smoking cessation group particularly addressing smokeless tobacco use if one is available.

Adolescent Sexuality

The journey to adulthood is seldom simple. Gender identification, sex role development, and adjustment to the emotions surrounding intimacy mark the tasks of adolescence. An individual's sexuality is defined on the basis of his behavior or how he fulfills each of these tasks. Sexual encounters often place the adolescent in a situation of conflicting loyalties, contradictory impulses, and confusing choices. Promiscuity, pregnancy, and venereal disease are particular concerns related to adolescent sexuality.[108]

TEENAGE PREGNANCY

The age of female adolescents experiencing sexual intercourse for the first time is decreasing as the number of pregnancies among this group continues to escalate.[109] By age 16, 29% of boys and 17% of girls have had sexual intercourse. By age 18, these figures increase to 65% for males and 51% for females.[110] In the United States over 1 million teenage girls in the 15 to 19 age category and 30,000 under 15 years become pregnant annually.[111] By their 18th birthdays, 22% of black females and 8% of white females have become mothers. Forty-one percent of black females and 19% of white females have had one or more children by age 20.[112,113]

Risks. Inherent risks related to teenage pregnancy are both social and medical. Pregnancy and subsequent parenting alter a teenager's social interaction with peers. As the teenager being to "show," she often feels like an outcast among her friends. She cannot participate in extracurricular activities and might be required to have a visiting teacher at home to continue her studies. Although many young women are currently choosing to remain unmarried rather than marry an individual who is not prepared to handle the responsibilities associated with marriage and raising a child, single parenthood can be stressful. In 1960, 15.4% of births to women under 20 were to single mothers; by 1983 the rate was 54.1%.[114] Unless a young woman's parents are supportive both emotionally and financially, the stresses placed on this adolescent are great. Where do I live? How can I afford to bring up a child? Where can I get a job? Do I finish school? Do I have this baby? Do I keep this baby? Will things ever be the same with my friends? and Will I ever have fun again? are some of the questions a teenage mother might ask herself. Frequently, teenage mothers do not finish high school and depend on welfare to survive.[115]

Medical risks for teenage pregnancy include (1) obstetric complications; (2) premature and low-birth-weight babies (usually associated with smoking and limited prenatal care, particularly early in the pregnancy); and (3) fetal, neonatal, and maternal morbidity and mortality, which might be related to infection with a communicable disease ranging from rubella to AIDS.

SEXUALLY TRANSMITTED DISEASES

An increase in teenage sexual activity has led to a significant increase in the rate of venereal disease among American youths.[115] Approximately one in four sexually active adolescents will become infected with a sexually transmitted disease before graduating from high school.[116] Presently, over 20 sexually transmitted disease (STDs) are known to occur in adolescents. Five common STDs among adolescents are chlamydial and gonorrhea infections, syphilis, herpes, and acquired immune deficiency syndrome (AIDS). The prevalence of a relatively new organism, human papilloma virus (genital warts) is increasing among college students and might shortly be recognized as the number one STD among teenagers. The following adolescent populations should be screened routinely for STDs:[117] those who are sexually active; victims of rape, incest, or sexual abuse; those who are pregnant; those who are promiscuous; those practicing prostitution; male homosexuals; those who have had or suspect contact with a person known to have a STD; those who are or have been imprisoned; males with leukocyturia; and those with recurrent venereal infections.

Chlamydia. An estimated 3 to 4 million Americans contract a Chlamydia trachomatis infection yearly. Sexually active women under 20 years of age have chlamydial infection rates 2 to 3 times higher than females over 20. Adolescents with chlamydial infections usually present with the following symptoms:[117] (1) mucopurulent urethral discharge, (2) dysuria with frequency and urgency, (3) bartholinitis, (4) cervicitis, (5) rectal pain, tenesmus, and diarrhea, (6) pelvic inflammatory disease (PID), (7) right hypochondrial pain (perihepatitis), (8) acute epididymitis, and (9) postpartum or postabortion endometritis. If an oral lesion is present it is primarily seen on the tongue and can be communicable to dental personnel. Adolescents with chlamydia are usually treated with tetracycline or erythromycin.

Gonorrhea. In 1984, 878,556 cases of gonorrhea were reported for a rate of approximately 375 cases per 100,000 population.[119] This disease is one of staggering proportions because the actual prevalence might be double the reported prevalence.[120] Adolescents accounted for 25% of documented gonorrhea cases in the United States during 1984. The 20- to 24-year age group accounted for 37.5% of documented cases.[119]

Gonorrhea is caused by Neisseria gonorrhoeae, a gram-negative diplococcus almost exclusively transmitted by sexual contact. The primary sites of infection are the genitalia, anal canal, and pharynx. Pharyngeal infection with the bacteria is found in about 20% of patients with gonorrhea.[121,122] Systemic signs usually occur in males within 1 week from becoming infected. Urethral discharge, urinary frequency and urgency, and pain are common. Females with gonorrhea can be asymptomatic or demonstrate vaginal or urethral discharge, dysuria with frequency, and urgency, backaches, and abdominal pain.[123] Intraoral manifestations associated with gonorrhea are relatively nondescript and can resemble various other lesions. One or more of the following can be observed: ulcerations, diffuse erythema, necrosis of interdental papillae, edema, spontaneous gingival bleeding, and a pseudomembrane. Gonococcal stomatitis can therefore leave the patient with a sore mouth, bad taste, and halitosis. Submandibular lymphadenopathy and fever can also be present.[124] The discomfort caused by these oral lesions should be treated palliatively with oral rinses or a topical anesthetic to assist the patient in maintaining the normal oral functions of eating, drinking, and speaking. With systemic treatment, usually involving the administration of tetracycline or some form of penicillin, infectiousness is rapidly reversed.

Syphilis. In 1984, 69,888 cases of syphilis were reported, yielding a rate of approximately 30 cases per 100,000 population.[119] Syphilis is most common in the 20-to-24 age bracket; the next highest prevalence rate is found among teenagers. Treponema pallidum is the organism responsible for syphilis. This anaerobic spirochete can be transmitted through sexual contact, contaminated blood, or contact with lesions harboring the organism.

Primary lesions usually occur within 2 to 3 weeks of exposure in the form of a painless chancre. As the lesion enlarges it either erodes on the surface or ulcerates. It is usually hemorrhagic, yellowish in color, and encrusted. Pain can occur if the lesion become secondarily infected. Lymphadenopathy accompanies the chancre. The lesion usually reduces in size within a month and can leave scarring. The perioral, genital, and anal regions are common sites for chancres to develop (Fig. 6-16). Secondary syphilitic manifestations appear 6 to 8 weeks after the initial exposure. The patient experiences malaise, generalized lymphadenopathy, and/or eruptions of the mucous membranes and skin. Oral manifestations include pharyngitis and a highly contagious mucous patch characterized by a painless, raised lesion with a central zone of erosion and covered with a grayish plaque[123] (Fig. 6-17). These clinical signs can last from several days to 1 year. Medical management of syphilis is extremely successful with the use of a parenteral long-acting antibiotic. Seroconversion to negative usually occurs within 1 year.

The latent or tertiary stage of syphilis results from untreated secondary syphilis. A person with secondary syphilis can be asymptomatic for a period of 20 or more years. In one-third of patients with a history of uncured syphilis, late signs of the disease appear. The manifestations of tertiary syphilis include (1) the gumma, a localized inflammatory granulomatous lesion of skin, mucous membranes, larynx, bone, nervous tissue, and viscera which is not infectious; (2) cardiovascular disease; and (3) sensory-motor nerve damage. Oral signs can consist of a gumma of the tongue or palate, glossitis (bald, wrinkled tongue), and leukoplakia.[123]

Approximately 250 cases of congenital syphilis occurred in 1984 from infected mothers transmitting the disease to their children in utero. Physical anomalies vary based on the time during gestation that the fetus was infected. Most fetal luetic infections are contracted during late pregnancy and involve the teeth, resulting in Hutchinson's incisors, which are peg-shaped permanent central incisors with a notching of the incisal edge, and morphologically de-

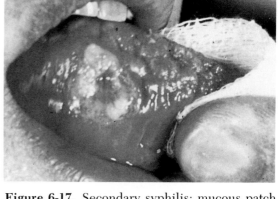

Figure 6-17. Secondary syphilis: mucous patch lesion on the lateral border of the tongue. Copyright of the American Dental Association. Reprinted with permission. Oral Manifestations of Bacterial, Viral, and Mycotic Infections—slide series, slide #60.

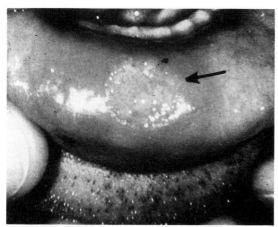

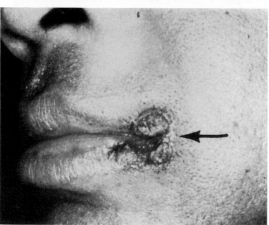

Figure 6-16. Primary syphilis. Chancre—intraoral and extraoral lesions. From Goldman, H. M.: Dermatologic Diseases Affecting the Oral Mucosa. Medcom, 1973, slide #63.

fective first permanent molars with several supernumerary cusps known as mulberry molars (Figs. 4-9, 4-10). The primary dentition is rarely affected since early fetal luetic infections, which occur during the formation of the crowns of these teeth, frequently result in abortion or stillbirth.

Herpes Simplex. Reported new cases of genital herpes number approximately 724,000 yearly in the United States, with a cumulative prevalence of over 20 million infected persons.[125] The etiology of herpes infections involves two different viruses—herpes simplex virus type I (HSV-I) and type II (HSV-II). Traditionally, it was said that herpetic lesions above the waist (mouth, nose, eyes, brain, and skin) were caused by HSV-I and those below the waist (genital) were caused by HSV-II. This distinction is no longer clear-cut, because although the majority of genital herpes lesions are caused by HSV-II, genital infections due to HSV-I are increasing. This increase can be accounted for based on the fact that (1) the primary type I lesion (herpetic gingivostomatitis) is often subclinical in nature, affecting a large percentage of the population unbeknownst to them; and (2) the secondary type I recurrent infection (herpes labialis or the "cold sore") is so common that many people do not realize they are infectious (Fig. 6-18). The practice of oral-genital

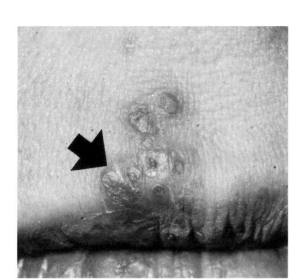

Figure 6-18. Secondary HSV I—herpes labialis or cold sore. Courtesy of J.E. Bouquot, DDS, MS, West Virginia University.

sex allows for the inoculation or crossover of the type I virus from the oral virus site of one individual to the genital area of another.

The clinical course of the disease is identical regardless of the virus type. Infection is initiated by direct contact with lesions, infected saliva, or respiratory secretions.[126] Vesicular lesions usually erupt after an incubation period of 2 days to 1 week and last clinically for approximately 10 to 14 days. On visual disappearance these viruses enter the nerve endings and migrate to the regional ganglia (HSV I—trigeminal, HSV II—sacral), where they remain dormant until stress, sunlight, trauma, menses, or intercourse reactivates them. Recurrent lesions are usually less severe than the primary form.[123] Regardless of the stages of a herpetic lesion (papular, vesicular, ulcerative, or encrusted) it should be regarded as highly infectious with the potential to be transmitted to others or to a new site on the patient, although autoinoculation occurs more frequently in the immunocompromised host. The dental professional can contract a herpetic infection (herpetic whitlow) through a break in the nail beds or the conjunctiva of the eye from aerosol or droplet inoculation. Although there is no cure for herpes, topical and systemic drugs, e.g., acyclovir, iododeoxyuridine, and lysine, have

been used, but with limited success in recurrent lesions.[123]

An estimated 3 to 5% of infants born through the infected birth canal of a mother with herpes acquire a neonatal herpes infection.[125] These infected infants have a mortality rate of 40 to 60%, and 50% of those who survive acquire neurologic or ocular lesions.[117]

AIDS. AIDS (acquired immunodeficiency syndrome) is caused by a virus known as human immunodeficiency virus (HIV). This virus infects T-lymphocytes, which are white cells important to normal immune response function. The infection destroys the T-cells, weakening the immune system. As of 1990 an estimated 1 million Americans are believed to be infected with the HIV virus.[127] In the United States, 95% of AIDS cases have been attributed to the following high-risk groups: homosexual or bisexual males, intravenous drug users, hemophiliacs, blood transfusion recipients, and those who have had heterosexual contact with persons with AIDS or at risk for AIDS.[128] Ninety percent of AIDS patients are between 20 and 49 years of age, which means many of these individuals were adolescents at the time of infection with the virus. Seroconversion or the presence of HIV antibody in the blood of an infected person can occur between 2 weeks and 6 months after exposure to the virus. Because of this time lapse, donated blood can be negative when tested yet highly infectious. Because antigens are produced prior to antibodies, antigen detection would further reduce HIV transmission through blood transfusions. Currently research is being conducted to develop a reliable HIV surface antigen test. The latency period between infection and overt clinical symptoms can be as short as 2 years, but it averages between 7 and 10 years in 30 to 50% of HIV-infected adults.[129] HIV has been isolated from the blood, semen, vaginal secretions, saliva, tears, urine, and breast milk of infected individuals. The known modes of transmission include blood, vaginal secretions, and semen. Transmission from an infected mother to her infant can occur during pregnancy or childbirth. Although contaminated blood poses a

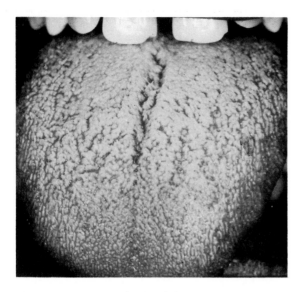

Figure 6-19. Hairy leukoplakia. Courtesy of J.E. Bouquot, DDS, MS, West Virginia University.

threat to the dental professional, the titer of the virus in saliva does not appear to be high enough to transmit the infection. Comparatively speaking, the risk of contracting hepatitis B virus from exposure to contaminated saliva is much greater. Additionally, HIV is sensitive and does not survive outside the body; therefore casual contact cannot be implicated in the spread of AIDS.

Oral manifestations of the disease include hairy leukoplakia (Fig. 6-19), Kaposi's sarcoma lesions (Fig. 6-20), candidiasis (Fig. 6-21), herpes, opportunistic bacterial infections that tend to prey on the immunocompromised host, acute necrotizing ulcerative gingivitis, and aggressive periodontal disease (Fig. 6-22). Common medical conditions found in the AIDS patient include hepatitis B, pneumocystis carinii pneumonia, and other STDs such as gonorrhea and syphilis.[130]

Presently there is no cure for AIDS. AZT (zidovudine, formerly azidothymidine) has shown promise in slowing down the disease process in some patients. The dental health educator might prescribe (1) acyclovir and suggest brushing the tongue for the treatment of the "cotton wool" feeling associated with hairy leukoplakia; (2) laser surgery, localized injections of chemotherapy, or radiation for an oral Kaposi's lesion; (3) nystatin for candidiasis; (4) acyclovir (Zovirax) for an initial perioral herpetic outbreak; (5) an oral prophylaxis with a povidone iodine sulcular lavage to decrease bleeding and discomfort during scaling; and (6) home care instructions consisting of chlorhexidine (Peridex) rinses twice daily along with meticulous oral hygiene to reduce the progression of periodontal disease.[131]

In summary, if a patient has a history or

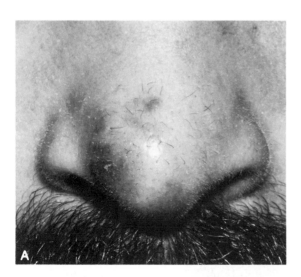

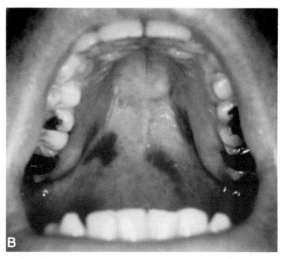

Figure 6-20. Kaposi's sarcoma. *A,* Extraoral lesion of the nose. *B,* Intraoral lesions of the palate. Courtesy of J.E. Bouquot, DDS, MS, West Virginia University.

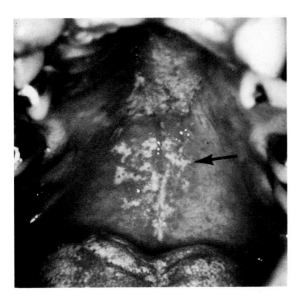

Figure 6-21. Candidiasis. Courtesy of R.I. Hart, DDS, West Virginia University.

is being treated for a sexually transmitted disease it is the role of the dental professional to contact the patient's physician to determine his current health status. As with most STDs, unprotected contact with an active lesion, blood, or blood products greatly increases the dental professional's risk for contracting the disease. Optimum infection control procedures must be practiced with all patients. These are referred to as "universal precautions." If a patient has signs or symptoms that cause the dental professional to suspect a STD and the patient is not being treated, elective treatment should be postponed and the patient should be referred to a physician for evaluation.[123] The patient

should be rescheduled within a reasonable period of time to assure him that he is not being abandoned, but it is necessary to reverse an infection before any elective dental care is accomplished. The dental professional has an ethical responsibility to treat the patient at the initial appointment if the patient requires emergency care.

CONTRACEPTION AND PREVENTION OF DISEASE

Pregnancy and infections with sexually transmitted diseases are increasing in epidemic proportions among the nation's adolescent population. Contraception and disease-prevention education and services need to be tailored to the developmental level of each adolescent, not his chronologic age. Human sexuality programs should include values, sex role and gender clarification, health and sex education, family life and planning, and effective decision-making.[132] Parents should begin discussing human sexuality issues with their children early in life, but many do not. Schools can help increase communication between parents and children through mutual sex education counseling. In order to have an effect on teenage pregnancy statistics, education must reach adolescents before they experience sex, not after.

No perfect method of contraception is available (Table 6-6).[133] The barrier methods of contraception (condoms or diaphragms with spermicidal foams or jellies) provide the best protection against STD.

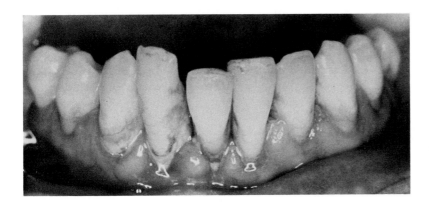

Figure 6-22. Aggressive periodontitis associated with HIV. Courtesy of J.E. Bouquot, DDS, MS, West Virginia University.

Table 6-6. Lowest Percentage of U.S. Women Expected to Experience an Accidental Pregnancy During the First Year of Consistent and Correct Use of a Particular Contraceptive Method

Method	Lowest Percent Expected
Chance	89
Spermicide (foam, cream, jelly, and vaginal suppositories)	3
Periodic abstinence	
Ovulation method	8
Symptothermal	6
Calendar	10
Postovulation	2
Withdrawal	4
Cap (with spermicidal cream or jelly)	5
Sponge	5
Diaphragm (with spermicidal cream or jelly)	3
Condom (without spermicide)	2
Intrauterine device (IUD)	
Medicated	1
Nonmedicated	2
Pill	
Combined	0.1
Progesterone only	0.5
Injectable progesterone	
DMPA	0.3
NET	0.4
Implant	
Capsule	0.3
Rod	0.2
Female sterilization	0.2
Male sterilization	0.1

Adapted from Breedlove, B., Judy, B., and Martin, N. (eds): Contraceptive Technology, 1988–89. 14th Ed. Atlanta, Printed matter, 1989, p. 151, which listed the following reference: Trussel, J., and Kost, K.: Contraceptive failure in the United States: A critical review of the literature. Studies in Family Planning, *18*, Tables 1 and 2, 1987.)

The birth-control pill, when taken correctly, is the best method for controlling fertilization. Unfortunately, contraceptive knowledge and use among adolescents are relatively low. Approximately half of American adolescents did not use any contraceptives the first time they had intercourse.[134] This poor utilization might be due to (1) a pattern of infrequent and spontaneous sexual encounters; (2) emotional difficulty such as shame, anxiety, or embarrassment in acknowledging to themselves and communicating to their sex partners the possibility of sexual activity and the need for protection; (3) limited access to contraceptive services; and (4) misinformation or a lack of knowledge related to contraceptive methods and techniques for use.[135] Substance abuse interferes with the cognitive and decision-making processes and can also be responsible for increasing the chance of unplanned sexual intercourse without the use of contraception.[109] Health education programs emphasizing contraception must focus on decreasing the use of ineffective methods of contraception and limiting sexual contact without the utilization of protective measures.[136] When attempts at contraception fail or no method is used, the likelihood of accidental pregnancy increases.

Prenatal education for pregnant adolescents is necessary to promote the health of the young mother and her child. Early prenatal counseling is critical, particularly in an age group in which infant mortality rates remain high.[137]

Among STDs, AIDS continues to surpass other diseases in terms of public concern. Unfortunately, the media remain the major source of information on AIDS for most adolescents. Media information is often inadequate or superficial, and youths can have difficulty fully understanding its meaning, often misinterpreting the intent of the message.[138] In the absence of a vaccine or treatment for AIDS and several other STDs, education remains the only effective method for control. A variety of organizations, informational packages, and audiovisual materials are available (see Appendix D) to enhance the educational process.[139]

ESTHETIC DENTAL CONCERNS

In contemporary society, oral health refers not only to the absence of pathology, but also to concern for the esthetic appearance of the teeth. Many people regard their smiles as their most important feature. The smile has frequently been referred to as the mirror of the soul. The mouth and teeth often create a first and lasting impression. A smile can open the lines of communication between two people; it can place an individual at ease and make him feel welcome. Unfortunately, many people dislike their smiles because they consider their teeth too large, too yellow, or too crooked.

Placement of tooth-colored restorations, correction of malocclusions, bonding of restorations to hypoplastic enamel and dentin, fabrication of esthetic prostheses and appliances to prevent damage to the dentition (e.g., thumbsucking deterrents and athletic mouthguards), bleaching of discolored teeth, and recontouring of morphologic defects are all dental services that enhance the patient's appearance or image.[140] The dental health educator functions by making patients aware of these esthetic techniques, describing the alternatives available and the procedures and costs involved. Although the patient can be reassured about his esthetic concerns, he should never be assured of perfection or an unrealistic outcome.

Composite Resins and Veneers

A patient's esthetic needs might be satisfied by conservative anterior composite resin and veneer restorations, which can be combined with bleaching and cosmetic contouring. Improvement is relatively immediate, decreasing the patient's chair time, and this approach is normally less expensive than more invasive procedures such as the placement of a crown.[141] Tooth-colored restorations are contraindicated when there are obvious signs of bruxism, clenching, or other abusive oral habits and when there is insufficient coronal dentin to provide retention.[142]

Bonding is a useful method for camouflaging stains, lightening a tooth's color, closing diastemas, and restoring chips. This technique requires no anesthetic, minimal tooth reduction, and produces an immediate result. Initially, the procedure is similar to sealant placement. The tooth is etched with a mild concentration of phosphoric acid before the liquid bonding material is applied to the tooth. The bonding agent is then light-cured or autopolymerized until it hardens. Additional layers of a more durable plastic composite material are then applied to the prepared tooth. Bonded restorations should be replaced every 3 to 8 years due to stain and wear.[143]

Veneers can also be used to lighten discolored teeth and eliminate spaces. Preformed plastic laminate veneers require limited contouring and are easy to polish, but like bonded restorations they can discolor or chip. Porcelain veneers are superior to plastic veneers because they do not stain or chip, and they are superior to traditional porcelain crowns because they do not irritate the gingival tissue. The tooth is etched, and the veneer is cemented into place with a composite material and cured. The major disadvantage of porcelain veneers is that they require some tooth reduction.

Composite resins are used to restore facial or interproximal caries, mainly on anterior teeth. With time they can stain, and they tend to wear more quickly than amalgam restorations.

Porcelain inlays and onlays are relatively new in the area of esthetic dentistry. Because these restorations are secured by a chemical bond to the tooth, they require less reduction than conventional gold inlays and onlays. The tooth is diminished by 0.5 mm both facially and lingually and 1 mm on involved cusps. This reduction requires the placement of a temporary filling until the laboratory finishes the inlay. With the invention of computer-aided design and computer-aided manufacturing (CAD-CAM), it is possible to construct these ceramic restorations chairside, during one appointment.[144] After the exposed dentin is lined with a shaded glass ionomer, the tooth is etched and bonded and the inlay is cemented with a color-compatible composite material. These restorations do not stain or irritate the tissues; they resist abrasion, reduce sensitivity, and rarely experience marginal leakage.[143]

Bleaching

Many intrinsic and extrinsic stains can be removed from teeth by one of three bleaching techniques: professional, professional/home bleaching, and at-home bleaching. Bleaching requires no reduction in tooth structure and no anesthetic. The six anterior teeth are those most commonly bleached, and the procedure is usually not performed on children because of the pain that can result from bleaching teeth with large pulp chambers.[143] Bleaching is also contraindicated for patients with hypersensitive teeth and thin, flaky enamel.

Prior to treatment, the teeth to be bleached should be radiographed and tested with the vitalometer. A baseline assessment of the proposed teeth and soft tissue is advised to determine the presence of side effects, when and if they arise. Preparing the teeth for office bleaching is the most important step in the process. Care must be taken to prevent leakage of the bleaching agent onto the tissues within the area to be treated. The soft tissue should be covered with a protective ointment, e.g., Orabase. The teeth are sealed off from the oral environment by placement of a thick rubber dam, followed by ligation of the teeth with waxed dental floss and painting of the cervical portion of the teeth with copalite varnish (Fig. 6-23). The current shade of the patient's teeth is determined and recorded with a standard shade guide. The teeth to be bleached should be pumiced (do not use a fluoride prophylaxis paste), thoroughly rinsed and dried, and etched with 37 to 50% phosphoric acid. The teeth must be thoroughly rinsed (1 min) to remove the acid and dried again prior to continuously saturating them with the chemical oxidizing agent, a 33% solution of hydrogen peroxide. If a light source is used to activate the bleaching process, the top of the beam is directed at the prepared teeth for 20 to 30 min on medium intensity; the intensity can be gradually increased as long as the patient feels comfortable. The light source should be 36 to 41 cm from the teeth, and the patient should be given protective goggles. Heat paddles can also be used. The paddle is applied to each tooth individually for approximately 2 to 3 min according to the patient's sensitivity level. Subsequent to treatment the teeth are polished to restore their luster.[145,146] The success rate for vital bleaching is about 75%, and most cases require 5 to 8 sessions to obtain a suitable result. Sessions should be spaced approximately 1 week apart, and the degree of color change should be evaluated during each visit. Periodic retreatment is necessary if regression occurs, but regression is rare after the first week of treatment.

Nightguard vital bleaching is less expensive because only two or three office appointments are warranted. If a patient has mild yellow, orange, or light brown tooth discoloration, an impression is taken on the first visit. The second appointment consists of trying-in the vacuum-formed soft plastic nightguard, which is similar to a custom athletic mouth protector but slightly thinner (Fig. 6-24). With the tray in place, the oc-

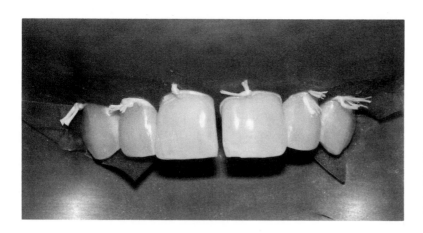

Figure 6-23. Rubber dam isolation in preparation for bleaching. Courtesy of G.L Dickinson, DDS, MS, West Virginia University.

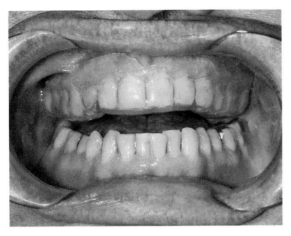

Figure 6-24. Nightguard bleaching. Courtesy of G.L. Dickinson, DDS, MS, West Virginia University.

clusion should be checked and the nightguard adjusted if necessary. The nightguard should completely cover the teeth while leaving the palate and gingival tissue as exposed as possible. Instructions for home bleaching are also given. A 355-ml (12-oz) tube of 10% carbamide peroxide is prescribed or dispensed to the patient, and the patient is advised to place 2 or 3 drops of the bleaching solution in each indentation in the nightguard that corresponds to the tooth to be lightened. The dental health educator must emphasize the importance of thorough brushing, flossing, and rinsing before inserting the nightguard each bedtime. The patient should expectorate excess liquid on insertion and wear the appliance throughout the night. The nightguard should be cleaned and rinsed each morning and immersed in cool water when not in use. Initial results might be noticed within 2 weeks, but optimal change usually requires about 6 weeks.[147]

Tooth bleaching strictly accomplished at home can be obtained from 10 known products currently on the market (Table 6-7).[148] The active ingredient in all brands is either carbamide peroxide or hydrogen peroxide. Some companies provide dispenser trays for delivery of the bleaching solution or gel, whereas others recommend brushing the agent on the teeth. In order to determine the efficacy and possible adverse effects of at-home bleaching and to compare delivery methods, Clinical Research Associates conducted studies of the kits currently marketed for home use. The CRA report concluded that (1) all products lightened teeth; (2) the best regimen consists of plaque removal, tray insertion for 3 to 4 h once or several times daily, and the replenishment of the bleach every hour due to swallowing and dilution with saliva; (3) enamel is not adversely affected by bleaching, but contact with dentin and resin restorative materials should be avoided; (4) most patients experienced no adverse effects; the occasional tooth hypersensitivity, tissue sloughing, nausea, and sore throat were resolved quickly when the treatment was discontinued; (5) patient compliance was good if verbal instructions preceded home use and office recalls were enforced; and (6) TMJ dysfunction associated with poorly designed trays was implicated as at-home bleaching's greatest drawback.[148] Because new products are being formulated and their contents adjusted on a daily basis, dental health educators must be responsible for keeping abreast of these changes so they can make recommendations to their patients and appropriately address their questions and concerns.

Mouth Protectors

Adolescents engaging in contact sports should wear mouthguards or protectors to prevent oral trauma. Wearing this appliance also provides the individual with a feeling of security, because the chances of tooth fracture or avulsion are greatly reduced.[149]

A custom mouth protector should fit snugly to prevent dislocation but should not impinge on the soft tissue, stimulate the gag reflex, or interfere with breathing or speaking. Inexpensive stock-type mouthguards can be found in some pharmacies and sporting goods stores.

Although all high school and college football programs in the United States require their athletes to wear mouth protectors, many other sports programs only recommend their use.[150–152] It is the role of the

Table 6-7. Home-Use Tooth-Bleaching Products

Product Name	Company	Active Ingredient	Relatively Rapid Bleach	Complete Kit Available	Bleach Sold Separately	DDS/PT Directions	PT Consent Form	Tray Instructions	Relatively Viscous	Sold only to DDS
Denta-Lite	Challenge	Carbamide peroxide 10%	X	X		X	X	X		X
Dentbright	Cura	Carbamide peroxide 10%			X	X	X	X	X	X
Gly-Oxide	Marion	Carbamide peroxide 10%			X					
Natural White	Aesthete	H_2O_2 6%	X	X		X		N/A	X	
Nu-Smile	M & M	Carbamide peroxide 15%	X		X	X	X			X
Peroxyl	Colgate/Hoyt	H_2O_2 1.5%			X				X	
Proxigel	Reed/Carnrick	Carbamide peroxide 10%	X		X				X	
Rembrandt Lighten	Den-Mat	Carbamide peroxide 10%	X	X	X	X	X	X	X	X
Ultra-Lite	Ultra-Lite	Carbamide peroxide 10%	X		X	X	X	X	X	X
White & Brite	Omnii	Carbamide peroxide 10%	X	X	X	X	X	X		X

Materials compiled from July 1989 and December 1989 CRA Newsletters published by Clinical Research Associates, Provo, UT 84604.

dental health educator to visit students in classrooms and speak to coaches and parents about the need for mouth protection on the field and court. Local dental offices, the dental school, or the public health department could sponsor preseason screening, mouthguard fabrication, and emergency treatment, if necessary, for those adolescents and young adults who are participating in organized sports.

COMMENTS

Adolescents battle routinely for their self-esteem. Such problems as acne, menstruation, and malocclusion can threaten the standards a teenager has set for himself and how he believes others perceive him. Suicide, teenage pregnancy, eating disorders, delinquency, and drug abuse are only a few of the many social problems that can emerge in an adolescent's effort to cope with his surroundings as he struggles to make the transition to adulthood. The adolescent can have a smoother, more productive journey to adulthood if he is provided with a firm but sensitive set of expectations and standards that provide opportunities for learning and progress. In the communities studied by Ianni, it was established that the adolescent remains attached to the cultural, ethnic, and social class lifestyles of his parents despite his quest for independence. If role models are effective, the adolescent's crises become less urgent and he comes to seek identity rather than independence.[153]

As a health professional, the dental health educator is responsible for recognizing problems, establishing open lines of communication, and providing intervention or help strategies for the adolescent. Assistance can consist of personal counseling or referral to an individual or agency equipped to help. The design and implementation of risk-reduction programs for adolescent health problems are enhanced by focusing on personal image and efficacy.[154,155] The dental health educator can assist the individual by teaching him to know what to do

and how to do it; motivating him to want to do it; and helping him believe he can do it (e.g., flossing, weight loss, and smoking cessation). Offering the teenager caring, feasible options, whether they involve dental esthetics or otherwise, can assist him in enhancing his self-satisfaction and improving his self-image. A heightened sense of worth enables an individual to believe in himself and his capabilities and make an informed decision to move forward or act. Health education is the best medicine.

REFERENCES

1. Pan American Health Organization: Health of Adolescents and Youths in the Americas. Publication No. 489, Washington DC, World Health Organization, 1985.
2. Lowrey, G. H.: Growth and Development of Children. 6th Ed. Chicago, Year Book, 1973.
3. Heisler, A. B., and Friedman, S. B.: Adolescence: Psychological and social development. J. Sch. Health, 50:381–385, 1980.
4. Pinkham, J. R., et al. (Eds.): Pediatric Dentistry: Infancy through Adolescence. Philadelphia, W.B. Saunders, 1988.
5. Alexander, A.: Adolescent health: Challenge of the 80s. J. Sch. Health, 50:47, 1980.
6. Inhelder, B., and Piaget, J.: The Growth of Logical Thinking from Childhood to Adolescence. New York, Basic Books, 1958.
7. U.S. Bureau of the Census: Current Population Reports: Population Estimates and Projections, 1989. Series P-25, No. 1018. Washington, DC, U.S. Government Printing Office, 1989.
8. Willgoose, C. E.: Health Teaching in Secondary Schools. 3rd Ed. Philadelphia, Saunders, 1982.
9. Palmer, C. A.: Reaching the terrible teens. Dent. Hyg., 49:364–367, 1975.
10. Mathewson, R. J., et al.: Fundamentals of Dentistry for Children. Chicago, Quintessence, 1982.
11. U.S. Public Health Service, National Institute of Dental Research: Caries Prevalence in U.S. Schoolchildren 1986–1987. National Institutes of Health. Publication #(PHS) 89-2247. U.S. Dept. of Health and Human Services, 1989.
12. McDonald, R. E., and Avery, D. R.: Dentistry for the Child and Adolescent. 5th Ed. St. Louis, C.V. Mosby, 1987.
13. Sutcliffe, P.: A longitudinal study of gingivitis and puberty. J. Periodontol., 7:52–58, 1972.
14. Page, R. C., et al.: Clinical and laboratory studies of a family with a high prevalence of juvenile periodontitis. J. Periodontol., 56:602–610, 1985.
15. Nizel, A. E., and Papas, A. S.: Nutrition in Clinical Dentistry. 3rd Ed. Philadelphia, W.B. Saunders, 1989.
16. Wilkins, E. M.: Clinical Practice of the Dental Hygienist. 6th Ed. Philadelphia, Lea & Febiger, 1989.
17. Graykowski, S. A., Barile, M. F., and Stanley, H. R.: Periadenitis aphthae: Clinical and histopathologic aspects of

lesions in a patient and of lesions produced in rabbit skin. J. Am. Dent. Assoc., 69:118–126, 1964.

18. Skip, I. I.: Epidemiologic aspects of recurrent aphthous ulcerations. Oral Surg., 33:400–406, 1972.

19. Wray, D., et al.: Recurrent aphthae: Treatment with vitamin B$_{12}$, folic acid and iron. Br. Med. J., 2:490–493, 1975.

20. Baker, K. A., and Helling, D. K.: Oral health products. *In* A Handbook of Nonprescription Drugs. 8th Ed. Washington, DC, American Pharmaceutical Association, 1986.

21. Linn, E. L.: Teenagers' attitudes, knowledge, and behaviors related to oral health. J. Am. Dent. Assoc., 92:946–951, 1976.

22. Rugg-Gunn, A. J., and MacGregor, I. D. M.: A survey of toothbrushing behavior in children and young adults. J. Periodontal Res., 13:382–389, 1978.

23. Pao, E. M., and Mickle, S. J.: Nutrients from meals and snacks, 1980. Agricultural Outlook Conference, Session 29, Washington, DC, 1981.

24. McBean, L. D., and Speckman, E. W.: Food faddism: A challenge to nutritionists and dieticians. Am. J. Clin. Nutr., 27:1071–1078, 1974.

25. Food and Drug Administration: A Study of Health Practices and Opinions: Final Report. Dept. of Health, Education and Welfare. Contract No. FDA 66-193, June 1972 and F.D.A. Talk Paper, October 6, 1972.

26. Gifft, H. H., Washbon, M. B., and Harrison, G. G.: Nutrition, Behavior and Change. Englewood Cliffs, NJ, Prentice-Hall, 1972.

27. Jalso, S., Rivers, J., and Burns, M.: Nutritional beliefs and practices. J. Am. Dietet. Assoc., 47:263, 1965.

28. Gross, K. B., Brough, K. M., and Randolph, P. M.: Eating disorders: Anorexia and bulimia nervosas. J. Dent. Child., 53:378–381, 1986.

29. Altshuler, B. D.: Anorexia and bulimia: A review for the dental hygienist. Dent. Hyg., 60:466–471, 1986.

30. Stege, P., Visco-Dangler, L., and Rye, L.: Anorexia nervosa: Review including oral and dental manifestations. J. Am. Dent. Assoc., 104:648–652, 1982.

31. Crisp, A. H., et al.: Clinical features of anorexia nervosa: A study of a consecutive series of 102 female patients. J. Psychosom. Res., 24:174, 1980.

32. Diagnostic and Statistical Manual of Mental Disorders DSM-III-R. 3rd rev. ed. Washington, DC, American Psychiatric Association, 1987.

33. Robin, P.: Anorexia nervosa: When dieting can lead to death. Co-Ed., 27:22, 1981.

34. French, R. N., and Baker, E. L.: Anorexia nervosa and bulimia. Indiana Med., 241–245, 1984.

35. Gandour, M. J.: Bulimia: Clinical description, assessment, etiology and treatment. Int. J. Eating Disorders, 3:3, 1984.

36. Renshau, D. C.: Dentists and bulimia/anorexia nervosa. Penn. Dent. J., 52:20–21, 1985.

37. Mitchell, J. E., and Pyle, R. L.: The bulimic syndrome in normal weight individuals: A review. Int. J. Eating Disorders, 1:61, 1982.

38. Lee, D. S.: Starving for beauty. Dent. Tmwk., 1:273–277, 1988.

39. Lucas, A. R.: Bulimia and vomiting syndrome. Contemp. Nutr., 6:1–2, 1981.

40. Russell, G.: Bulimia nervosa: An ominous variant of anorexia nervosa. Psychol. Med., 9:429–448, 1979.

41. Abrams, R. A., and Ruff, J. C.: Signs and symptoms of bulimia. J. Am. Dent. Assoc., 113:761–764, 1986.

42. Harrison, J. L., George, L. A., Cheatham, J. L., and Zinn, J.: Dental effects and management of bulimia nervosa. Gen. Dent., 33:65–68, 1985.

43. Walsh, B. T., Croft, C. B., and Katz, J. L.: Anorexia nervosa and salivary gland enlargement. Int. J. Psychiatry Med., 11:255–261, 1982.

44. Roberts, M. S., Li, Shou-Hua: Oral findings in anorexia nervosa and bulimia nervosa: A study of 47 cases. J. Am. Dent. Assoc., 115:407–410, 1987.

45. Johnson, D. L., and Rue, V. M.: The bulimic dental patient: Recognition and recommendations. Dent. Hyg., 59:372–377, 1985.

46. Mallick, M. J.: Anorexia nervosa and bulimia: Questions and answers for school personnel. J. Sch. Health, 54:299–301, 1984.

47. Ruff, J. C., and Abrams, R. A.: Preventive dental prosthesis for the patient with bulimia. Sp. Care Dent., 7:218–220, 1987.

48. U.S. Dept. of Health and Human Services: Disease Prevention and Health Promotion: The Facts. Palo Alto, Bull. Publishing, 1988.

49. Trends and Current Status in Childhood Mortality, United States, 1900–1985. Vital and Health Statistics, Series 3, No. 26, DHHS Publication No. PHS 89-1410, Hyattsville, MD, National Center for Health Statistics, 1989.

50. Finch, S. M., and Poznanski, E. O.: Adolescent Suicide. Springfield, IL, Charles C Thomas, 1971.

51. Mishara, B. L.: The extent of adolescent suicide. Psychiatric Opinion, 12:32–37, 1975.

52. McKenry, P. C., Tishler, C. L., and Christman, K. L.: Adolescent suicide and the classroom teacher. J. Sch. Health, 50:130–132, 1980.

53. Curran, B. E.: Suicide. Pediatr. Clin. North Am., 26:737–745, 1979.

54. Goldberg, E. L.: Depression and suicide ideation in the young adult. Am. J. Psychiatry, 138:35–39, 1981.

55. Green, A. H.: Self-destructive behavior in battered children. Am. J. Psychiatry, 135:579–581, 1978.

56. Garfinkel, B. D., Froese, A., and Hood, J.: Suicide attempts in children and adolescents. Am. J. Psychiatry, 139:1257–1261, 1982.

57. Hayes, P. A., Prince, M. T., and Hayes, K.: The suicidal adolescent. J. Dent. Child., 55:133–136, 1988.

58. American Association of Suicidology, 2459 South Ash Street, Denver, CO 80222.

59. National Institute on Drug Abuse: National household survey on drug abuse: Population estimates 1988. DHHS Publication No. ADM 89-1636, Washington, DC, U.S. Government Printing Office, 1989.

60. Wagner, B. J.: Intervening with the adolescent involved in substance abuse. J. Sch. Health, 54:244–246, 1984.

61. Johnston, L. D., O'Malley, P. M., and Bachman, J. G.: Illicit drug use, smoking, and drinking by America's high school students, college students, and young adults, 1975–1987. DHHS Publication No. ADM 89-1602, Washington, DC, U.S. Government Printing Office, 1988.

62. Rosengard, J. R.: Marijuana. Science Digest, 83:71–77. 1978.

63. Young, B. F.: Drug abuse: What dental professionals should know. Dent. Hyg., 60:546–550, 1986.

64. Streit, F.: Parents and Problems: Through the Eyes of Youth. Highland Park, NJ, Essence, 1978.

65. Goodstadt, M. S.: School-based drug education in North America: What is wrong? What can be done? J. Sch. Health, 56:278–281, 1986.

66. The first lady's drug awareness campaign: Questions and answers from Mrs. Nancy Reagan. J. Sch. Health, 55:79–81, 1985.

67. Tarlon, A. R., and Rimel, R. W.: Drug abuse prevention—the sponsoring foundations' perspective. J. Sch. Health, 56:358, 1986.

68. Koop, C. E.: The quest for a smoke-free young America by the year 2000. J. Sch. Health, 56:8–9, 1986.

69. Botvin, G. J. and Eng, A.: A comprehensive school-based smoking prevention program. J. Sch. Health, 50:209–213, 1980.

70. Evans, R. I.: Smoking in children: Developing a social-psychological strategy of deterrence. J. Prev. Med., 5:122–127, 1976.

71. Newman, I. M.: Capturing the energy of peer pressure: Insights from a longitudinal study of adolescent cigarette smoking. J. Sch. Health, 54:146–148, 1984.

72. Coan, R. W.: Personality variables associated with cigarette smoking. J. Pers. Soc. Psychol., 26:86–104, 1973.

73. Matarazzo, J., and Matarazzo, R.: Smoking. In International Encyclopedia of the Social Sciences. Edited by D. Sills. New York, Macmillan and Free Press, 1968.

74. Fracchia, J., Sheppare, C., and Merlis, S.: Early cigarette smoking and drug use: Some comments, data and thoughts. Psychol. Rep., 34:371–374, 1974.

75. McKennell, A.: British research into smoking behavior. In Smoking, Health and Behavior. Edited by E. Borgatta and R. Evans. Chicago, Aldine, 1968.

76. Matarazzo, J., and Saslow, G.: Psychological and related characteristics of smokers and nonsmokers. Psychol. Bull., 57:493–513, 1960.

77. Williams, A. F.: Personality and other characteristics associated with cigarette smoking among teenagers. J. Health Soc. Behav., 14:374–380, 1973.

78. Newman, I. M.: Ninth grade smokers-two years later. University of Illinois, anti-smoking educational study. J. Sch. Health, 41:497–501, 1971.

79. Klein, J. A., et al.: A smoking cessation program that really works. Dent. Tmwk., 2:9–14, 1989.

80. Borden, P. S., Christen, A. G., McDonald, J. L., and Klein, J. A.: A smoking cessation program for the oral health care practice. Dent. Hyg., 62:339–343, 1988.

81. U.S. Department of Health and Human Services, Public Health Service: The Health Consequences of Smoking for Women: A Report of the Surgeon General. Washington, DC, Government Printing Office, 1980.

82. Christen, A. G., and Glover, E. D.: Tobacco education and "quit smoking" program in the dental office and community: The why's and wherefore's. Gent. Dent., 75:83–87, 1985.

83. Christen, A. G., et al.: Nicotine gum: Can it help your patients quit smoking? Mod. Med., 52:226–234, 1985.

84. Christen, A. G., et al.: Efficacy of nicotine chewing gum in facilitating smoking cessation. J. Am. Dent. Assoc., 108:594–597, 1987.

85. Sadles, M. C.: Smokeless tobacco: A review of the literature for dental hygienists. Dent. Hyg., 61:360–364, 1987.

86. Connolly, G. N.: Tobacco and snuff: Growing health threats. Nation's Health, April 6, 1985.

87. Harper, S.: In tobacco where there's smokeless fire. Ad. Age, 51:85, 1980.

88. Hunter, S. M., et al.: Longitudinal patterns of cigarette smoking and smokeless tobacco use in youth: The Bogalusa heart study. Am. J. Pub. Health, 76:193, 1986.

89. Marty, P. J., McDermott, R. J., and Williams, T.: Patterns of smokeless tobacco use in a population of high school students. Am. J. Pub. Health, 762:190, 1986.

90. Greer, R. O., and Poulson, T. C.: Oral tissue alterations associated with the use of smokeless tobacco by teenagers: I. Clinical findings. Oral Surg., 56:275, 1983.

91. Guggenheimer, J., et al.: Changing trends of tobacco use in a teenage population in western Pennsylvania. Am. J. Pub. Health, 76:196, 1986.

92. U.S. Department of Health and Human Services: The Health Consequences of Using Smokeless Tobacco: A Report of the Advisory Committee to the Surgeon General. No. 86-2874, Bethesda, NIH Publication, 1986.

93. American Academy of Pediatrics, Committee on Environmental Hazards Report: Smokeless tobacco—a carcinogenic hazard to children. Pediatrics, 76:1009, 1985.

94. U.S. Department of Health and Human Public Health Service: The Health Consequences of Using Smokeless Tobacco. A Report of the Surgeon General. Washington, DC, Government Printing Office, 1986.

95. Schinke, S. P., et al.: Health effects of smokeless tobacco. JAMA, 257:781, 1987.

96. Offenbacher, S., and Weathers, O. R.: Effects of smokeless tobacco on the periodontal, mucosal, and caries status of adolescent males. J. Oral Pathol., 14:169, 1985.

97. Poulson, T. C., Lindenmuth, J. E., and Greer, R. O.: A comparison of the use of smokeless tobacco in rural and urban teenagers. CA, 34:248–249, 1984.

98. Squier, C. A.: Smokeless tobacco and oral cancer: A cause for concern? CA, 34:242–247, 1984.

99. Heth, J.: Kids think it's macho to chew. Des Moines Register, June 6, 1982.

100. Winn, D. M., et al.: Snuff dipping and oral cancer among women in the southern United States. N. Engl. J. Med., 304:745–749, 1981.

101. Johnson, R., and Herzog, A.: Oral effects of smokeless tobacco use. Dent. Hyg., 61:354–359, 1987.

102. Squires, W. G., et al.: Hemodynamic effects of oral smokeless tobacco in dogs and young adults. Prev. Med., 13:195–206, 1984.

103. Shroeder, K. L., and Chen, M. S.: Smokeless tobacco and blood pressure. N. Engl. J. Med., 312:919, 1985.

104. McDermott, R. J., Clark, B. J., and McCormack, K. R.: The reemergence of smokeless tobacco: Implications for dental hygiene practice. Dent. Hyg., 61:348–353, 1987.

105. Schroeder, K. L., Chen, M. S., and Kuthy, R. A.: Smokeless tobacco: The new thing to chew on. Ohio Dent. J., 59:11, 1985.

106. Schroeder, K. L., et al.: Bimodal initiation of smokeless tobacco usage: Implications for cancer education. J. Ca. Educ., 2:15–21, 1987.

107. American Dental Association: Guide to Dental Health. J. Am. Dent. Assoc., Special Issue, 1986.

108. Silber, T. J.: Adolescent sexuality: Developmental and ethical issues. In The Health of Adolescents and Youths in the Americas. Pan American Health Organization. Publication No. 489, Washington, DC, World Health Organization, 1985.

109. Proctor, S. E.: A developmental approach to pregnancy prevention with early adolescent females. J. Sch. Health, 56:313–316, 1986.

110. Moore, K. A.: Facts at a Glance. Washington, DC, Child Trends, 1988.

111. Office of Promotion Affairs: The Adolescent Family Life Demonstration Projects: Program and Evaluation Summaries. Washington, DC, 1986.

112. Unpublished data from the National Institute of Child Health and Development: Bethesda, National Institutes of Health, 1985.

113. U.S. Bureau of the Census: Current Population Reports, 1985.

114. National Institute of Child Health and Development: Adolescent pregnancy and childbearing-rates, trends, and research findings. In U.S. Bureau of the Census, Current Population Reports, 1986.

115. Gans, J. E., et al.: America's Adolescents: How Healthy Are They? Chicago, American Medical Association, 1990.

116. Shafer, M. A., and Moscicki, A. B.: Sexually transmitted diseases in adolescents. In The Health of Adolescents.

Edited by W. R. Hendee. San Francisco, Jossey-Bass, 1990.

117. Silber, T. J., and Woodward, K.: Sexually transmitted diseases in adolescence. *In* The Health of Adolescents and Youths in the Americas. Pan American Health Organization. Publication No. 489. Washington, DC, World Health Organization, 1985.

118. Centers for Disease Control: Chlamydia trachomatis infections: Policy guidelines for prevention and control. Morbidity and Mortality Weekly Report Supplement, 1985.

119. Centers for Disease Control: Sexually Transmitted Disease Statistics Calendar Year 1984. Atlanta, Center for Prevention Services, 1985.

120. Hook, E. W., and Holmes, K. K.: Gonococcal infections. Ann. Intern. Med., *102*:243–299, 1985.

121. Feldman, Y. M., and Nikitas, J. A.: Pharyngeal gonorrhea. N.Y. State J. Med., *80*:957–959, 1980.

122. Karus, S. L.: Incidence and therapy of gonococcal pharyngitis. Sex. Transm. Dis., 6:143–147, 1979.

123. Little, J. W., and Falace, D. A.: Dental Management of the Medically Compromised Patient. 2nd Ed. St. Louis, C.V. Mosby, 1984.

124. Chue, P. W. Y.: Gonorrhea: Its natural history, oral manifestations, diagnosis, treatment and prevention. J. Am. Dent. Assoc., *90*:1297–1301, 1975.

125. Guinan, M. E., Wolinsky, S. M., and Reichman, R. C.: Epidemiology of genital herpes simplex virus infection. Epidemiol. Rev., 7:127–146, 1985.

126. Woodall, I. R., et al.: Comprehensive Dental Hygiene Care. 3rd Ed. St. Louis, C.V. Mosby, 1989.

127. Centers for Disease Control: AIDS Indices/Facts 7/31/90. Atlanta, Center for Disease Control, 1990.

128. U.S. AIDS Activity Center for Infectious Diseases: Acquired Immunodeficiency Syndrome (AIDS) Weekly Surveillance Report. Atlanta, Centers for Disease Control, 1986.

129. American Dental Association: AIDS: The disease and its implications for dentistry. J. Am. Dent. Assoc., *115*:395–403, 1987.

130. Roberts, M. W., Brahim, J. S., and Rinne, N. F.: Oral manifestations of AIDS: A study of 84 patients. J. Am. Dent. Assoc., *116*:863–866, 1988.

131. Winkler, J. R., Murray, P. A., Grassi, M., and Hammerle, C.: Diagnosis and management of HIV-associated periodontal lesions. J. Am. Dent. Assoc., Supplement 25–34, 1989.

132. Kapp, L., Taylor, B. A. and Edwards, L. E.: Teaching human sexuality in junior high school: An interdisciplinary approach. J. Sch. Health, *50*:80–83, 1980.

133. Breedlove, B., Judy, B., and Martin, N.: Contraceptive Technology 1988–1989. 14th Ed. Atlanta, Printed Matter, 1989.

134. Hofferth, S. L., and Hayes, C. D. (Eds.): Risking the Future: Adolescent Sexuality, Pregnancy, and Childbearing. Vol. 2. Washington, DC, National Academy Press, 1987.

135. Chesler, J.: Twenty-seven strategies for teaching contraception to adolescents. J. Sch. Health, *50*:18–21, 1980.

136. Kirby, D.: The effects of school sex education programs: A review of the literature. J. Sch. Health, *50*:559–563, 1980.

137. Timberlake, B., Fox, R. A., Baisch, M. J., and Goldberg, B. D.: Prenatal education for pregnant adolescents. J. Sch. Health, *57*:105–108, 1987.

138. Price, J. H., Desmond, S., and Kukulka, G.: High school students' perceptions and misperceptions of AIDS. J. Sch. Health, *55*:107–109, 1985.

139. Fulton, G. B., Metress, E., and Price, J. H.: AIDS: Resource materials for school personnel. J. Sch. Health, *57*:1987.

140. Nash, D. A.: Professional ethics and esthetic dentistry. J. Am. Dent. Assoc., *117*:7E–9E, 1988.

141. Weinstein, A. R.: Anterior composite resins and veneers: Treatment planning, preparation, and finishing. J. Am. Dent. Assoc., *117*:38E–45E, 1988.

142. Christensen, G. J.: Tooth-colored inlays and onlays. J. Am. Dent. Assoc., *117*:12E–17E, 1988.

143. Saunders, J. F.: More than just pretty. R.D.H., 7:29, 38–39, 45, 1987.

144. Leinfelder, K. F., Isenberg, B. P., and Essig, H. E.: A new method for generating ceramic restorations: A CAD-CAM system. J. Am. Dent. Assoc., *118*:703–707, 1989.

145. Feinman, R. A., Goldstein, R. E., and Garber, D. A.: Bleaching Teeth. Chicago, Quintessence, 1987.

146. Sheets, C. G.: A conservative technique for treating discolored teeth. Dent. Tmwk., 2:168–170, 1989.

147. Haywood, V. B., and Heymann, H. O.: Nightguard vital bleaching. Quintessence International, *20*:173–176, 1989.

148. Clinical Research Associates: Tooth bleaching, home-use products. Newsletter, *13*, July, Dec., 1989.

149. Everett, M. S.: Mouth protectors. Dent. Hyg., 56:27–33, 1982.

150. Turner, C. H.: Mouth protectors. Brit. Dent. J., *143*:3, 1977.

151. Going, R. E., et al.: Mouthguard materials: Their physical and mechanical properties. J. Am. Dent. Assoc., 89:132–138, 1974.

152. Garon, M. W., Merkle, A., and Wright, J. T.: Mouth protectors and oral trauma: A study of adolescent football players. J. Am. Dent. Assoc., *112*:663–665, 1986.

153. Ianni, F. A.: Providing a structure for adolescent development. Phi Delta Kappan, *70*:673–682, 1989.

154. O'Rourke, T., Smith, B. J., and Nolte, A. E.: Health risk attitudes, beliefs and behaviors of students grades 7–12. J. Sch. Health, *54*:210–214, 1984.

155. Lawrence, L., and McLeroy, K. R.: Self-efficacy and health education. J. Sch. Health, *56*:317–321, 1986.

Chapter 7

DENTAL HEALTH IN ADULTS

*Considering the increased perplexities of life, the
fragmentary nature of our knowledge, the
accidentalness of adult existence, the
unavoidable errors we make, the situation of the
adult is by no means as different from that of
the child as it is generally assumed. Every adult
is in need of help, of warmth, of protection, in
many ways differing and yet in many ways
similar to the needs of the child.*

Erich Fromm
The Sane Society

OROFACIAL DEVELOPMENT

The adult facial skeleton is approximately
twice as large as the skeletal dimensions of
the newborn's face; whereas the cranium of
the adult differs in size by only 50%.[1,2] By
adulthood (≥age 18 years), all of the permanent teeth have fully completed their
formation except for the roots of the third
molars, which usually finalize their development by age 25 years.[1]

THE ADULT DENTAL PATIENT

"Adults" are rarely discussed in the literature as a particular group with specific
dental health care needs. Instead, this age
group of 18 or 21 to 64 years is considered
the general population. Statistics on caries
or periodontal disease for example, often
generalize their findings over some 46 years

of man's existence. This chapter attempts to
identify dental health concerns typical to
adults at certain periods of time during the
adult life span and elaborate on them.

Dental Fear

As discussed in Chapter 3, low finances
is one of the major reasons people do not
seek routine dental treatment.[3] In addition,
however, approximately 8 to 15% of the
adult population admit avoiding dental care
because of feelings of extreme anxiety. Surveys also indicate that nearly half of the
American people report fear of dentistry at
varying levels.[4,5] There are three main fears:
fear of pain, fear of loss of control, and fear
of dismemberment or destruction. Patients
who experience dental fear and avoidance
are commonly those who have had negative
or unpleasant dental experiences in the
past. Fear can also be engendered by accounts of the unfortunate dental experiences of others and by media parodies of
dental care.[6] The distorted depictions of

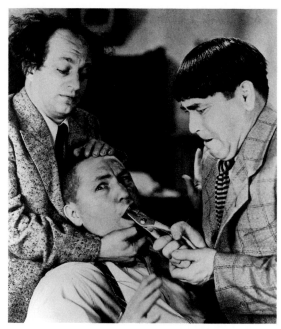

Figure 7-1. Comedic portrayal of fear as it relates to dentistry. Copyright 1990 Norman Mauer Productions, Inc. Columbia Pictures Industries, Inc. All Rights Reserved. The Three Stooges is a trademark of Norman Mauer Productions, Inc.

pain and fear in dentistry by W. C. Fields and the Three Stooges (Fig. 7-1) are classic examples.

ABNORMAL BEHAVIOR PATTERNS

Seven types of psychosomatic tendencies can be manifested by the fearful patient:

1. *Anxiety* involves varying degrees of apprehension. The severely anxious patient feels vulnerable to bodily danger and might require sedation. The moderately anxious patient needs constant reassurance by being informed of the dental procedure(s) each step of the way. The mildly anxious patient is relatively calm and denies fearful episodes during previous dental appointments. Keep this patient informed.
2. *Chronic complaining* is usually a manifestation of the elderly or the denture patient. A sympathetic but firm approach is required to help the patient accept what cannot be changed.
3. *Uncontrolled behavior or hysteria* is a learned response to a fearful situation. A firm, sympathetic approach can help to ease the patient's stress, but the patient rarely relaxes. Appointments should be short and premedication might be necessary.
4. *Obsessiveness* is a characteristic of the patient who questions every facet of treatment. This individual tries to cover his insecurities by acting as though he knows it all. He is usually a difficult patient.
5. *Paranoia* is exhibited by suspicion. The patient continually requires reassurance during treatment because he is sure that there is a problem with his treatment. The dental health educator must be calm and reassuring.
6. *Compulsive behavior* can be noted in patients who engage in exaggeratedly meticulous plaque removal. Many of these individuals are also compulsive handwashers. Meticulous cleaning habits satisfy an urge to rid the body of unclean thoughts or actions. Compulsive toothbrushers often feel plaque removal is all that is necessary to maintain their teeth.
7. *Self-pity* is typified by the individual who focuses on his own insecurities. Pathetic statements (e.g., "I doubt you can fix my teeth, they're so ugly," or "My teeth are decayed because I've inherited soft teeth; I care for my teeth the best I can") are common. Patience, kindness, and firmness are helpful but will not cure the patient.[7]

TREATMENT METHODS

A variety of behavioral methods have been developed to help fearful patients overcome their anxiety. The objective of these coping mechanisms is to modify (1) how threatening the patient perceives the dental appointment or (2) how incapable the patient feels he is to manage an anxiety-producing situation, e.g., a visit to the dentist. Behavioral coping techniques include iatrosedation, relaxation, desensitization, imagery, cognitive restructuring, biofeedback, hypnosis, electroanesthesia, acupuncture, and acupressure.

Iatrosedation. The dental health educator and the patient meet in a nonclinical environment to discuss the patient's fears.

Relaxation Techniques. Muscular and mental relaxation procedures are designed to help the patient manage his anxiety. Progressive relaxation involves alternating the contraction and relaxation of various muscle groups from the head to the feet to release tension. Relaxation response links relaxation to the reciting of a key word such as "one," to alleviate any mental distractions. The practitioner or the voice on the tape conducting the relaxation exercises should be slow, consistent, and low-pitched.

Systematic Desensitization. Each step of an anxiety-provoking situation is replaced with relaxation. The patient is first taught to subdivide the stressful event into a series of scenes leading from the least to the most fearful, e.g., making a dental appointment on the telephone, driving to the dental office, sitting in the waiting room, getting into the operatory chair, and receiving a dental anesthetic. When a patient can imagine the first scene without experiencing anxiety, he is allowed to visualize the next scene. If unthreatened, he progresses toward the high-fear end of the hierarchy until he can review the entire series of events without experiencing anxiety or fear.

Imagery. A self-control technique is recommended that evokes pleasant thoughts that are incompatible with those of fear or anxiety, e.g., imagining a moon-drenched beach enhanced by the echoing of sleek, gentle waves and the warmth of a midnight breeze.

Cognitive Restructuring. Cognitive self-control techniques are designed to change a patient's beliefs about the who, what, when, where or whys that influence his fears. What one says to oneself about an event guides how he behaves or reacts. For instance, an impacted, dilacerated tooth requires a hemi-section during an extraction. The procedure requires additional time and discomfort to the patient. The patient responds, "I knew I shouldn't have had this done, I knew it would hurt. I'll never go back to the dentist again." Therapeutic self-statement modification restructures the patient's thoughts concerning the event. He perceives the procedure as more difficult than the norm, but he is glad that he had the oral surgery to prevent future complications from occurring.

Biofeedback. Through the use of special monitoring equipment, persons are taught to identify internal cues for anxiety, such as a rise in blood pressure. Once the patient is aware of his physiologic response to stressful stimuli, he can control it through relaxation.[8]

Hypnosis. A trance-like mental state is induced through verbal suggestion in order to manage pain and anxiety. Hypnosis is often used with systematic desensitization.

Electroanesthesia. Local anesthesia is produced by an electric current. The method is relatively painless.

Acupuncture and Acupressure. Pain relief can be achieved by the insertion of needles or application of pressure to certain areas of the body.

Pharmacologic methods permit provision of dental care with minimal patient-management effort, but they do not address patient fear. Methods such as the combination of local anesthesia and nitrous oxide permit treatment of patients with moderate dental fear by blocking pain while only slightly depressing the patient's level of consciousness. Deep sedation involves a depressed consciousness and prevents the patient from responding to verbal instructions. General anesthesia, which creates a total loss of consciousness, must be used for the dental phobic with extensive dental needs. Unfortunately, because these methods block the fear (by removing the patient's control) they also block learning. The most successful long-term therapies for dental fear have been derived from the behavioral approach.[8]

Although fear is a multifaceted problem, it is most successfully managed with one tool, communication. The dental health educator should call a patient by name to put him at ease and allow him some control by giving him the option to raise his hand if he experiences discomfort. It is advisable to observe a patient's nonverbal cues such as movements or facial expressions and talk to him about his fears if he is willng. If he withdraws, the educator should not push him; letting him maintain his control is essential.[9,10] The dental health educator should avoid (1) unnecessary use of words with negative connotations such as pain or shot; (2) technical language which might confuse a patient or make him anxious; and (3) misleading assurances that a procedure is painless when in fact the patient will experience pain. Being truthful with a patient enhances trust and reduces fear and anxiety.[11]

Certain aspects of the dental environment trigger fears, e.g., the smell of alcohol or rubber base materials, the sound of the high-speed handpiece, the feel of the rubber cup during polishing, the taste of a topical anesthetic, the sight of needles or blood. Whatever the source of fear, if the dental health educator is aware of it, certain measures or precautions can be taken to minimize the stimuli that elicit the fear response.[9,10] Research indicates that dentist behaviors that significantly reduce a patient's anxiety are dedication to the prevention of pain, friendliness, ability to work quickly, calmness, and the provision of moral support.[12]

Several medical centers, hospitals and universities across the country have established clinics to treat the fearful dental patient. Some of the more prominent dental anxiety clinics are listed in Appendix E.[5]

Periodontal Disease

The incidence of periodontal disease increases with age as a result of the cumulative effects of various causal factors. The American Academy of Periodontology classifies adult periodontitis into four major categories:[13]

1. *Slight*—gingival inflammation has progressed into the deeper periodontal structures and alveolar bone crest, with slight bone loss. The usual periodontal probing depth is 3 to 4 mm.

2. *Moderate*—a more advanced state displaying increased destruction of the periodontal structures and noticeable loss of bone support, possibly accompanied by an increase in tooth mobility. There might be furcation involvement in multirooted teeth.

3. *Advanced*—further progression of periodontitis with major loss of alveolar bone support, usually accompanied by increased tooth mobility. Furcation involvement in multirooted teeth is likely.

4. *Rapidly progressive*—includes several unclassified types of periodontitis characterized either by rapid bone and attachment loss, or slow but continuous bone and attachment loss, and resistance to normal therapy. It is usually associated with gingival inflammation and continued pocket formation.

Although bacterial plaque is the major causal factor in gingival inflammation and subsequent periodontal disease, several other contributing and predisposing factors increase the adult's likelihood of developing infections of the oral soft tissue. Poor oral hygiene, particularly in areas of malalignment or around rough, poorly contoured restorations, can cause plaque to accumulate. Xerostomia produced by certain drugs, diseases, or treatments decreases oral lubrication, self-cleaning, immunity, pH, and remineralization as well as affecting speech, taste, and digestion. The patient with a reduction in salivary flow is therefore more prone to developing periodontal disease and dental caries. Reliance on a soft diet, which results in disuse of the periodontium, and oral habits that overstimulate the periodontium in a localized area are both detrimental to these structures. Periodontal manifestations can also be initiated or complicated by systemic disease (e.g., diabetes), drug therapy (e.g., dilantin), and hormonal disturbances (e.g., pregnancy, menopause).[14]

Hormonal Influences. Throughout a woman's adult life, estrogen levels undergo numerous peaks and valleys. The menstrual cycle, pregnancy, and menopause are the three major phases responsible for these fluctuations. Normal estrogen and progesterone levels change significantly during gestation. These hormonal changes have been shown to produce an exaggerated gingival response when associated with local irritants such as plaque. Because women taking oral contraceptives experience similar hormonal alterations that mimic pregnancy, they can also exhibit a "drug-induced pregnancy gingivitis" in response to bacteria.[15]

The dental health educator must apprise the patient taking oral contraceptives of their potential for altering the oral tissue. A study performed by Knight and Wade concluded that a "small but significant" loss of attachment was experienced by oral contraceptive users.[16] This slight increase in pocket depth was reported in individuals taking oral contraceptives longer than 18 months. Similar increases in gingival crevicular flow were also found in women taking "the pill." These increases were significant only during the first 6 months of oral contraceptive use.[17] Other oral findings associated with use of the pill include a 30% increase in xerostomia,[17] radiopacities of mandibular bone,[18] gingival pigmentation in women with light complexions,[19] and an increased incidence of localized osteitis or dry socket following mandibular third-molar extractions.[20] Patients taking oral contraceptives should be advised to practice meticulous oral hygiene and use additional methods of contraception when concurrent antibiotic premedication or therapy is prescribed. Patients should also be made aware of the contraindications for oral contraceptive use such as smoking, impaired liver function, and history of breast carcinoma or thrombophlebitis.[14]

Menstruation usually ceases between the ages of 42 and 55 years; the cessation is referred to as menopause. As ovarian function declines, estrogen secretion diminishes. Many women require estrogen replacement therapy to counteract the changes the body may undergo such as hot flashes, body sweats, headaches, heart palpitations, and sleeplessness.[14] Virtually no research has been conducted to assess the effect of estrogen replacement therapy on the periodontium. It is hypothesized that periodontal changes in response to plaque occur in postmenopausal women receiving estrogen replacement therapy similar to those experienced by women taking oral contraceptives.

Hypersensitive Teeth

Many adult patients complain of tooth sensitivity, particularly in the cervical area, during instrumentation or the application of air. Cervical hypersensitivity is frequently related to the accumulation of plaque in areas where cementum and dentin remain exposed. Such exposure can be due to gingival recession resulting from age, periodontal disease (pathologic), trauma (toothbrush abrasion), or surgery (apically repositioned flap); anatomic exposure of dentin at the cementoenamel junction; or loss of enamel or cementum from wear, abrasion, or dental caries.

In order to alleviate a patient's discomfort from mechanical stimuli (toothbrushing, instrumentation), chemical stimuli (plaque, acidic foods), or thermal stimuli (hot or cold food, beverages, air), certain guidelines must be followed. The patient should be taught flossing and a correct toothbrushing method with a soft brush to thoroughly remove plaque from exposed cervical areas. Specific acidic or sour foods that cause sensitivity should be avoided. Office desensitization procedures should be considered, which include the application of sodium or stannous fluoride desensitizing pastes, iontophoresis, calcium hydroxide, and bonding adhesives and resins.[14] Numerous patient-applied commercial desensitizing pastes are also available; they must be used daily for at least 4 weeks before a noticeable improvement is achieved.

Radiographic Assessment

Approximately 90% of the United States population admits to some type of radiographic examination each year. Dental offices are potentially responsible for a large portion of the public's exposure to radiation because over half of all radiographic equipment is located in dental offices and clinics.[21]

Patient protection is of primary importance. American Dental Asociation exposure recommendations state that

Radiation for diagnostic purposes should be kept to a minimum and should be used only after careful consideration of the dental and general health of the patient. Radiographic examinations should not be an automatic part of every dental exam. Professional judgment rather than a time interval should determine the frequency and extent of each radiographic exam.[22]

Initially, a complete radiographic survey is requested of asymptomatic patients to obtain baseline information for analyzing future changes. When symptoms present, additional radiographs, usually periapicals, can be taken. Bitewing radiographs should be taken routinely to assess interproximal and subgingival conditions that cannot be seen clinically.

Reducing the frequency of radiation exposure is not the only means of protecting a patient from overexposure. Equipment and patient shielding and film and technique precautions are also required. All patients should wear a lead apron and thyroid collar during exposure to radiation. If these precautions are complied with universally, pregnant patients are at no greater risk than any other patient. Between uses, lead aprons should be hung to prevent damage to the lead material. Open-ended and lead-lined position-indicating devices or cones and collimation and filtration devices must be standard. High-speed, high-quality film also decreases the patient's exposure. After intraoral placement of the film, the cone should be positioned as close to the patient as possible. By decreasing the tube-to-film distance, one can virtually eliminate scatter radiation.[23]

Frequently adult patients express concern over radiographic exposure and technique. The dental health educator should be prepared to address patients' questions regarding risk and assure them of the protective measures designed to ensure their safety. Personalizing an explanation of the advantages of radiographs in delivering a diagnosis in each particular case is suggested. Prior to placing the film in the patient's mouth, the educator should instruct the patient in how the procedure is performed and how to breathe to avoid gagging. If some discomfort is expected due to the presence of exostoses or the small size of the patient's mouth, the film should be bent slightly and the patient should be reassured that the procedure will be brief. After film processing, the dental health educator should review the mounted films with the patient and include him in the treatment plan phase. Good rapport can be established if the dental health educator is skillful in his radiographic technique and displays concern over the patient's protection, comfort, and oral health needs.

PREVENTION OF DENTAL DISEASE

Oral Hygiene

As discussed in Chapter 2, the adult patient comes to the dental health educator with a growing reservoir of experiences that affect his ability to learn. The dental health educator must refer to the adult patient's educational, social, and psychological background when providing dental health instruction. Adults tend to resist learning that is incongruent with their self-concept as responsible, autonomous individuals capable of making their own decisions. It is therefore imperative that emphasis be placed on the knowledge, skill, and responsibility required to perform and self-evaluate oral hygiene practices. The oral physiotherapy aids recommended must be readily available to the patient to minimize frustration. Self-evaluation devices such as disclosing agents and diet diaries must also be easily obtainable. Adults must be encouraged to participate in the dental health process by reviewing radiographs with the dental health educator or observing the activity of their own plaque under a phase microscope. Oral health care tasks designed through the co-operative efforts of the educator and patient are clearer and more meaningful to the patient, and it is more likely that oral hygiene goals will be attained.[24,25]

Care of Prostheses

Fixed partial dentures are prostheses cemented in position to replace one or more natural teeth; They are also referred to as fixed bridges. A pontic or an artificial tooth crown restores the function of a previously lost tooth and is supported or anchored in place by an abutment tooth. The fixed bridge can improve occlusion and prevent drifting of adjacent teeth or supereruption of opposing teeth. To appear esthetic, each pontic must resemble an individual tooth that looks as though it is erupting from the gingiva.[26]

Fixed partial prostheses are relatively easy to clean if the patient has been instructed properly and given the proper equipment. Flushing debris from beneath the pontics and around the abutments with an oral irrigator can be helpful. Actual plaque removal requires sulcular brushing and a floss threader to cleanse the proximal surfaces of abutment teeth and the gingival surface of pontics[14] (Fig. 7-2).

Removable partial dentures are prostheses that can be removed at will and serve to replace one or more (but not all) natural teeth. Hygiene procedures involve maintaining the prosthesis, the abutment teeth and surrounding gingiva, and the mucosa of edentulous areas. Procedures for cleansing are similar to those required for various other dental prostheses, but special attention must be paid to the metallic parts. Rinsing after meals, immersion in denture cleaners overnight or for several hours daily to remove stains and debris while allowing the tissues to rest, and brushing to remove bacterial plaque are recommended. A specially designed clasp brush should be adapted to the inner surfaces of clasps to remove plaque and protect the supporting teeth from bacterial exposure[14] (Fig. 7-3).

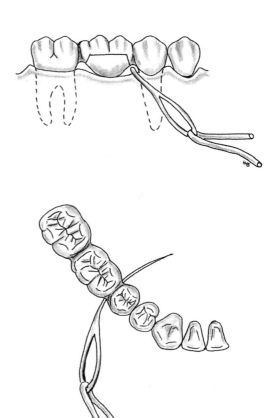

Figure 7-2. Use of a floss threader to slide floss under pontics and against the sides of abutment teeth to remove bacterial plaque. Redrawn by H.J. Bianco, Jr., D.D.S., M.S., West Virginia University, from Wilkins, E.M.: Clinical Practice of the Dental Hygienist. 6th Ed. Philadelphia, Lea & Febiger, 1989.

The edentulous areas should be gently brushed and circulation stimulated by the use of frequent digital massage. Abutment teeth and other remaining natural teeth require meticulous plaque-control measures. Healthy supporting teeth ensure the longevity of the appliance, and a clean appliance promotes oral health.[14]

Implants and Their Maintenance

An implant consists of a metallic anchor (usually titanium) surgically inserted or

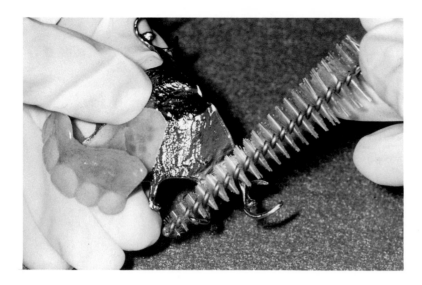

Figure 7-3. Clasp brush designed to remove bacterial plaque from the inside surfaces of clasps. The prosthesis should be held carefully over a soft surface to avoid accidental breakage.

grafted into intact tissue to support an abutment with a porcelain replacement tooth or an overdenture.[26] There are three basic types of implants, subperiosteal, transosteal, and endosseous.[27-29] *Subperiosteal* implants are placed beneath the gingiva and periosteum but over the bone itself. These thin frame-shape devices are best suited for the patient with an atrophied mandible who is unable to tolerate a conventional denture. Subperiosteal implants in the maxilla have been met with varying degrees of success (Fig. 7-4). *Transosteal* implants are placed through the bone from the inferior border to the alveolar crest. These staple-type implants are indicated for the edentulous mandible with a minimal alveolar ridge height of 8 to 9 mm (Fig. 7-5). *Endosseous* or osseointegrated implants are inserted into the bone and require proliferation of bone up to or into the implant for anchorage similar to that of natural teeth. Endosseous implants consist of three types: blade, ramus frame, and cylinder. Blades are used with natural teeth to support fixed partial prostheses or complete prostheses retained by a metal superstructure (Fig. 7-6). Ramus frames support complete dentures (Fig. 7-7). Cylinder implants provide more versatility in that a series of two or more implants can support the replacement of a complete prosthesis, one or more implants with natural teeth can support a fixed restoration, and one cylinder

alone can serve as a single tooth replacement (Fig. 7-8).

Implant success depends on the technique of implant placement, the physical health of the patient, adequacy of alveolar bone support, and the absence of infection. Because the implant is surrounded by a soft tissue sulcus, microbial accumulation can cause inflammation just as gingivitis develops around natural teeth exposed to plaque. Long-term inflammation can result in reduction of marginal bone height, compromising the support of the implant. Meticulous oral hygiene is the key to securing the longevity of the implant. Patients should be instructed about the design and function of their implant and must actively participate in the oral hygiene procedures necessary prior to, during, and after placement of the prosthesis.[14,26,29]

A home care kit developed for Branemark System users consists of a soft toothbrush, flat and tapered endtufted toothbrushes, proxabrushes, dental mirrors, disclosing tablets, dental floss, and an instruction booklet (Fig. 7-9).[30] Some practitioners recommend oral irrigators, an electric toothbrush, a rubber interdental stimulator, Super Floss, and mouthrinses such as Listerine or Peridex.[31-38] Whatever aids patients use, care must be taken to use them correctly and avoid implements (e.g., pipe cleaners) or dentifrices that contain hy-

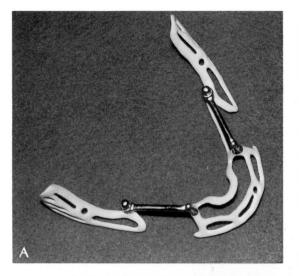

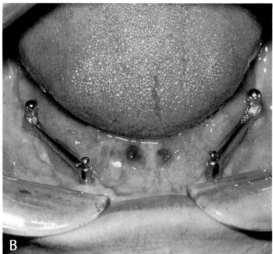

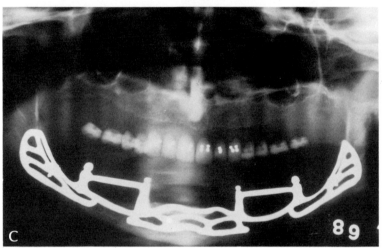

Figure 7-4. *A.* Mandibular subperiosteal implant. *B.* A clinical view. *C.* A radiographic view. Courtesy of H.J. Bianco, Jr., D.D.S., M.S., West Virginia University.

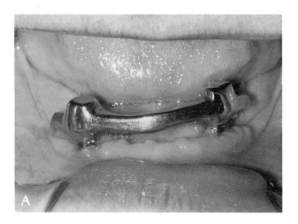

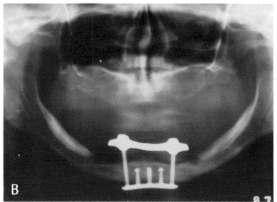

Figure 7-5. *A.* Mandibular transosteal (staple type) implant as it appears clinically; *B.* Radiographic view of the staple implant. Courtesy of H.J. Bianco, Jr., D.D.S., M.S., West Virginia University.

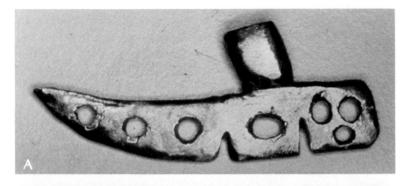

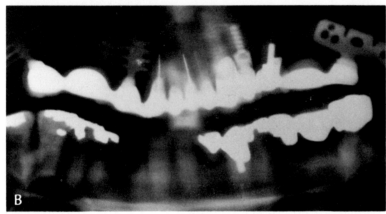

Figure 7-6. *A.* The blade— a type of endosseous implant. *B.* Radiographic view of two types of blade implants on the maxilla used to support the fixed partial prostheses pictured. Courtesy of H.J. Bianco, Jr., D.D.S., M.S., West Virginia University.

drated silica or other abrasives, which can scratch or mar the titanium. Directing the oral irrigator into the sulcus and excessive water pressure can cause bacteremia and can damage the junctional epithelium.[39] The implant patient should avoid chewing on ice or hard candy.

In addition to home care procedures a routine oral prophylaxis is recommended. Plastic instruments, although bulky and better suited for supragingival instrumentation, have been designed to remove calcarious deposits without scratching the titanium-coated implant[40] (Fig. 7-10).[30] Calculus is removed by placing the blade apical to the deposit and using a rapid flicking motion.[38] The 1989 Proceedings of the World Workshop in Clinical Periodontics recommended the manufacture of a Teflon or thinner plastic curette that could be used subgingivally without changing the surface topography of the implant. Removal of plaque, stain, and materia alba is best accomplished by toothbrushing, rubber-cup polishing with tin

oxide,[29] or the use of an air-powder abrasive system (Prophy-jet) at the lowest setting.[38] Use of the Prophy-jet is prohibited for contact lens wearers and persons with respiratory disorders or hypertension.[41] Ultrasonic cleaning is contraindicated because it can scratch the implant and dislodge it from the alveolar bone.[29]

Assessment is an important component of implant maintenance. The periodontium surrounding the implant should be evaluated for gingival deviations in color, consistency, and spontaneous bleeding and for bony status as exhibited by a radiographic examination. Healthy, stable implants possess a normal trabecular bone pattern that remains in close contact with the implant surface. Mobile implants do not display this contact, and a radiolucency is seen surrounding the implant.[29] For the first year after implant placement, radiographs should be taken every 3 months; they should be taken once yearly thereafter.[42,43]

Periodontal probing of implants is not es-

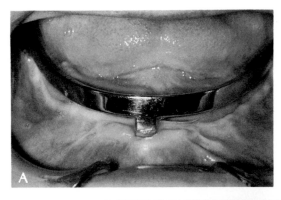

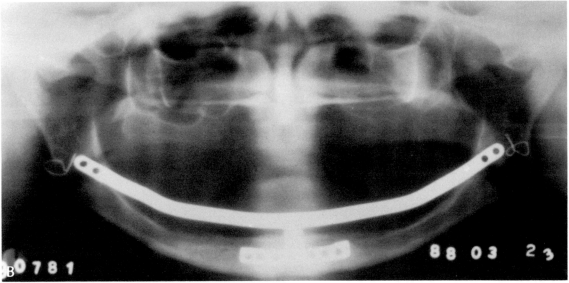

Figure 7-7. *A.* The ramus frame, a type of endosseous implant, as it appears clinically; *B.* Radiographic view of the ramus frame. Courtesy of H.J. Bianco, Jr., D.D.S., M.S., West Virginia University.

sential because necessary information regarding bone height should be ascertained at regular intervals with radiographs. If probing is incorporated into the tissue assessment, a plastic probe should be used (Pro-Dentec Perio-Probe). Only light pressure should be exerted to prevent penetration of the fragile epithelial attachment. Such penetration could result in damage to the bone/implant attachment, and bacteria could be introduced into the epithelium.[44,45] If the patient is experiencing pain with a hollow sensation, looseness of the implant can be further confirmed. If percolation (bubbles along the gingival line of the implant) occurs on application of pressure on the occlusal surface of the prosthesis, loose or fractured screws, abutments, or fixtures are the cause. If left untreated, a loose superstructure can lead to eventual failure of the total implant.[37]

Fluoride and Dental Caries

Fluorides, particularly in the drinking water, are the primary reason that dental caries claims fewer teeth among the young. When a person resides in a fluoridated community throughout life, the benefits continue.[14,46] Unlike its systemic effect in children, fluoridated water has its major effect locally in the adult by diffusing through the minute spaces between enamel crystals. In a 1951 study, adults aged 20 to 44 years living in fluoridated Colorado Springs exhibited 60% less caries experience than adults in Boulder, where fluoride was not made

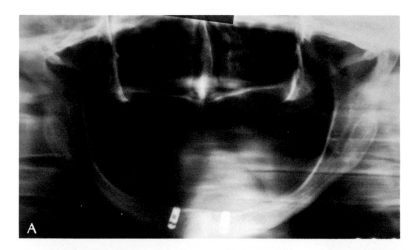

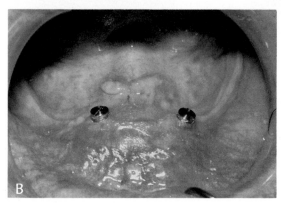

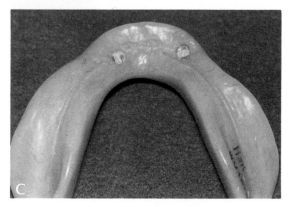

Figure 7-8. Implants. *A.* The cylinder, a type of endosseous implant, as it appears radiographically; *B.* Two cylinder implants are magnetized to support a complete prosthesis as shown in *C.* Implants (cont.).

available. In fluoride-deficient Boulder, adults had three to four times as many permanent teeth extracted due to caries.[47] Comparisons between fluoridated and nonfluoridated areas are less dramatic today; caries reductions range from 17 to 38%. The smaller difference between areas can be explained by patient use of multiple fluoride therapies, e.g., dentifrices, rinses, supplements, and home care gels in fluoride-deficient communities.

Because people now keep their teeth longer, more emphasis must be placed on prevention of periodontal disease and control of the more vulnerable tooth surfaces. Usually beginning at age 50, there is a marked increase in root caries where gingival recession has taken place.[48] Stamm and Banting found a lower rate of root caries in communities that were fluoridated.[49] Advanced research, both in vivo and in vitro, has shown that teeth with root caries can be remineralized with fluoride.[50-52] Certainly

the routine application of an office fluoride treatment and a daily fluoride rinse are advisable. Adult patients are also prime candidates for recurrent or secondary caries at the margins of restorations and would benefit from these various forms of topical fluoride delivery. Fluoride in variable doses has also been prescribed therapeutically for the treatment of osteoporosis.[53]

Nutrition

The United States Food and Drug Administration recognizes five food groups based on their nutritional content: fruit and vegetable; bread and cereal; dairy; meat, poultry, fish, and beans; and fats, sweets, and alcohol. It is recommended that adults consume four servings each from the fruit-and-vegetable and bread-and-cereal groups and two servings each from the dairy and

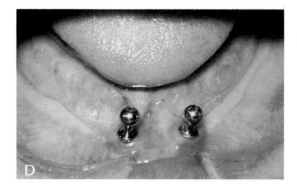
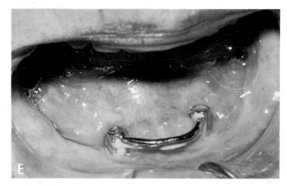

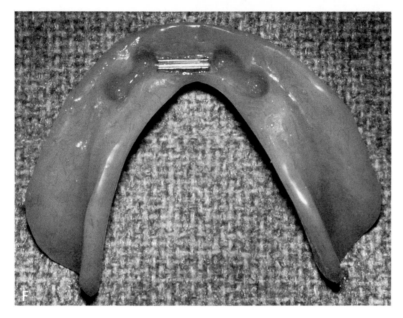

Figure 7-8. *D.* Ball cylinders also improve denture fit and retention. *E.* Two cylinders can be used to support a bar (note the calculus on the right implant). *F.* The prosthesis is fabricated with a clip that attaches to the bar for retention. Courtesy of H.J. Bianco, Jr., D.D.S., M.S., West Virginia University.

meat groups. If foods from these food groups are eaten in the amounts indicated, intake will be approximately 1200 calories, with adequate proteins, vitamins, and minerals. No servings are recommended for the fifth group; this group is highly caloric and has no nutritional value. Although most adults need at least 1200 calories daily, physical activity requires an additional supply of calories for energy. Pregnant, lactating, and premenopausal women must also receive iron beyond that which is supplied by the four food groups.[54]

FOOD LABELING

The labeling of foods enables the consumer to make informed choices about the nutrient content of foods and the ingredients in a product. The ingredients found in highest concentrations are listed first. Net weight and the name and location of the manufacturer are also listed on the label. Such information allows a consumer to compare different brands of the same product for nutritional value and cost per weight, count calories, and select foods for special restrictive diets such a low-sodium, low-cholesterol, or no-sugar.[54]

A dental health educator providing nutritional instruction to a patient must teach the individual how to read labels. Even if the patient's problem relates solely to a reduction in fermentable carbohydrates, the general nutritional knowledge gained by the patient can be transferred to meet the needs of his family also. Diet counseling in caries prevention generally deals with sucrose

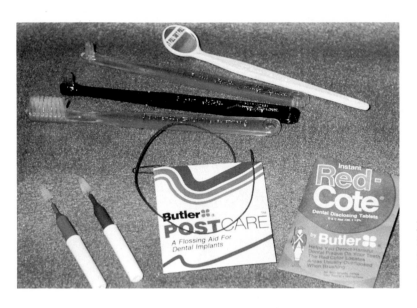

Figure 7-9. A home care kit for implant maintenance. Courtesy of Nobelpharma USA, Inc.: Chicago, Nobel Industries Sweden.

(table sugar) because of its high concentration in foods referred to as sweets. Nevertheless, the dental health educator must teach the patient to recognize other forms of sugar that are also cariogenic. A 1983 survey conducted by Good Housekeeping and the Food and Drug Law Institute found that consumers depended heavily on food labels to avoid certain ingredients such as sugar.[55] Yet another consumer study indicated that 32% of the surveyed felt honey was not a sugar and that 16% believed the same of molasses.[56] These findings suggest that though the public might read labels, they are basically uninformed about the different types of sugars, e.g., dextrose, sucrose, lactose,

and fructose.[56] Many people believe that sugars from natural sources and brown sugar are healthful alternatives.

The dental health educator must remember that the total sugar content of a foodstuff is not the major factor in determining cariogenicity. Although sucrose is usually considered the major offender, it has about the same caries-producing activity as fructose and glucose. The cariogenicity of foodstuffs is primarily influenced by (1) the physical nature of the sugar when ingested (retentive vs. nonretentive), (2) the rate of clearance of the sugar from the oral cavity (sticky foods have a slower oral clearance), and (3) the sugar concentration of the food. Concentra-

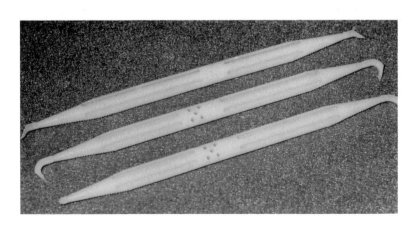

Figure 7-10. Plastic instruments developed to scale calculus that has adhered to the implant without scratching the implant surface itself. Courtesy of Nobelpharma USA, Inc.: Chicago, Nobel Industries Sweden.

tion is the ratio of sugar mass to total mass of the food. An apple with a sugar content of 16 grams is less cariogenic than a serving (approximately 28 g) of a sugar-coated cereal with a sugar content of 17 g. The apple has about the same sugar content as the cereal, but because of the high water content of the apple, its sugar concentration is only 11%—too weak to penetrate plaque. Conversely, the sugar concentration in the frosted cereal is approximately 57%;[54] a high enough concentration that when the cereal contacts the plaque, the plaque pH drops below 5.5, and tooth demineralization occurs.

FOOD PREPARATION

Adults responsible for food preparation either at home or as employees should be familiar with the nutrient loss associated with cleaning, cutting, and cooking foods. The outer leaves and skin of many fruits and vegetables are rich in nutrients. Cleaning and soaking these foods results in a loss of water-soluble vitamins. This loss is compounded when fruits and vegetables are chopped or sliced. Cutting causes some nutrients to become unstable so it is necessary to eat the food immediately, or freeze or refrigerate it to preserve its nutritional value and prevent spoilage.[54]

Both the type of cooking method and the vessel used are significant factors related to nutrient loss. When one boils food, water should barely cover the food, the vessel should be covered and should not be copper. Baking soda to preserve the green color of vegetables should not be added. Pressure cooking retains nutrients almost twice as well as boiling at atmospheric pressure. Nutrients are also removed less readily by steaming than by boiling. Because vegetable-cooking water becomes a reservoir for nutrients, the water should be saved and used as stock.

Baking foods in a conventional oven destroys heat-sensitive nutrients. In frying, nutrient loss is proportional to time. Microwaving is probably the ideal method for preserving vitamins and minerals because of the short cooking time and the minimal use of water.[54]

OTHER ADULT HEALTH CONCERNS

Alcoholism

In Chapter 6, adolescent alcohol use and abuse are discussed. The prevalence of alcoholism—a chronic dependency on alcohol—is greater for adults than for adolescents. Several social factors are probably related to this phenomenon. For example, Public Law 98-363, signed into law in July 1984, adopted 21 years of age as the uniform drinking age.[57] No questions are asked of a legal adult; drinking is acceptable. Social and business obligations and the increasing pressures of adult life might actually induce an alcoholic dependency. The National Drug and Alcoholism Treatment Utilization Survey of 1982 found approximately 300,000 clients in treatment for alcoholism; 95% were over 18 years of age, 78% were male, and 71% were white.[58]

Drinkers are labeled according to frequency of alcohol ingestion and amount ingested, from social drinkers and moderate and heavy drinkers to those dependent on alcohol. It is believed that approximately 10% of the U.S. population is addicted to alcohol. Over 90% of alcoholics are employed; over half of these individuals hold managerial or professional positions. Unfortunately, many of these individuals are members of the dental profession. Annually, alcoholism costs American society $117 billion in lost production, medical expenditures, and hospitalization.[59]

SYMPTOMS

Although alcoholic patients are not always recognizable as such, it is important for the dental health educator to be aware of signs which may be indicative of a patient with alcoholism. Symptoms and signs and conditions related to alcoholism include:

1. Physiologic—hypertension, cirrhosis of the liver, esophageal varicies, nutritional deficiencies, leukopenia, frequent urination (over six times daily), frequent thirst for water, sexual and reproductive dysfunction, blackouts (temporary amnesia) while drinking, and dementia. Oral complications can involve poor oral hygiene and severe gingival inflammation. If jaundiced, the gingiva can appear yellowish-brown. The tongue might be shiny and red, and the patient might exhibit angular cheilosis and swollen glands.[14,59]
2. Psychological—an obsessive desire to drink surpasses all other concerns. The patient often denies he has a drinking problem and views alcohol as a "friend."[59]
3. Behavioral—the patient is fearful, anxious, and combative when confronted about his drinking problem; he might make loud and lascivious advances to mere acquaintances or strangers; he might have difficulties with close personal relationships; and he might have a record of arrest(s) for drunk driving (often accident-related), absenteeism, and poor job performance.[14,58]

The alcoholic patient is often difficult to anesthetize. The onset, penetration, and the duration of the anesthetic can be diminished because of the patient's elevated blood alcohol level. Postoperative healing time is also increased due to the patient's lowered immunity and susceptibility to infection. General anesthesia is not recommended.[7]

INTERVENTION

When an alcoholic has tried to control his behavior alone and can't, he becomes depressed and vulnerable to intervention. The dental health educator can be instrumental in intervention for the heavy problem drinker by directing him to seek professional help. A private consultation is advised, in which the dental health educator suggests to the patient that he believes a problem exists. When dependency is apparent, open confrontation in the dental office is usually not recommended. Most alcoholics will deny their addiction and become hostile. The dental health educator should contact family and other important persons in the patient's life and suggest that they meet with trained professionals and counselors to determine a method of intervention. Ignoring the signs and symptoms of alcohol dependence in a patient, friend, or loved one is often easier than confrontation, but the risk must be taken. Alcoholism is a disease that requires treatment.[59] Appendix F provides a list of chemical dependency organizations for the alcoholic and his significant others.[14]

Smoking

The percentage of adult smokers in the United States has declined since 1965, with the number of males who smoke decreasing from an estimated 53% in 1964 to less than 33% in 1985. The percentage of female adult smokers has decreased from 34% in 1965 to 28% in 1985,[60] but the mortality rate for lung cancer among women has increased. A male smoker aged 30 to 40 years who smokes an average of 2 packs of cigarettes per day loses an estimated 8 years of his life when compared to nonsmokers of the same age and sex.[61]

Cigarette smoking acts synergistically with excessive alcohol consumption to increase the incidence of oral and laryngeal cancer.[62] The numerous health risks associated with smoking are outlined in Chapter 6.

Oral Cancer

Oral cancer accounts for approximately 4% of all cancers in males and 2% in females. Over 90% of oral cancers occur in individuals over 40 years of age who both smoke heavily and consume large amounts of alcohol.[63] If oral carcinomas are detected early as localized lesions, survival rates are substantially higher. In addition to the stage

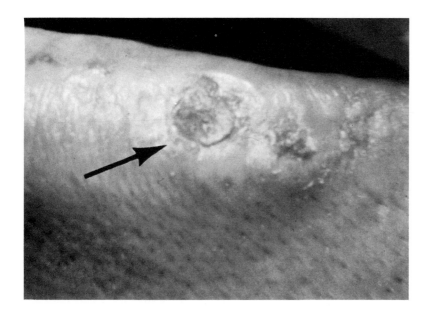

Figure 7-11. Squamous cell carcinoma of the lower lip. Courtesy of J.E. Bouquot, D.D.S., M.S., West Virginia University.

of the cancer at the time of diagnosis (as judged from its size, evidence of involved lymph nodes, and metastasis), the survival rate depends on the site or location of the cancer, the type or tissue origin of the cancer, and the treatment available.[64]

Survival rates are usually based on 5-year increments. The first 5 years is usually the most critical and is considered a major milestone for most oncology patients. Five-year survival refers to a patient who has gone 5 years without symptoms after treatment. The 5-year survival for carcinoma of the lip is about 84%, whereas pharyngeal carcinoma has a 5-year survival rate of only 22%.[63] This stands to reason, because a lesion on the lip is readily seen and usually diagnosed early (Fig. 7-11).

DESCRIPTION

Ninety percent of all malignant oral neoplasms are of the squamous cell or epidermoid type (Fig. 7-12). Generally, squamous cell carcinomas in the anterior segment of the mouth are well differentiated histologically, produce keratin, and grow slowly. More aggressive, immature tumors have a poorer prognosis. They affect posterior sites more predominantly, such as the posterior tongue or tonsils. The most frequent sites of occurrence for oral carcinomas are the lateral borders of the tongue and the floor of the mouth.[65] This cancer-prone area is often referred to as the "cancer trough" (Fig. 7-13).[64] Lesions most frequently observed in the oral cavity are usually white (leukoplakia), red (erythroplakia), or white with red areas within them (speckled leuko-

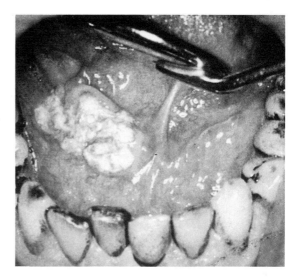

Figure 7-12. Squamous cell carcinoma of the floor of the mouth. Courtesy of J.E. Bouquot, D.D.S., M.S., West Virginia University.

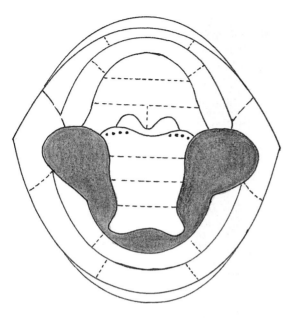

Figure 7-13. "Cancer trough" (shaded area) denotes the location of the majority of oral cancers. Redrawn by H.J. Bianco, Jr., D.D.S., M.S., West Virginia University, from American Cancer Society: Diagnosis of Oral Cancer. *In* Oral Cancer: Diagnosis, Treatment, and Rehabilitation, 1973.

plakia). Speckled leukoplakia has the greatest malignant potential.[66] Approximately one-third of oral cancers are flat, one-third are lobulated masses, and one-third present as ulcerations.

INTERVENTION

The dental health educator's role in early cancer detection is vital to saving lives. All anatomic intraoral and extraoral structures must be thoroughly examined using visual, radiographic, and tactile procedures.[67] One should first examine the patient visually, examining the head and neck for variations in color, texture, and symmetry and for abnormal masses or growths. A radiograph might be indicated. Palpating the head and neck area for abnormalities is an integral part of cancer assessment. The types of palpation include

1. Bimanual—tissue is pressed gently between the fingers of two hands, as is done for the floor of the mouth.

2. Bidigital—tissue is pressed and gently rolled between fingers of the same hand as is done with the gingiva, lips, tongue, buccal mucosa, thyroid, and cervical lymph nodes. The patient should turn his head to each side, making the sternocleidomastoid muscle on the opposite side of the neck more prominent for examination.

3. Bilateral—two hands are used simultaneously to examine the same structures on each side of the head and neck, as is done for the temporomandibular joint and the pre- and post-auricular nodes, for example (see Fig. 7-14).

Teaching the patient how to conduct his own oral cancer assessment is a valuable adjunct to the professional screening.[68] It has been reported that 85% of all oral carcinomas can be seen either directly or indirectly with a mirror.[69] A step-by-step oral cancer self-examination guide is shown in Figure 7-15.[70] This instructional model should be practiced at home. All that is required are two mirrors (mouth and vanity), good vanity and mouth lighting, and gauze or a washcloth. During the instruction phase, the patient should be shown pictures of normal and abnormal oral structures. Then, using the step-by-step format, he should be taught to explore his own mouth for inconsistencies. These procedures should be reviewed and reinforced during each recall oral screening. The patient should also be in-

EXTRAORAL PALPATION SITES

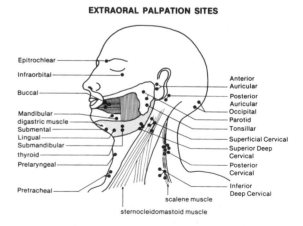

Figure 7-14. Lymph nodes of the head and neck.

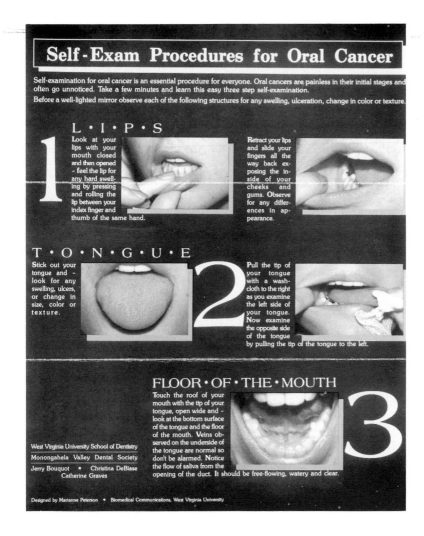

Figure 7-15. An instructional pamphlet for patients to reinforce self-examination procedures for oral cancer.

structed to contact his dentist or physician if he notes any unfamiliar or abnormal findings of the head or neck. Treatment modalities for cancer are discussed in Chapter 9.

Orthodontics

Adults currently receive 25 to 30% of all orthodontic treatment.[26] Because tooth movement slows with age, orthodontic rehabilitation usually takes longer for adults than for children.

The dental health educator must not take for granted that the adult orthodontic patient is familiar with the necessary oral care procedures. The patient should be taught about the significance of plaque around orthodontic appliances and teeth, the types of oral physiotherapy aids for cleaning around orthodontic appliances and their use, the components and importance of a multiple fluoride program and the techniques for administration, and the importance of frequent orthodontic, caries, and periodontal evaluations.[14]

Orthognathic Surgery

Orthognathic surgery, performed primarily on adults, might be required if a mandible or maxilla is too large or too small or a combination of these deviations exists. This hospital procedure entails repositioning the jaws and wiring them into proper alignment. Intraoral incisions are made so no facial scars are visible. Plastic materials can be used to augment the chin or cheek-bones. Orthodontics is required to reposition the teeth. The range of treatment is usually from 1 to 3 months, and the outcome is permanent. Although this surgery is relatively expensive, the dental health educator should advise a prospective candidate of the chances for improved speech, mastication, and esthetics.[26]

Temporary postoperative numbness, edema, and pain are common for the patient who has undergone orthognathic surgery, as well as the patient who has had surgical correction of a fractured jaw. Because the patient's teeth are wired in place for 6 to 8 weeks, a meticulous oral hygiene regimen is imperative to prevent infection. Irrigation and toothette swabbing is advised for the first few days after surgery, until the tenderness subsides. Toothbrushing in conjunction with oral irrigation should follow. Saline or chlorhexidine and fluoride mouthrinses enhance the effectiveness of the regimen in the prevention of gingivitis and caries. A liquid/soft diet is also indicated. These foods should be high in vitamins and protein to promote tissue growth and repair. The patient can be fed through a straw or through a nasogastric feeding tube. Table foods pureed with a blender, baby foods, fruit juice, milk, and soup are all nutritious and can be easily swallowed.[14]

Temporomandibular Joint Dysfunction

Many Americans experience some form of temporomandibular joint (TMJ) dysfunction. The mass media have increased general awareness of this disorder, and many people with symptoms have sought the advice of their private dentists.[71]

Assessment of the condition is accomplished by multidirectional arthrotomograms of the joint. Clinical examination of the patient's occlusion and the opening and closing mechanism is also indicated. If the patient's lateral pterygoid muscle is sensitive, if he experiences pain or crepitus on opening and closing, if wear facets are observed on several teeth, if the patient awak-

ens with a headache or jaw pain, or if the patient has a limited opening or a large deflection to one side on opening, a TMJ disorder is likely.[72] Selective grinding of occlusal surfaces, splinting, electric stimulation, physical therapy, and muscle relaxants are routinely accepted as initial modes of treatment across the country for TMJ dysfunction. Surgery is classically the last resort for the correction of a disk or joint problem.

THE MULTIDIMENSIONAL ADULT

The U.S. population is steadily growing older; the median age is 31.5 years. By the year 2030, this figure could rise to 40.8 years.[73] Adult needs therefore dictate the direction that dental care takes and will take in the future.

Adults are probably the most involved patients in the scope of dental practice. When the dental health educator addresses the needs of a child with caries or the adolescent using smokeless tobacco, he must also communicate with the parents, who are responsible for supervising the youngster's oral hygiene and lifestyle practices.

Adults, of course, have their own dental concerns and fears as outlined in this chapter. In addition, many adults function in a third capacity, as caregivers to family members outside the nuclear family or to individuals or groups in an employee-client relationship. Some of these persons are responsible for performing daily mouth care on the developmentally disabled, medically compromised, or the elderly residing at home or institutionalized. The dental health educator must be cognizant of the adult's three potential levels of operation (parent, adult, and caregiver) and interact accordingly.[74]

REFERENCES

1. Pinkham, J. R., et al. (Eds.): Pediatric Dentistry: Infancy through Adolescence. Philadelphia, W.B. Saunders, 1988.

2. Lundstrom, A.: Introduction to Orthodontics. New York, McGraw-Hill, 1960.
3. Bailit, H. L., and Manning, W.: The need and demand for periodontal services: Implications for dental practice and education. J. Dent. Educ., *52*:458-462, 1988.
4. Scott, D. S., and Hirschman, R.: Psychological aspects of dental anxiety in adults. J. Am. Dent. Assoc., *104*:27-31, 1982.
5. McCann, D. (Ed.): Dental phobia: Conquering fear with trust. J. Am. Dent. Assoc., *119*:593-598, 1989.
6. Milgrom, P., Weinstein, P., Kleinknecht, R., and Getz, T.: Treating Fearful Dental Patients: A Patient Management Handbook. Englewood Cliffs, NJ, Prentice-Hall (Reston), 1985.
7. Stoll, F. A.: Dental Health Education. 5th Ed. Philadelphia, Lea & Febiger, 1977.
8. McBride, B.: How can you help all those frightened patients? R.D.H., *6*:14-18, 41, 1986.
9. St. Germain, A. G.: Handle with care. R.D.H., *9*:12-13, 15, 1989.
10. Hull, R. H.: Managing the fearful dental patient. D.H. News, *2*:9-10, 1989.
11. Fong, C.: The dental hygienist's role in alleviating dental fear and anxiety. Dent. Hyg., *60*:66-69, 1986.
12. Corah, N. L., et al.: The dentist-patient relationship: Perceived dentist behaviors that reduce patient anxiety and increase satisfaction. J. Am. Dent. Assoc., *116*:73-76, 1988.
13. American Academy of Periodontology: Current Procedural Terminology for Periodontics. 5th Ed. Chicago, American Academy of Periodontology, 1987.
14. Wilkins, E. M.: Clinical Practice of the Dental Hygienist. 6th Ed. Philadelphia, Lea & Febiger, 1989.
15. Vennetti, C. M., and Miller, S. S.: Oral contraceptive therapy: Effects on the oral tissues. Dent. Hyg., *61*:168-171, 1987.
16. Knight, G. M., and Wade, A. B.: The effects of hormonal contraceptives on the human periodontium. J. Periodontal Res., *9*:18, 1974.
17. El-Ashiry, G. M., et al.: Effects of oral contraceptives on the gingiva. J. Periodontol., *42*:273, 1971.
18. Lorio, G. P.: Effects of oral contraceptives on oral structures: A review. Gen. Dent., *30*:140, 1982.
19. Hertz, R. S., Beckstead, P. C., and Brown, W. J.: Epithelial melanosis of the gingiva possibly resulting from the use of oral contraceptives. J. Am. Dent. Assoc., *100*:713, 1980.
20. Das, A. K., Bhowmick, S., and Dutta, A.: Oral contraceptives and periodontal disease. J. Indian Dent. Assoc., *43*:47, 1971.
21. Burger, P. A.: X-rays . . . benefits and hazards. R.D.H., *8*:19-23, 1988.
22. Council on Dental Materials, Instruments and Equipment: Recommendations in radiographic practices. 3rd Ed. Chicago, American Dental Association, 1984.
23. Wuehrmann, A. H., and Manson-Hing, L. R.: Dental Radiology. 3rd Ed. St. Louis, C.V. Mosby, 1973.
24. Peterson, M.: Treating adult patients as partners in dental health education. Dent. Hyg., *60*:346-349, 1986.
25. Knowles, M., et al.: Andragogy in Action. San Francisco, Jossey-Bass, 1984.
26. Saunders, J. F.: More than just pretty. R.D.H. *7*:29, 38-39, 45, 1987.
27. Buchs, A. U.: Dental implants: An overview of recent developments. Dent. Impressions, *5*:1-4, 1988.
28. Hartell, W. J.: Dental implants: No longer just skin deep. Dent. Tmwk., *2*:49-51, 1989.
29. Muzzin, K. M. B., Johnson, R., Carr, P., and Daffron, P.: The dental hygienist's role in the maintenance of osseointegrated dental implants. Dent. Hyg., *62*:448-453, 1988.
30. Nobelpharma USA, Inc.: Clinical Guidelines for Hygiene Maintenance of Patients Treated with the Branemark System. Chicago, Nobel Industries Sweden.
31. Schaeken, M. J. M., DeJong, M. H., Franken, H. C. M., and van Der Hoeven, J. S.: Effects of highly concentrated stannous fluoride and chlorhexidine regimens on human dental plaque flora. J. Dent. Res., *65*:57, 1986.
32. Tryggve, L., and Enersen, M.: Effects of chlorhexidine gel in a group of maintenance care patients with poor oral hygiene. J. Periodontol., *57*:364, 1986.
33. Lang, N. P., et al.: Effects of supervised chlorhexidine mouthrinses in children—a longitudinal trial. J. Clin. Periodontal Res., *17*:101, 1982.
34. Cancro, L. P., Paulovich, D. B., Klein, K., and Picozzi, A.: Effects of a chlorhexidine gluconate mouthrinse on dental plaque and calculus. J. Periodontol., *43*:687, 1972.
35. Mankodi, S., Ross, N. M., and Mostler, K.: Clinical efficacy of Listerine in inhibiting and reducing plaque and experimental gingivitis. J. Clin. Periodontol., *14*:285-288, 1987.
36. Fine, D. H., Letizia, J., and Mandel, I. D.: The effect of rinsing with Listerine antiseptic on the properties of developing dental plaque. J. Clin. Periodontol., *12*:660,666, 1985.
37. Gordon, J. M., Lamster, I. B., and Seiger, M. C.: Efficacy of Listerine antiseptic in inhibiting the development of plaque and gingivitis. J. Clin. Periodontol., *12*:697-704, 1985.
38. Stefani, L. A.: The care and maintenance of the dental implant patient. Dent. Hyg., *62*:447, 464-466, 1988.
39. James, R. A.: Perio-implant considerations. Dent. Clin. North Am., *24*:415, 1980
40. Balshi, T. J.: Hygiene maintenance procedures for patients treated with the tissue integrated prosthesis (osseointegration). Quintessence International, *17*:95, 1986.
41. Orton, G. S.: Clinical use of an air powder abrasive system. Dent. Hyg., *61*:518, 1987.
42. Collings, G. J.: Insertion of a Ramus frame implant. Dent. Clin. North Am., *24*:571, 1980.
43. Branemark, P. I., Zarb, G. A., and Albrektsson, T: Radiographic Result, In Tissue-Integrated-Prosthesis. Chicago, Quintessence, 1985.
44. Deporter, D. A., et al: A clinical and radiographic assessment of a porous-surfaced titanium alloy dental implant system in dogs. J. Dent. Res., *65*:1071, 1986.
45. Shulman, L. B., Rogott, G. S., Savitt, E. D., and Kent, R. L.: Evaluation in reconstructive implantology. Dent. Clin. North Am., *30*:327, 1986.
46. Jackson, D.: An epidemiological study of dental caries prevalence in adults. Arch. Oral Biol., *6*:80, 1961.
47. Russell, A. L., and Elvove, E.: Domestic water and dental caries VII. A study of the fluoride-dental caries relationship in an adult population. Pub. Health Rep., *66*:1389, 1951.
48. Jong, A. W. (Ed.): Community Dental Health. 2nd Ed. St. Louis, C.V. Mosby, 1988.
49. Stamm, J. W., and Banting, D. W.: The occurrence of root caries in adults with a lifelong history of fluoridated water consumption. J. Dent. Res., *57*:149, 1978.
50. Johansen, E., et al.: Remineralization of carious lesions in elderly patients. Gerodontics, *3*:47, 1987.
51. Featherstone, J., et al.: Remineralization of artificial caries-like lesions in vivo by a self-administered mouthrinse or paste. Caries Res., *16*:235, 1982.
52. Johansen, E., Taves, D. R., and Olsen, T. O.: Continuing evaluation of the use of fluorides. Am. Assoc. Adv. Sci., *11*:61, 1979.
53. Reutler, F. W., et al.: In Fluoride in Medicine. Edited by T.L. Vischer. Bern, Hans Huber, pp. 143-152, 1971.
54. Nizel, A. E., and Papas, A. S.: Nutrition in Clinical Dentistry. 3rd Ed. Philadelphia, W.B. Saunders, 1989.

55. McNutt, K. W., Sloan, A. E., and Powers, M.: Consumer perceptions of consumer protection. Food Drug Cosm. Law J., *39*:86, 1984.

56. McNutt, K. W., Sloan, A. E., Shields, B., and Powers, M. E.: Consumer attitudes and behaviors related to foods and dental health. Dent. Hyg., *60*:350-356, 1986.

57. National Highway Traffic Safety Administration: Facts on Alcohol and Highway Safety. U.S. Department of Transportation, 1985.

58. U.S. Department of Health and Human Services; Alcohol, Drug Abuse and Mental Health Administration: National Drug and Alcoholism Treatment Utilization Survey, Executive Report, 1983.

59. Wilkinson, C.: The chemically dependent patient. Dent. Tmwk., 2:199-202, 1989.

60. U.S. Department of Health and Human Services: Prevalence of Cigarette Smoking: 30 Years of Change. Office on Smoking and Health, unpublished report, 1985.

61. U.S. Department of Health and Human Services: Smoking and Health: A Report of the Surgeon General, 1984. Rockville, MD, Office on Smoking and Health. DHEW Pub. No. (PHS) 7950066, 1979.

62. U.S. Department of Health and Human Services: The Health Consequences Smoking for Women: A Report of the Surgeon General, 1980. Rockville, MD, Office on Smoking and Health, 1980.

63. American Cancer Society: Cancer Statistics. CA, *40*:9-26, 1990.

64. Baker, H. W.: Diagnosis of oral cancer. *In* Oral Cancer: Diagnosis, Treatment, and Rehabilitation. American Cancer Society, 1973, pp. 2-10.

65. Spouge, J. D.: Oral Pathology. St. Louis, C.V. Mosby, 1973.

66. Mashberg, A., and Samit, A. M.: Early detection, diagnosis, and management of oral and oropharyngeal cancer. CA, 39:67-88, 1989.

67. Barnes, C. M., Nelson K. W., and Conover, G. H.: Results of head and neck examination. Dent. Hyg., *59*:504-506, 1985.

68. Tolle, S. L., and Allen, D. S.: Oral cancer self-examination. Dent. Hyg., *59*:356-360, 362, 1985.

69. Laskin, D.: The challenge of oral cancer. J. Oral Surg., 32:247, 1974.

70. Bouquot, J., DeBiase, C. B., and Graves, C. E.: Self-exam procedures for oral cancer. (Patient education pamphlet.) Morgantown, West Virginia University, 1988.

71. American Dental Association: Dentistry in the 80's: A changing mix of services. J. Am. Dent. Assoc., *116*:617-624, 1988.

72. Woodall, I. R., et al: Comprehensive Dental Hygiene Care. 3rd Ed. St. Louis, C.V. Mosby, 1989.

73. Tacker, B. S.: Dual career couples. R.D.H., 7:12-15, 1987.

74. Boundy, S. S., and Reynolds, N. J. (Eds.): Current Concepts in Dental Hygiene. St. Louis, C.V. Mosby, 1977.

Chapter 8

THE DISABLED

There is another and perhaps greater danger involved in this matter of accepting the limitations of others. Sometimes we are apt to regard as limitations qualities that are actually the other person's strength. We may resent them because they are not the particular qualities which we may want the other person to have. The danger lies in the possibilities that we will not accept the person as he is but try to make him over according to our own ideas.

Eleanor Roosevelt
You Learn By Living

PROFESSIONAL RESPONSIBILITY

Although the American Dental Association was organized in 1859, it was not until 1927 that the American Society for the Promotion of Children's Dentistry was formed. In 1941, this same organization was renamed the American Society of Dentistry for Children. Many of the practitioners who promoted dental care for youngsters were the same professionals who were treating the handicapped. By the time the American Academy of Pedodontics was established in 1948, it was an accepted fact that the pedodontist was also responsible for providing "comprehensive oral care for the emotionally, mentally, or physically handicapped and chronically ill patient."[1]

In 1952, the Academy for the Oral Rehabilitation of Handicapped Persons (changed in 1957 to the Academy of Dentistry for the Handicapped) was created for the purposes of (1) promoting and maintaining high standards of dental care for physically and mentally handicapped persons, (2) encouraging and assisting dental professionals in gaining the preparation necessary to treat the mentally and physically handicapped, and (3) stimulating dental research in care for the physically and mentally handicapped patient.[1]

Unfortunately, for many years dental care has been labeled as the greatest unmet health need of the handicapped.[1] It has only been in the last two decades that the dental profession has seriously addressed the dental needs of the handicapped. Several barriers have prohibited members of the dental health profession from successfully providing comprehensive care to these individuals. These obstacles include[2,3]

1. Office inaccessibility
2. Insufficient factual information concerning the care and needs of the handicapped patient
3. Inadequate curricula in dental schools and professional training programs
4. Apathy of parents or legal guardians toward dental needs

5. Noninclusion of dental professionals in total health care planning teams
6. Poor acceptance or unfavorable attitudes regarding preventive dentistry for the disabled in the school or professional dental environment
7. Lack of a coordinated effort by members of health professions on a national, state, and local level
8. Inadequate funding

Efforts at alleviating these impediments have been met with significant success. In 1968, Title I, Part B of Public Law 88-164, established funds for the development of university-affiliated facilities (UAFs). These centers offered specialized training in the comprehensive care of the disabled. Several years later, Section 504 of the Rehabilitation Act of 1973 was passed, which stated that it was both illegal and discriminatory for health care providers to deny services to an individual, solely on the existence of a handicapping condition. Federal regulations regarding this act have detailed suggestions for the development of health care programs for the disabled in institutions of dental education, private dental offices, and other treatment facilities.[3,4] People with disabilities were deinstitutionalized and placed in a variety of "normal" home, educational, and employment settings as a result of this act.

Special Care in Dentistry, a periodical sponsored by the Academy of Dentistry for the Handicapped and published by the American Dental Association, has made information pertaining to handicapping conditions and their dental management available to the profession. In 1973, 11 dental schools received funding totaling $4.7 million from the Robert Wood Johnson Foundation to design programs to train dental students in care of the nonhospitalized special patient.[5] The success of this pilot program led to the establishment of specific dental and dental hygiene curricular guidelines for dental care for the disabled population.[6,7] The Education of All Handicapped Children Act (Public Law 94-142), enacted in 1975, provides for free, appropriate education for all children, despite the presence of a handicap.[8]

The dental health educator has the professional responsibility to treat all patients as equal in their rights to dental care. The ultimate goal of all dental health interventions for the disabled should be to assist the individual in assuming responsibility for his own oral health as dictated by his physical and mental capabilities. Caregivers can be taught to provide oral hygiene services to the dependent person.

WHO IS HANDICAPPED? DISABLED?

A handicapped person, as defined by sections 503 and 504 of the Rehabilitation Act of 1973, refers to any individual who[9]

1. has a physical or mental impairment which substantially limits one or more major life activities such as caring for one's self, performing manual tasks, walking, seeing, hearing, speaking, breathing, learning, and working.
2. has a record of such an impairment (has a history of or has been misclassified as having a condition that limits major life activities).
3. is regarded as having such an impairment.

More recently, the distinction between a handicap and a disability has become an important issue. A disability is an impairment or defect in a person's physical or mental functioning that can be measured and described objectively. Conversely, a handicap is an obstacle that imposes a limitation in functioning. A disability can be viewed as a part of the person, whereas a handicap is what others do to the disabled when they limit their growth through physical or social barriers.[10]

A handicapped person might have one or a multiplicity of disabilities involving physical, mental, medical, behavioral, sensory, or learning impairments. The severity of these conditions varies from one individual to another, ranging from temporary to permanent, and from a minor disability to total dependence. Even a severely disabled person is not necessarily handicapped. For example, a wheelchair-dependent person is not handicapped if he can function as an employee in the workplace and a parent and spouse at home. Everyone experiences a temporary disability at some period during his life, such as a broken arm or a loss of voice associated with laryngitis. Although many disabled persons are medically compromised and/or elderly, they should not be considered handicapped solely on the basis of their disease or age. Therefore the medically compromised and the elderly are addressed separately in Chapters 9 and 10 respectively.

Disabling conditions are normally grouped into four categories: developmental disabilities; sensory disabilities; orthopedic, central nervous system, and muscular disorders; and learning and behavior disorders. Specific disabilities under each category are discussed in relation to their description, epidemiology, classification, etiology, medical management, orofacial manifestations, and dental and oral hygiene treatment considerations.[7]

DEVELOPMENTAL DISABILITIES

A developmental disability is one that is either present at birth (congenital) or occurs during the developmental period (prior to 18 years of age). Congenital anomalies can be inherited, acquired during gestation, or inflicted during parturition. Some birth defects are not evident at birth; and appear years later. Most developmental disabilities persist throughout the life of the individual, but many can be effectively treated. The major disorders in this category are mental retardation, cerebral palsy, epilepsy, and autism.[11]

Mental Retardation

The American Association on Mental Deficiency defines mental retardation as "significantly sub-average intellectual functioning which exists concurrently with deficits in adaptive behavior, and is manifested during the developmental period." "Significant sub-average intellectual functioning" refers to an intelligence quotient of 2 or more standard deviations below the average. This means that an individual with an IQ of 70 or below would be classified as mentally retarded. "Existing concurrently with deficits in adaptive behavior" signifies that an individual does not possess the personal independence and social responsibility expected of someone his age and cultural background. A mentally retarded child does not demonstrate the language skills or social interaction of a normal child the same age. By adulthood, the retardate has a limited chance of earning a minimum wage, maintaining a family, and becoming an integral member of society. "During the developmental period" denotes that the deficit becomes apparent before the age of 18 years.

EPIDEMIOLOGY

Approximately 3 to 4% of the U.S. population are considered mentally retarded.[12] This figure more accurately represents persons with low intelligence levels, because IQ continues to be used as the main determinant in the diagnosis of mental retardation. When low IQ is combined with impaired adaptive behavior, however, it has been said that the prevalence is only 1%, particularly among adults.[13] Older retardates are less visible because of death and successful assimilation of some of these individuals into the general population.

Mental retardation appears to be slightly more frequent in males than in females; approximately 55% of the mentally retarded are males. Eight-five percent of the mentally retarded reside at home, and the remaining 15% live in institutions, hospitals, or prisons. Of those living at home, about 18% are on waiting lists for institutional care.

CLASSIFICATION

Mildly retarded individuals score between 51 and 70 on the IQ test and account for 89% of all retarded persons. With proper education and habilitation, the mildly retarded can function at the third to sixth grade level and are often placed in a synonymous category known as *educable. Moderately retarded* individuals have IQ scores in the 36 to 50 range and comprise approximately 6% of the mentally retarded population. With intensive training, they can achieve the abilities of a first to second grade child. The *severely retarded* account for 3.5% of the retardate population. They have IQ scores between 20 and 35. The term *trainable* is given to moderately to severely retarded individuals in the 25 to 49 IQ range. Trainable mentally retarded persons can usually be taught a manual skill in a sheltered workshop setting. The *profoundly retarded* possess IQ scores below 20. They respond minimally to their environment, have multiple medical problems, and are usually institutionalized; they require supervision or are totally dependent on a caregiver for their personal needs. The profoundly retarded constitute only 1.5% of the total retardate population.[3]

ETIOLOGY

Approximately 25% of mental retardation is acquired or inherited. An individual can acquire brain damage prenatally, perinatally, or postnatally at some point during the developmental period. Inherited metabolic or chromosomal aberrations can also have an adverse effect on an individual's intellectual potential. A list of the common causes of mental retardation during each stage of development is presented in Table 8-1.[12] In the majority (75%) of individuals labeled mentally retarded, no specific cause can be identified.

MEDICAL MANAGEMENT

Due to recent advances in medical diagnosis, prevention, and treatment techniques, health education for the expectant mother can be extremely successful in the prevention of mental retardation. Informing women about the detrimental effects of alcohol, drugs, and poor diet on the health of their unborn children can make a difference. Parents receiving genetic counseling can be advised not to have children or to limit the number of pregnancies due to risks related to their carrier status for genetic disorders that can cause mental retardation and other disabling conditions or chronic diseases. Pregnant women with a suspected risk can undergo amniocentesis; fetal cells

Table 8-1. Causal Factors Associated with Mental Retardation

Prenatal (Conception to the onset of labor)	Perinatal (Labor and delivery)	Postnatal (After delivery to age 18 years)
Viral infection	Trauma	Infections
Rubella	Difficult deliveries	Meningitis
Influenza	Anoxia	Encephalitis
Cytomegalovirus	Prematurity	Prolonged high fevers
Syphilis		Physical injury and accidents
Injuries		Social deprivation
Trauma		Lead poisoning
Rh incompatibility		
Alcohol consumption		
Poor nutrition		
Toxemia		
Drug use and abuse		
Inherited (genetic) defects		
Metabolic disorders, e.g., PKU		
Chromosomal aberrations, e.g.,		
Down syndrome, Klinefelter syndrome		

are aspirated via the abdominal wall to determine the existence of a genetic disorder. Some disorders diagnosed with this technique can be treated, but others cannot. When treatment options are not available, the parent(s) can elect abortion in some states.[12]

The majority of severely to profoundly retarded persons are identified at birth or shortly thereafter. Most retardates in the mild to moderate range, however, are not recognized until they enter school. The peak period of identification for this group is between 6 and 16 years. As soon as a determination is made, an individualized educational plan (IEP) must be created for each child.[14]

Mental retardation rarely exists as an entity in itself. The retardate population as a whole has a higher percentage of emotional disturbances, sensory defects, language disorders, neuromuscular forms of impairment (e.g., cerebral palsy), seizures (e.g., epilepsy), leukemia, infectious hepatitis, and other physical anomalies such as congenital heart disease.[15]

OROFACIAL MANIFESTATIONS

The most common dental problems associated with mental retardation are periodontal disease and untreated carious lesions. These problems are not inherent to the disability but correspond primarily to dental neglect (See Fig. 8-1).[16] Structural abnormalities in the oral cavity are often related to disturbances in growth patterns. Retarded persons who exhibit craniofacial syndromes or Dilantin hyperplasia frequently have a malocclusion of some form.[17] Patients with Down syndrome display a wide variety of orofacial anomalies such as (1) a large, fissured tongue; (2) a short, con-

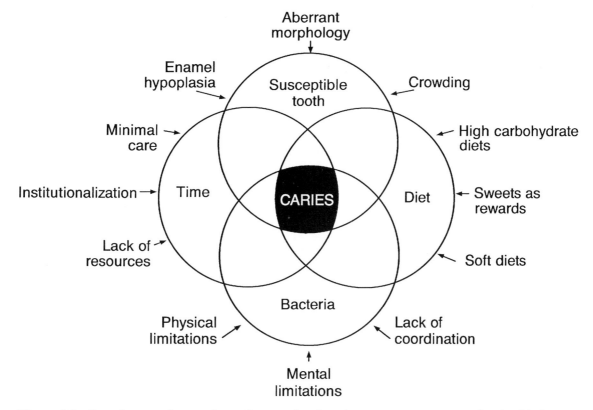

Figure 8-1. Complicating factors that influence the dental caries process among the disabled population. From Nowak, A.J.: Dentistry for the Handicapped Patient. St. Louis, C.V. Mosby, 1976, and Newbrun, E.: Cariology, San Francisco, University of California Press, 1975.

Table 8-2. Ten Cardinal Signs of Down Syndrome

Sign	Frequency (%)
Hypotonia	80
Poor moro reflex	85
Hyperflexibility of joints	80
Excess skin on back of short, thick neck	80
Flat facial profile	90
Obliquely slanted eyes, narrow palpebral fissures (Fig. 8-2)	80
Small, low ears	60
Dysplasia of pelvis	70
Clinodactyly of 5th finger (Fig. 8-3)	60
Simian crease (Fig. 8-3)	45

Modified slightly from Nowak, A.J.: Dentistry for the Handicapped Patient. St. Louis, C.V. Mosby, 1976, p. 47.

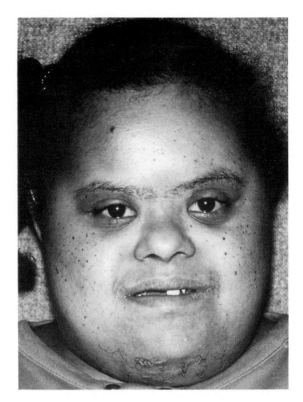

Figure 8-2. The eyes of a person with Down syndrome are characterized by an oblique slant, and narrow palpebral fissures. Median epicanthal folds persist in about half of the younger patients and one-third of adults with Down syndrome.

stricted palate occurring concomitantly with an underdeveloped maxilla, tendency toward class III malocclusion, and a posterior crossbite or an anterior openbite; (3) delayed and unsequential exfoliation and eruption of teeth; and (4) small cone-shaped teeth with hypoplastic enamel. Although periodontal disease is largely attributed to local factors, the relatively frequent occurrence of acute necrotizing ulcerative gingivitis and the premature loss of mandibular incisor teeth, particularly in Down's patients, leads the dental health educator to believe that the causes might be more complex. Defective neutrophil chemotaxis,[18] elevations in parotid enzyme activity,[19] and a metabolic block in collagen maturation have been implicated as causal factors.[20]

Down syndrome caused by the existence of three number 21 chromosomes (trisomy 21) is the most common genetic defect associated with mental retardation and therefore deserves additional attention by the dental health educator. This disorder has an incidence of 1:600 live births; the risk increases proportionally with maternal age. The 10 cardinal signs of Down syndrome are listed in Table 8-2.[21] In addition to these signs, the individual is usually stocky and short in stature and has a waddling gait[1,20] and characteristic face (Fig. 8-2) and hands (Fig. 8-3).

Mentally retarded persons also frequently exhibit destructive oral habits. They include tongue-thrusting, bruxism, clenching, drooling, and self-injurious behavior for stimulation (e.g., head banging, biting, and scratching). Lesch-Nyhan syndrome is a condition dominated by self-mutilation behaviors.[22] Pica (a craving for nonfood substances such as dirt, cigarette butts, and hair) is also common in the mentally retarded.

DENTAL AND ORAL HYGIENE TREATMENT CONSIDERATIONS

Documentation of a complicated medical history and assessment of the retarded patient's levels of cognitive and motor functioning are critical prior to the initial dental

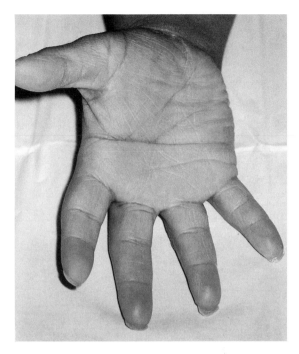

Figure 8-3. The hands of a person with Down syndrome are characterized by short, stubby fingers, curvature inward of the little finger (clinodactyly), and a single transverse line across the palm (simian crease).

appointment. This might require the dental health educator to consult with the patient's physician. Antibiotic premedication might be advised for a congenital heart valve defect, for example. A list of the patient's medications might also reveal an anticonvulsive drug (e.g., Dilantin for seizures) and psychotropic drugs for behavioral and emotional disorders.

It is also important for the dental health educator to determine if the patient has been to the dentist previously and what type of behavior he displayed. Maladaptive behavior can usually be prevented by the dental health educator through kind, patient communication. Touching and frequent smiling make the patient feel more comfortable. Many retarded persons try very hard to please someone who conveys a sincere interest in them.

Because the retardate generally has a short attention span and becomes easily frustrated, the dental health educator should schedule brief, early morning appoint-

ments. Instructions should be given slowly, at the patient's cognitive level of understanding. The tell, show, do method must be employed for each procedure performed.

Concomitant neuromuscular disorders might require wheelchair adaptations and/ or physical restraints during dental treatment. (Wheelchair and restraining management techniques are discussed later in this chapter.) Physical restraints are used only when absolutely necessary to prevent injury to the patient during the dental appointment because of poor behavior or poor muscle control. Restraints should not be used as a punishment or merely for the convenience of the dental staff. Restraints require the consent of a guardian or caregiver and should not cause the patient any physical discomfort.[23] People restraints are also a viable option (Fig. 8-4). Chemical restraints such as general anesthesia should only be considered when all other treatment modalities fail.

The patient's caregiver should be present during the review of oral hygiene, whether he is responsible for simply reinforcing home care in the higher-functioning patient or actually performing daily plaque removal on the lower-functioning individual. Disclosing solution is a useful adjunct to enhance the visualization of plaque. Mouth props can also be helpful to gain access to the dentition (Fig. 8-5). For the retardate who performs his own plaque removal but lacks fine motor coordination, the dental health educator can modify toothbrushes to suit the patient's individual needs (Fig. 8-6). Some companies have fabricated uniquely designed toothbrushes that require less dexterity (Fig. 8-7).[24] Floss holders (Fig. 8-8) are ideal tools for the disabled with limited dexterity. They also offer special assistance to caregivers who are responsible for flossing the teeth of individuals with more severe disabilities.

Diet counseling is also indicated for the individual who consumes excessive amounts of soft, cariogenic foods, is bottle fed, or receives fermentable carbohydrates in the form of tokens or reinforcers for performing desired behaviors. The dental health educator must conduct sessions with

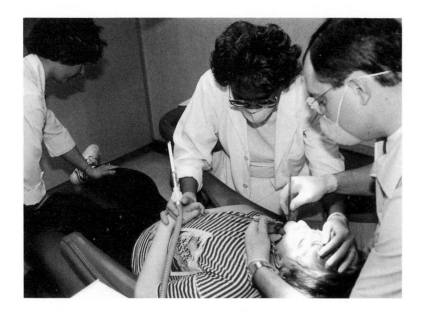

Figure 8-4. Restraining a patient's undesirable movements solely by the use of one or more persons.

the parent or caregiver to ensure that daily dietary practices are not contributing to dental caries. Unsweetened cereals, stickers, and stars are ideal reinforcers or rewards.

Dental office procedures should involve frequent prophylaxes, fluoride treatments, routine radiographs, and sealants for the young. A dental health educator who provides comprehensive, routine dental care to the retarded improves their quality of life by reducing their chances for infection, enabling them to enjoy mastication, and enhancing their self-image through an improved appearance and the elimination of mouth odor.[25]

Cerebral Palsy

The term cerebral palsy was coined by Dr. Winthrop Phelps[10] and has been in common usage since the 1930s. Cerebral palsy is defined as a disorder of movement and posture resulting from a permanent nonprogressive defect or lesion of the immature brain. The lesion classically produces motor distur-

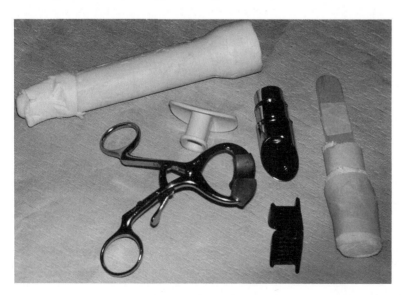

Figure 8-5. An array of mouth props designed to keep the mouth ajar during dental procedures.

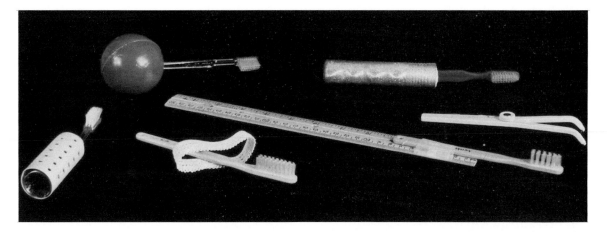

Figure 8-6. Toothbrush modifications individualized to suit a variety of dexterity problems.

bances as a major clinical symptom. This motor deficit can manifest as muscular paralysis, weakness, incoordination, or other aberrations of motor function caused by a pathology in the motor control center of the brain. Brain damage such as this can occur prenatally, perinatally, or postnatally before the central nervous system reaches maturity.[1]

EPIDEMIOLOGY

Cerebral palsy (CP) is the most common of nonprogressive disabilities and occurs in 7 out of every 100,000 people in the United States. Five to seven thousand infants are born each year with cerebral palsy, and an additional 1500 people develop the disorder

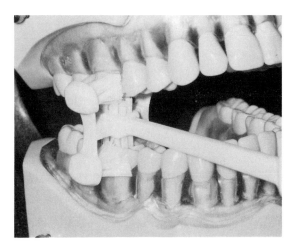

Figure 8-7. A commercially designed toothbrush that requires minimal dexterity and shortens brushing time by cleaning buccal, lingual, and occlusal surfaces on both the maxillary and mandibular arches simultaneously. Courtesy of OMNIA-dent USA, Lawrence Welk Drive, Escondido, CA 92026.

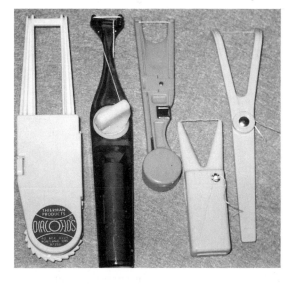

Figure 8-8. A variety of floss holders are available to aid the patient with limited dexterity or the caregiver who prefers not to insert his fingers into the mouth of a patient who bites. Courtesy of C. A. Spear, B.S.D.H., M.S., West Virginia University.

as a result of various types of head trauma.[26] Although there are no reports on the sex-related prevalence of cerebral palsy, males tend to be affected more frequently than females.[12]

Although not fatal, cerebral palsy is also not curable. Approximately 80% of CP patients can benefit from well-organized specialized treatment involving physical or surgical intervention; 10% are so mildly affected that no definite treatment is necessary, and the remaining 10% require institutionalization due to the severity of their disability.[27]

CLASSIFICATION

The extent and location of the damage to the central nervous system determine the degree of involvement and the clinical symptoms that a person experiences.[1] Phys-iologic and topographic classification systems for individuals with CP have been devised on the basis of the motor disorder and the limbs involved. These classification systems are outlined in Table 8-3.[12]

ETIOLOGY

Cerebral palsy is caused by numerous factors, all of which involve injury to the central nervous sytem at some time during development. Approximately 90% of cerebral palsy cases have their origin in the prenatal and perinatal periods.

Prenatal. A large number of CP cases have their genesis at this time due to the rapid growth rate that the brain undergoes between the second and fourth months of intrauterine life. Fetal or maternal anoxia, uterine bleeding after the fifth month of gestation, infections contracted during the first

Table 8-3. Common Physiologic and Topographic Classifications of Cerebral Palsy

Classification	Location of Brain Lesion	Percent of Cerebral Palsy Patients	Physical Characteristics/Limb Involvement
Physiologic			
Spasticity	Cortical	50–75	Minor stimulation causes exaggerated contractions; hyperirritability of muscles; poor head control; inability to use arms and legs; impaired speech, chewing, and swallowing; drooling
Athetosis	Basal ganglia	15–25	Involuntary muscle contractions; twisting, contorted movements; difficulty keeping balance or remaining upright; impaired speech, chewing, and swallowing
Ataxia	Cerebellum	10	Muscles respond incompletely to stimuli, resulting in a partial contraction; impaired balance and coordination; difficulty grasping
Mixed	Two or more areas	5–10	Combination of two or more types of CP in same person
Topographic			
Monoplegia		rare	One limb involved
Diplegia		10–20	Lower limbs predominately involved; upper limbs have minor involvement
Triplegia		rare	Three limbs involved
Paraplegia		10–20	Lower limbs only involved
Quadriplegia		15–20	All four limbs involved
Hemiplegia		35–40	Both limbs on the same side involved

Adapted from Lange, B.M., Entwistle, B.M., and Lipson, L.F.: Dental Management of the Handicapped: Approaches for Dental Auxiliaries. Philadelphia, Lea & Febiger, 1983, p. 126.

trimester (e.g., rubella, chicken pox, mumps, measles, influenza, and syphilis), premature birth, maternal diabetes, and exposure to radiation during the first trimester have all been implicated as causal factors. A condition with severe neural symptoms that include athetoid CP is known as kernicterus. This disorder results from high levels of circulating bilirubin in the infant's blood, secondary to an Rh incompatibility. This is one of the few causal factors that can be prevented. Inheriting cerebral palsy is rare, but when it does occur it is usually the result of a genetically transmitted defect in the basal cell nuclei.

Perinatal. The common causes of CP during labor and delivery are mechanical trauma and hypoxia. Both can be prevented by the physician paying particular attention to a woman's past medical history in regard to previous pregnancies and related complications. Fetal asphyxia can occur from a mechanical respiratory obstruction such as aspirated fluids or mucus, or from respiratory depression caused by excessively premedicating or anesthetizing the mother during labor. Fetal cerebral hemorrhage usually results from a prolonged or traumatic delivery. Neonatal fever over 3 days in duration also has a high correlation with development of cerebral palsy.

Postnatal. Cerebral palsy acquired during the postnatal period can be caused by carbon monoxide poisoning; high-altitude anoxia; cerebral vascular hemorrhage (e.g., from car accident, gunshot wound, or contact sports); cerebral infections (e.g., meningitis, encephalitis, and brain abscesses); toxemia related to the ingestion, inhalation or injection of toxic amounts of substances; and brain tumors, either through their progression or as a result of their removal.

No definite cause has been established in approximately 40% of cerebral palsy cases, and unfortunately no methods exist currently that can accurately diagnosis CP until after birth, when the child displays signs of delayed development.[12]

MEDICAL MANAGEMENT

In addition to their motor disability, most individuals stricken with cerebral palsy suffer associated disorders. Approximately 40% of those with CP also exhibit mental retardation, seizures, and vision problems; 60% have speech and language disorders; and 20% experience hearing difficulties.[11] Behavioral disorders only serve to further complicate matters.

The treatment for cerebral palsy can entail physical therapy, braces, occupational therapy, orthopedic surgery, speech therapy, medications, and supportive care for other related disabilities such as hearing loss, visual impairment, and seizures. Minimizing uncontrolled movements while strengthening functional movements is the goal of therapy.[12]

Because many individuals with cerebral palsy possess normal intelligence they frequently become frustrated with their limited ability to direct their movements and control their speech. Because of their appearance, however, persons with CP are often assumed to be mentally retarded and encounter social, educational, and emotional prejudices. These biases frequently create feelings of embarrassment and low self-esteem leading to anger, depression, and behavioral disorders. Psychological counseling and medication might be required.

OROFACIAL MANIFESTATIONS

Enamel hypoplasia of the primary teeth is common in children with cerebral palsy. This enamel defect can be correlated to the time the cerebral injury took place in utero. A slightly higher rate of caries and periodontal disease through adulthood is primarily due to neglect and a decreased self-cleansing ability related to the poorly functioning oral musculature. Abnormal functioning of the tongue, lips, and cheeks can make oral clearance of food more difficult, causing the prolonged retention of plaque and food debris in the mouth. Semisoft high-carbohydrate diets, which also tend to be cariogenic, seem to predominate because of the difficulty these patients experience in eating and swallowing. Dilantin-induced gingival hyperplasia can also contribute to

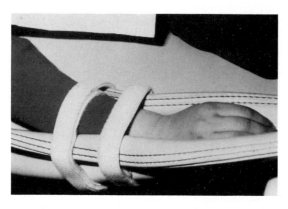

Figure 8-9. Restraining device. Adhesive tape, Velcro straps, or soft cloth strips can be placed over the wrists, ankles, or where needed to limit body movements or provide support for paralyzed limbs. Courtesy of D. Holmes, D.D.S., M.S., West Virginia University, and R. Mangello, B.S.D.H., Uniontown, PA.

the increased incidence of periodontal disease. A higher incidence of destructive oral habits, which include tongue thrusting, bruxism, and mouth breathing, also appear to contribute to the risk of dental disease in the CP patient. Excessive drooling due to hypotonicity of the lip muscles and predominance of mouth breathing fosters increased production of calculus and gingival inflammation.[12]

Class II malocclusion coupled with a high narrow palatal vault are also prevalent. Athetoid cerebral palsied persons seem to exhibit this occlusion more often because of the hypotonicity of the orbicularis oris muscle and excessive tongue thrusting. Fractures of the maxillary anterior teeth are not uncommon due to unstable ambulation and seizures which may lead to frequent falling.

DENTAL AND ORAL HYGIENE TREATMENT CONSIDERATIONS

Introductory information necessary for dental management of the cerebral palsied patient is similar to that required for a patient with mental retardation. A thorough medical history must be obtained that also documents the severity of the patient's

motor dysfunction and his mode of ambulation.

Muscle control associated with involuntary movements of the arms, legs, head, neck, mouth, and tongue is critical to the provision of dental care. Several restraining techniques can be used: (1) soft restraining cloths wrapped around the patient's arms and legs and secured around the dental chair stabilize the limbs (Fig. 8-9); (2) a Pediwrap or a sheet draped around the patient can also control involuntary arm and leg movements (Fig. 8-10); (3) the moldable bean bag chair placed on the dental chair or a bean bag apron molded over the patient provides comfort and stabilization[28] (Fig. 8-11); (4) the papoose board secures the head and body with Velcro straps (Fig. 8-12); and (5) wheelchair modifications that do not require transferring the patient to the dental chair. Wheelchair modifications include the use of adjustable wheelchair headrests, the

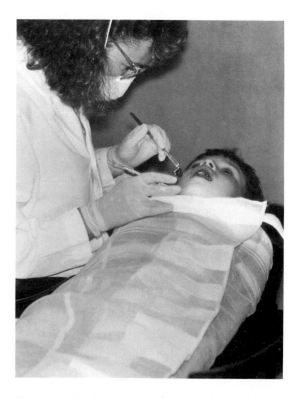

Figure 8-10. Restraining device. The Pediwrap is a nylon mesh drape that stabilizes movement by enclosing the patient from his neck to his ankles.

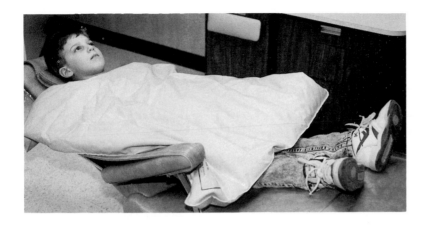

Figure 8-11. Restraining device. The bean bag can be placed over the patient or on top of the dental chair, with the patient's body molded into it to restrict uncontrolled movements.

positioning of the patient's back to the back of the dental chair and reversing the headrest of an older model dental unit, and a hydraulic lift specifically designed for wheelchairs (Fig. 8-13).[29]

The dental health educator might discover that the more eager the CP patient is to cooperate, the more uncoordinated his movements become. Morning appointments, a relaxed atmosphere with soft music and gentle, honest communication with frequent pats of assurance are advised.[25,30] Other suggestions for the dental health educator include (1) padding stiff limbs (contractures) that cannot be straightened, (2) cradling the patient's head to control slight movements of the head and neck (Fig. 8-14), (3) propping the mouth open to prevent an involuntary bite reflex (Fig. 8-5), and (4) using a rubber dam and proper suctioning

while keeping the patient in a partially upright position to avoid gagging, choking, and aspiration as a result of the patient's impaired swallowing mechanism.[25]

The oral manifestations of CP outlined in the previous section suggest a regimen of (1) oral physical therapy, (2) frequent plaque removal by toothbrushing and flossing, (3) frequent debridement of food from the palate and vestibule, (4) daily fluoride gel applications, and (5) dietary modifications.[11,12,31-34]

Cerebral palsied children can be defensive or intolerant of someone trying to touch their mouths. Desensitization through exercises that stimulate the mouth might be necessary before introducing plaque removal. Oral physical therapy can also help to calm the child and improve the functioning of the oral musculature.[35]

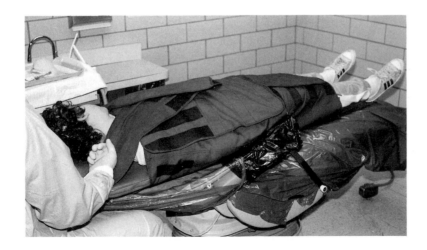

Figure 8-12. Restraining device. The papoose board is a stabilizing board with cloth wraps attached to it. Three wraps (lower, middle, and upper body) and a cloth forehead strap (for optional use) are folded over the patient and secured with Velcro. The wrists are secured beneath the middle wrap before it is closed.

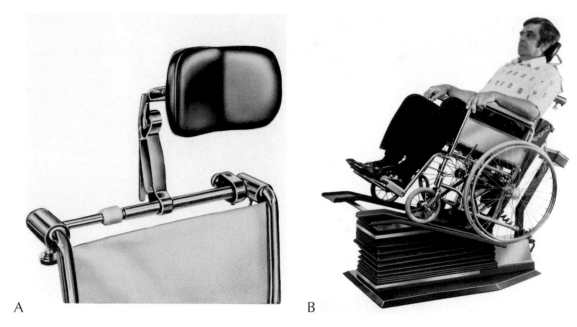

A   B

Figure 8-13. *A.* Adjustable wheelchair headrest. *B.* Hydraulic lift converts wheelchair into a dental chair. Courtesy of Metal Dynamics Corporation, 9324 State Road, Philadelphia, PA 19114.

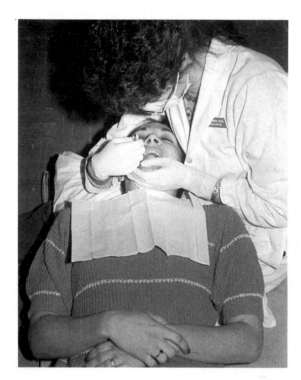

Figure 8-14. Cradling of the patient's head to prevent slight movements that could endanger the patient during treatment.

Modified toothbrushes (Fig. 8-6) are particularly beneficial for CP patients with impaired motor coordination, and they can be constructed easily and inexpensively. Bending toothbrushes under hot water (Fig. 8-15) or the use of an electric toothbrush can also be helpful (Fig. 8-16). For many cerebral palsied patients, brushing their own teeth will never be possible. Therefore parents or caregivers must be trained to perform plaque removal procedures while (1) controlling the patient's head and body movements; (2) gaining good visibility, and adequate lighting; and (3) maintaining patient comfort. Many operator/patient positions possess these characteristics (Figs. 8-17 to 8-20).[36]

Impaired oral functioning has classically been responsible for the consumption of softer, less nutritious foods by the CP patient. Often these foods are retentive and high in fermentable carbohydrates, increasing the individual's susceptibility to dental caries. Feeding skills, diet restrictions, and food preferences must be considered when designing a menu. The recent literature suggests coarsely grated and chopped fibrous foods at mealtime and the avoidance of tra-

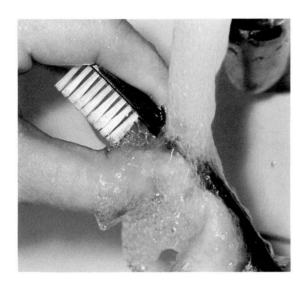

Figure 8-15. Toothbrushes can be bent under hot water to provide better angulation for plaque removal.

ditional snacks like popcorn, carrots, nuts, and pretzels, which are too hard in consistency.[12]

Epilepsy

Historic references to epilepsy have described seizures as acts of possession by demons or witchcraft.[11] Even today, many people are afraid of epilepsy because of the writhing movements that often take place during a seizure. Because people do not understand epilepsy, they often shun or discriminate against those who have it; epilepsy is still believed by some to be contagious. The terms epilepsy, recurrent convulsive disorder, and seizure disorder are all synonymous. Epilepsy is not a disease; it is a variable symptom complex characterized by recurrent paroxymal attacks of unconsciousness or impaired consciousness, usually accompanied by tonic or clonic spasms (alternating involuntary contraction and relaxation of skeletal muscle) or other abnormal behaviors, e.g., an alteration in sensory perception or balance.

EPIDEMIOLOGY

Epilepsy affects approximately 17% of the U.S. population. The actual prevalence is probably higher, but because of the stigma that is often associated with the condition and inadequate reporting methods, it is difficult to ascertain the exact prevalence. Studies suggest a prevalence between 2 and 22 per 1,000 population.[12]

Males appear to be affected slightly more than females. Most epileptics experience their first seizure during childhood or adolescence: about half occur before age 5 and 90% before the age of 20. Puberty is a common period for seizures to emerge.

CLASSIFICATION

Epilepsy is normally classified according to the type of seizure activity manifested.

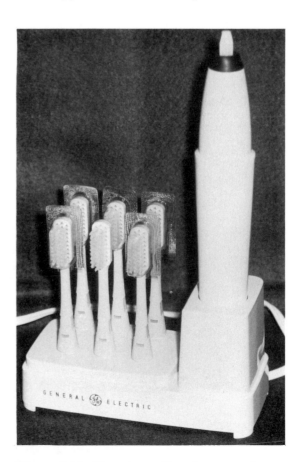

Figure 8-16. Electric toothbrushes assist the patient with poor manual dexterity.

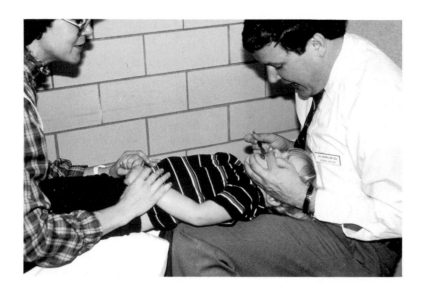

Figure 8-17. Patient positioning. The reclining patient is placed between two persons seated facing each other. One caregiver holds the patient's hands, and the other removes plaque.

Grand mal seizures are the most common type, and they can occur at any age. Grand mal is a classic term that refers to a generalized tonic-clonic seizure episode. Usually the seizure is preceded by an aura, which is an abnormal sensory response such as a peculiar smell, a strange sound, or a tingling sensation. The individual then loses consciousness, collapses, and undergoes a complete contraction of the muscles. An epileptic cry is produced when air is forced out of the lungs during contraction of the diaphram. Repetitious alternating contractions and relaxations (jerking motions) follow.

The tongue can be bitten and the teeth can fracture as a result of the rapid contraction of the jaw muscles. Bowel and bladder incontinence can occur as well as dyspnea, cyanosis, excessive salivation, profuse perspiration, and dilation of the pupils. The entire action might last from 1 to 3 min, and the patient might remain unconscious for up to 30 min thereafter. The patient frequently recovers confused, disoriented, and tired and might sleep for several hours after the episode.

Petit mal seizures are characterized by a transient loss of consciousness of 5 to 30 s.

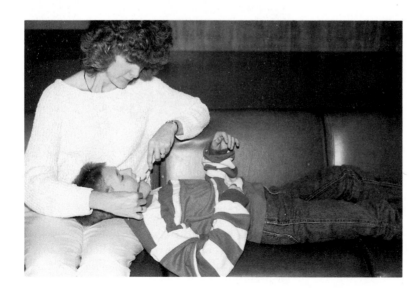

Figure 8-18. Patient positioning. The patient reclines on the couch with his head on the lap of the caregiver. A mouth prop can be used to increase visibility of the oral cavity.

Jacksonian or focal motor seizures consist of an involuntary twitching of one part of the body that travels to other parts of the body on the same side in a specialized sequence. For example, the focus of these clonic movements might begin at one corner of the mouth and then affect the cheek, eye, and neck on the same side. The seizure originates in the frontal lobe.[1,11,12]

ETIOLOGY

No cause is known for approximately 50 to 75% of patients with epilepsy. Identifiable causal factors can be described for about 25 to 50% of epileptics, relative to the time period during which the insult occurred (Table 8-4).[12]

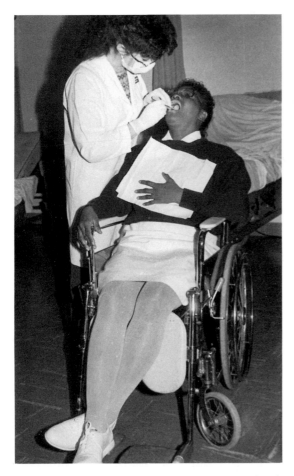

Figure 8-19. Patient positioning. For wheelchair patients, the caregiver can perform oral hygiene procedures by locking the chair wheels and standing next to the patient.

The individual can have a blank gaze or become unconscious without losing his posture. Resumption of activities usually occurs following an episode, with no recollection of the event. About 50% of youngsters 10 to 13 years of age with petit mal seizures develop the grand mal form.

Psychomotor seizures usually begin in the temporal lobe. The affected person exhibits repetitious, stereotypic behavior, e.g., picking at clothing, lip-smacking, or walking around in circles. This form of seizure can last from a few minutes to several hours and can be preceded by an aura. The frequency of psychomotor seizures increases with age and, they are the most difficult type to treat medically.

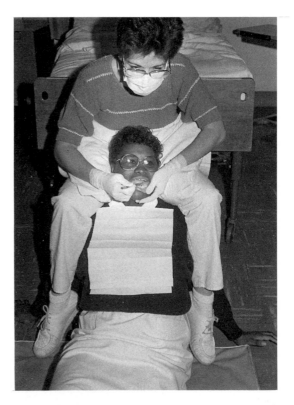

Figure 8-20. Patient positioning. Patient with uncontrolled arm movements sits on the floor. The caregiver sits in a chair behind the patient with her legs over the patient's shoulders to stabilize undesirable movements and performs oral hygiene procedures.

Table 8-4. Causes of Epilepsy

Conception to 2 Years	Three to 18 Years	Adulthood through Old Age
Prenatal and Perinatal		
Maternal trauma	Head trauma	Head trauma
Premature labor	Whooping cough	Brain tumor
Rubella	Lead encephalopathy	Vascular sclerosis
Complicated birth, e.g., breech, forceps delivery, anoxia	Allergy	
Undetected infections	Infectious diseases	Late evidence of birth injury
Congenital anomalies	Brain tumor	
Rh incompatibility	High fever	Other
Inherited metabolic disorders	Late evidence of birth injury	
Postnatal		
High fever	Other	
Postnatal trauma		
Infections		
Allergy		
Whooping cough		
Lead encephalopathy		
Other		

Adapted from Lange, B.M., Entwistle, B.M., and Lipson, L.F.: Dental Management of the Handicapped: Approaches for Dental Auxillaries. Philadelphia, Lea & Febiger, 1983, p. 108.

MEDICAL MANAGEMENT

Because seizures are the result of abnormal and uncontrolled activity of cerebral neurons and in most cases the disorder is idiopathic, treatment is palliative and therefore aimed at suppression of the abnormal activity. Drug therapy is the treatment of choice for about 70% of the epileptic population.[37-39] Anticonvulsant medications (e.g., phenytoin, phenobarbital, primidone, carbamazepine, ethosuximide, valproic acid, acetazolamide, phensuximide, methsuximide, and trimethadione) appear to completely control seizure activity in about one-half of patients.[40] Although drugs cannot cure epilepsy, they provide the only practical long-term treatment for the majority of patients with this condition.[41] Many of these prescribed anticonvulsants possess side effects, which can range from drowsiness to the initiation of a blood dyscrasia in a patient taking them.[12,30] Treatment with drugs usually continues for 2 to 3 years from the cessation of seizure activity.[37,42] Approximately 50% of patients sustain remission after a gradual withdrawal from medi-

cation.[43] Dietary restrictions and surgery are also plausible modes of treatment.

To reduce the probability of seizure, the epileptic is advised to avoid illegal drugs, missing medications, alcohol, fatigue, and stress. The patient frequently requires psychologic counseling to help him cope with his condition. Psychologic turmoil can increase the frequency of seizures, which in turn raises the dosage of the anticonvulsant needed.

OROFACIAL MANIFESTATIONS

Phenytoin (Dilantin)-induced gingival hyperplasia is related to the dosage of the drug and the presence of plaque and other irritants. Tuberous sclerosis and gingival fibromatosis can mimic phenytoin hyperplasia. A differential diagnosis can be made on the basis of the patient's medical history. Tissue overgrowth is pale and fibrous, and in younger patients it is generally more predominant in the anterior and buccal portions of the mouth. Approximately 25% of patients taking phenytoin experience gingival hy-

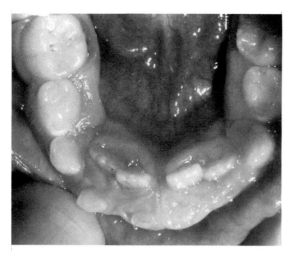

Figure 8-21. Phenytoin-induced gingival hyperplasia.

perplasia.[44] The overgrowth can be so extensive that the teeth are totally covered and essentially nonfunctional (Fig. 8-21). The initial signs of overgrowth can commence as early as two weeks from the onset of phenytoin therapy.[11]

Meticulous oral hygiene is paramount in the prevention and treatment of phenytoin hyperplasia. Although the excess gingival tissue can be excised during a gingivectomy, this procedure is futile without plaque control and possibly a change in medication. If the patient must remain on phenytoin for seizure control, a rubber appliance that exerts a positive pressure on the gingiva and is worn nightly at the very least has been shown to be effective.[45] If the fibrous overgrowth is allowed to continue untreated, malpositioning of teeth, impaired chewing, retained primary teeth, and poor esthetics will result.[11,12]

Trauma, primarily to the maxillary incisors, is another common orofacial manifestation of seizure disorders. Both the soft tissue and hard structures can be affected. Falls related to seizure activity can cause soft tissue lacerations and chipped, fractured, and avulsed teeth. Radiographs should be taken to determine the extent of the damage. Location of a tooth or tooth fragment is also essential to prevent aspiration. A dental treatment plan for such injuries should suggest fixed instead of removable appliances for replacement of teeth and the fabrication of head and mouth protectors to prevent further complications from falls. More flexible resin materials rather than ceramics are recommended for restorative procedures because they can withstand the forces of clonic activity.[46]

DENTAL AND ORAL HYGIENE TREATMENT CONSIDERATIONS

Careful assessment of a patient's seizure activity during a dental appointment should include the following questions: When did the patient's last seizure occur? What type of seizure was it? What factors precipitated the seizure? Was there an aura? How long did the seizure last? How frequently do the seizures occur? How are the seizures controlled? If medication has been prescribed to control the seizures, what was it, how much was given, and when?

If the patient experiences a grand mal seizure while in the operatory, the dental health educator should (1) not panic; (2) remove harmful objects surrounding the patient and from the patient's mouth; (3) loosen the patient's clothing and recline the dental chair to the supine position close to the floor if the individual is seated; (4) not attempt to restrain movements; (5) stay with the patient during and after the seizure to reorient him to his environment; (6) allow the patient to rest and freshen up before leaving; (7) reschedule the patient, if necessary; and (8) summon emergency medical assistance if the patient experiences status epilepticus—continuous seizures lasting longer than 5 min. The most common cause of status epilepticus is the abrupt discontinuance of routinely taken anticonvulsant medication. All seizure activity should be documented in the patient's health record and discussed with a parent or caregiver and the patient's physician.

Other modifications in dental treatment include short early-morning appointments and avoidance of anxiety or stress-provoking stimuli that might increase the patient's risk of seizure activity.

Autism

The first descriptions of autism as a developmental disability were those of Kanner in 1943.[47] Because the symptoms occurred in early infancy, the syndrome was termed early infantile autism. The National Society for Autistic Children (NSAC) defined autistic children as "all persons, regardless of age, with severe disorders of communication and behavior, whose disability becomes manifest during the early developmental stages of childhood."[48] The autistic child appears to suffer primarily from an impairment of his cognitive and/or perceptual functioning, the consequences of which are manifested by a limited ability to understand, learn, and communicate. Autistic persons can be aphasic (defective or an absence of language) and echolalic (meaningless repetition of words). They refer to themselves in the third rather than the first person.[49] A disturbance in the capacity to relate to people, objects, and events also exists. Autistic individuals seem to associate better with inanimate objects than people and display extreme social and emotional detachment. Stereotypic, repetitious, ritualistic play and a strong desire for consistency are dominant features of the autistic personality.[11]

EPIDEMIOLOGY

The prevalence of infantile autism is 4 to 5 per 10,000 population.[50] This translates to approximately 60,000 autistic children under 18 years of age in the United States. Boys are usually affected four to five times as often as girls.[11,51] Autism occurs internationally; it is not bound by race or socioeconomic status.

ETIOLOGY

Although the causes of autism are unknown, several theories concerning its causation have been postulated over the years. They include (1) inappropriate child-rearing and environmental stimuli; (2) heredi-

tary influences; and (3) organic disturbances related to physiologic, chemical, or neurologic abnormalities of the brain[1,11,51] A dysfunction of the reticular formation of the brain stem, producing a general state of arousal, has been implicated.[52,53]

MEDICAL MANAGEMENT

Infantile autism generally persists into adulthood. Many affected individuals also exhibit mental retardation and epilepsy. Approximately two-thirds to three-fourths of all autistic children can be expected to perform at some level of retardation throughout life; about 30% develop epilepsy.[54]

The signs and symptoms of autism are behavioral in nature and benefit from education, behavior modification, play, and speech therapy.[55] A structured learning environment coupled with social involvement in community activities is believed to be the most effective treatment available for autism.[11] Nevertheless, autism is rarely cured.

If overactive, aggressive, or self-injurious behavior is displayed by an individual with autism, psychotropic drugs might be indicated, but most authorities in the field prefer to use these medications as a last resort or as an adjunct to behavioral therapy.

OROFACIAL MANIFESTATIONS

Autistic persons do not exhibit any unique dental or oral soft tissue anomalies.[51] Patients with autism who have epilepsy might experience gingival hyperplasia from the medication phenytoin in conjunction with poor oral hygiene. The prevalence of dental caries might be slightly higher than in ordinary children because of several factors: a fixation on diet; a preference for soft, sweet-tasting foods; poor tongue coordination resulting in food retention;[1,51] poor manual dexterity interfering with oral hygiene practices; and the possibility of a drug-induced xerostomia elicited by psychotropic drug therapy.

DENTAL AND ORAL HYGIENE TREATMENT CONSIDERATIONS

The behavioral characteristics of autism present numerous challenges to the dental health educator. Although the tell, show, do method is generally an effective form of behavior modification, the dental health educator might experience difficulty with the tell and show aspects of instruction, primarily because the autistic child is impassive and opposes eye contact.

Suggested strategies for reaching the autistic child in a positive manner so that dental treatment can be accomplished include

1. *Rehearsals* should be conducted in the home by the parent to prepare the child for the dental appointment, and previsits to the dental office to get the child accustomed to the dental environment are helpful.[51]
2. *Eye contact* with the dental health educator should be reinforced by praise and tangible rewards such as unsweetened cereal. Brief periods of eye contact can be sustained if the dental health educator gently holds the child's chin and directs him so that they are face-to-face. Gradually longer intervals of eye contact must pass prior to reinforcement. If the child desires to be rewarded, he must wait while maintaining eye contact. This technique, referred to as shaping, is defined as the process of modifying an existing behavior by requiring successive approximations of the desired behavior before reinforcement is provided.[1]
3. *Constant repetition* of dental procedures is advised. Because the child relates to the repetition of words, the dental health educator might initiate the oral examination by playing a singing game such as "Now we are going to count your teeth, count your teeth, count your teeth."[49] The autistic child must be given instruction in small steps, giving him time to learn one concept before moving on to the next.[56]
4. *Consistency* in the dental environment to prevent the autistic child from becoming disturbed over alterations in his daily routine is highly recommended. In addition to the rehearsals outlined in #1, it is also important to keep dental appointments as consistent as possible. Therefore, when the autistic child returns to the dental office for subsequent appointments, he should see the same personnel, in the same operatory.
5. *Avoidance of loud voices and bright lights* is advised to prevent the child from getting upset and becoming unresponsive.
6. Use of *50% nitrous oxide–50% oxygen analgesia* has been reported as successful.[49,51] General anesthesia is usually chosen as a last resort for autistic persons with extensive dental needs, when all other attempts at routine therapy have failed.

Other Developmental Disorders

Other developmental disorders that might be of particular interest to the dental health educator because they possess orofacial manifestations include cleft lip and palate, mandibulofacial and craniofacial dysostosis, and ectodermal dysplasia.[1]

Cleft lip and palate affects 1:700 to 1:800 live births in the United States. Males are afflicted twice as often as females except for isolated clefts of the palate. If a cleft is unilateral, the left side is most common. In about half of the cases, clefts are associated with other developmental anomalies. Clefts can be classified as those involving either the primary palate (lip and alveolar process) or the secondary palate (hard, soft, and submucosal). Impaired speech, feeding, and swallowing imposed by the cleft can affect growth and development. Orodental characteristics can consist of facial defects, supernumerary teeth, missing teeth, malocclusion, poor muscle coordination, poor oral hygiene, caries, upper respiratory infections, and fever-induced hypoplasia.

Mandibulofacial dysostosis and craniofacial dysostosis are genetic defects that result in facial deformities affecting oral structure. In mandibulofacial dysostosis or Treacher Collins syndrome, the mouth has a fishlike appearance due to mandibular and zygomatic hypoplasia. Malocclusion and dental hypoplasia are common. Craniofacial dysostosis or Crouzon disease is the result of premature closure of the sutures of the skull. Crossbite, severe maxillary arch length deficiency, and a high narrow palatal vault are typical.

Ectodermal dysplasia is transmitted from mothers to their sons. This condition results in a deficiency of structures derived from ectoderm such as skin, mucosa, sweat glands, hair, and tooth enamel. Complete or partial anodontia with conical teeth is characteristic.

SENSORY DISABILITIES

Most people would agree that an individual's five senses are vital for communication and for normal existence. When an individual experiences a sensory disability such as deafness or blindness, the communication apparatus becomes impaired, but normal existence is still possible. An individual with a sensory deficit learns to rely on his remaining senses, which become highly acute to compensate for the loss.

Hearing Impairment

The term *hearing impaired* describes the individual who has defective but functional hearing, with or without the assistance of a hearing aid. *Deafness* refers to an inability to understand speech even with the use of a hearing device. Hearing impairment can be more accurately defined by the level of decibel loss, timing of the insult, and anatomic location of the defect.[1]

EPIDEMIOLOGY

In the U.S., approximately 14 million persons have hearing impairment.[57] Figures for those labeled deaf range from 13%[57] to 22%[58] of the total hearing-impaired population. In the latter study identifying a 22% overall deafness rate among hearing-impaired persons nationally, approximately 13% of this group were found to have lost their hearing before the age of 19.[58] One-third of the U.S. population over age 65 are considered hearing impaired.[12]

CLASSIFICATION

The intensity of sound is measured in decibels (dB), ranging from 1 to 100. Normal conversation at a distance of about 3 feet usually has an intensity of 60 dB. Hearing loss can be defined in terms of decibel loss as follows:[1,12]

Slight—a decibel loss in the 15 to 25 range; treatment is rarely necessary.
Partial—mild to moderate loss in the 30 to 65 decibel range; conversation is usually heard, but some amplification of sound can be helpful.
Severe—a decibel loss in the 65 to 95 range; conversations must be at close proximity to the affected person and must be spoken loudly. Severe hearing loss requires amplification and lip reading.
Profound—a decibel loss of 95 or above; speech is not heard even with amplification, but often a few sounds can be detected with a hearing aid. Training in lip reading and signing is advised.

Hearing loss can also be classified according to the time of the insult, which can occur prenatally, perinatally, or postnatally. The individual born with a hearing disability is said to have congenital hearing impairment; the individual who has an acquired disability is one who was born with normal hearing but whose hearing became impaired later in life.

The anatomic location of the defect is the third alternative for categorizing hearing loss. Conductive hearing loss results when injury or disease such as blocked eustachian tubes, allergies, or abnormalities that interfere with normal movement of the bones of the middle ear affect the conduction of sound waves through the outer and middle ear; the inner ear remains unaffected. Sensorineural hearing loss is usually developmental and results when the cochlea or cochlear nerves of the inner become damaged, inhibiting the transmission of heard messages to the brain. Consequently, speech discrimination also becomes impaired. Some individuals experience a combination of conductive and sensorineural hearing loss.[1,12]

ETIOLOGY

Numerous factors can damage the auditory mechanism. Prenatal and perinatal causal factors include (1) congenital anomalies, e.g., cleft palate, cerebral palsy, Down syndrome, and craniofacial anomalies that involve abnormal auditory nerve or ear structure;[59-61] (2) herpes simplex and cytomegalovirus infections, as well as rubella (maternal German measles infection of the fetus producing multiple congenital anomalies, e.g., hearing loss, visual impairments, mental retardation, and cardiac defects); (3) trauma or anoxia related to labor and delivery; (4) prematurity; (5) blood incompatabilities such as Rh factor (which is declining due to the Rhogam vaccine); (6) heredity (only 10% of hearing-impaired children are born to hearing-impaired parents);[62] and (7) unknown causes. Postnatal causes usually consist of (1) heredity; (2) infections, particularly chronic otitis media, high fevers, meningitis, or mumps; (3) trauma; (4) drugs; (5) cortical lesions; (6) environment such as prolonged exposure to a noisy atmosphere; and (7) aging.[63] Meniere's disease, which begins during middle age, is characterized by hearing loss and vertigo.[1]

MEDICAL MANAGEMENT

Treatment is usually determined on the basis of type and degree of hearing loss and patient age at onset. It includes modalities such as surgery, amplification by use of a hearing aid, and educational programs designed to teach communication skills, e.g., speech, written and diagrammatic language, lip-reading, sign language or manual communication, and use of a telecommunications device.

Lip-reading is one of the most difficult forms of communication and is only about 26% efficient.[64] Many words and sounds look similar on the lips and require intense concentration to discern. Words can also be camouflaged by facial gestures or moustache hair.

American sign language (ASL) is the major form of communication among the deaf in the United States.[65] Sign language consists of both fingerspelling (26 signs, one for each letter of the alphabet, with each word spelled out; see Fig. 8-22[66]) and signing. Fingerspelling is a supplement to signing. Signing is the portrayal of words, such as depicting cold by shivering. Another aid to communication for the hearing-impaired is the teletypewriter (TTY) or telecommunications device (TDD). These machines enable the person to communicate over the phone providing both participants have the device. TDD permits the transmission of written communication. The message is displayed on a screen, allowing the individual freedom of communication without assistance.

OROFACIAL MANIFESTATIONS

Dental defects are rarely directly associated with hearing impairments but have been reported in patients who exhibit hearing loss related to such conditions as cleft lip and palate, ectodermal dysplasia, prematurity, and rubella. It is also common for individuals with sensory disabilities to grind their teeth. Bruxism might serve as a source of stimulation to replace that which is lacking as a result of the sensory deficit.

DENTAL AND ORAL HYGIENE TREATMENT CONSIDERATIONS

When a patient with hearing loss is scheduled for a dental appointment it is important for the dental health educator to obtain information regarding type, severity, and age

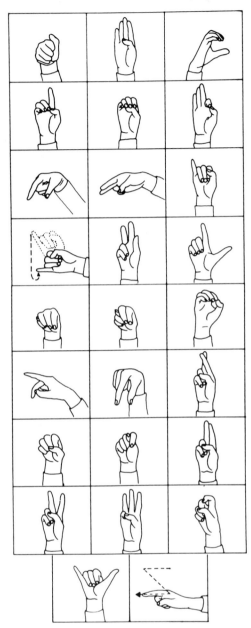

Figure 8-22. American Manual Alphabet. From Riekehof, L. L.: The Joy of Signing. 2nd Ed. Springfield, MO, Gospel Publishing House, 1987.

health educator does not know how to sign, the educator should become familiar with some basic signs prior to the dental appointment e.g., open, close, brushing, flossing, daily, radiographs (Figs. 8-23 and 8-24).[67] Signing should always be accompanied by the verbal counterpart for the symbol. Diagrams drawn in advance or pictures that represent possible complications of an undesired behavior (e.g., smokeless tobacco use) or a sequence of treatment (e.g., implant procedures) are ideal supplements to written messages. If one is totally unprepared, a pad and pencil can serve as the major tools for communication.

Whatever the form of communication, the

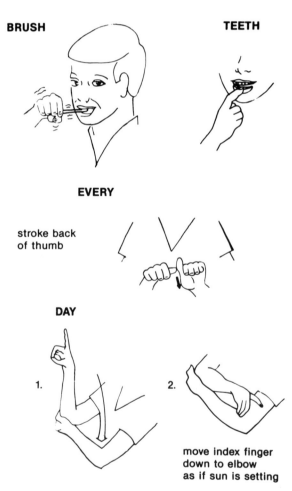

Figure 8-23. Sign language for instructing the hearing-impaired patient to brush his teeth every day. From Mueller, K., and Gantt, D.: Communicating with the deaf patient. J. Dent. Handic., 3:22–25, 1978.

at onset of the hearing impairment. Determining how the individual communicates will assist the dental health educator in preparing a plan that will enhance the dialogue between the two parties.

If sign language is the patient's preferred method of communication and the dental

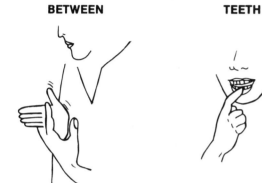

USE

move hand in
vertical circles

FLOSS

wiggle little finger
out from fist

BETWEEN

TEETH

wiggle hand sideways
between fingers

Figure 8-24. Sign language for instructing the hearing impaired patient to use floss between his teeth. From Mueller, K., and Gantt, D.: Communicating with the deaf patient. J. Dent. Handic., 3:22–25, 1978.

dental health educator must observe certain guidelines when caring for an hearing-impaired patient:[1,68-70]

1. Relax and don't panic; a kind and patient demeanor is most helpful for making the individual feel comfortable in the dental environment.
2. If the patient has had limited dental experience, allow him to observe another patient in the office who is having a similar procedure done.
3. Alert the staff as to the patient's communication skills and make a notation in the chart.
4. Avoid communication in front of a window or bright light to prevent glare in the patient's eyes; the speaker's mouth should be completely visible during communication.
5. Speak naturally; voice volume should not be increased or exaggerated by excessive, pronounced lip movements.
6. Keep communication accurate yet simple.
7. Communicate with a pencil and paper when wearing a mask.
8. Avoid background noise, particularly when conversing. Hearing aids should be removed or the volume decreased during treatment.
9. Never talk about the patient in his presence without including him.
10. Recommend the patient bring an interpreter if the necessary communication skills to interact effectively with the patient are inadequate; smooth-flowing dialogue enhances the rapport between practitioner and patient. As the relationship develops, the interpreter should assume a more passive role.
11. Tell, show, do should be used consistently throughout treatment to keep the patient aware of events before they occur so as not to startle him.
12. Send the patient home with written instructions and follow-up appointment cards to alleviate the possibility of missed information by the patient during the appointment.
13. Give the patient the opportunity to ask questions before the conclusion of the appointment.

Resources for deaf persons can be found in Appendix G.[10,57]

Visual Impairments

Unlike the hearing-impaired, the visually impaired person is more readily recognizable because of the white cane he might carry, the dark glasses he might wear, or the guide dog that might accompany him.

Limitations in sight range from a slight impairment in vision to complete blindness with no perception of light.[69] A person is considered legally blind when even after the best optical correction he sees at 20 feet what a person with normal vision can see at 200 feet (a visual acuity of 20/200). Legal blindness also refers to alterations in peripheral vision in which the visual field is no wider than 20°. Visually impaired refers to the person who has some loss of peripheral vision or a visual acuity of no better than 20/70 in the best eye after optical correction.[12,71]

CLASSIFICATION

Vision disorders can take numerous forms. They include (1) amblyopia—dimness of vision from nonuse of eyes, (2) aniseikonia—a difference in the size and shape of an image perceived by each eye, (3) astigmatism—distortion resulting from imperfect curvature of the cornea, (4) cataract—an opacity of the lens causing a blockage of light perception, (5) color blindness—inability to distinguish one or more primary colors, (6) diplopia—double vision, (7) glaucoma—partial or total blindness resulting from intensive destructive pressure of fluids inside the eye, (8) hyperopia—farsightedness, (9) macula degeneration—loss of central vision, (10) myopia—nearsightedness, (11) nyctalopia—night blindness, (12) retinitis pigmentosa—degeneration of the retina causing an inability of the eye to transmit images to the brain, and (13) transient blindness—temporary blindness resulting from fluctuations in the blood pressure of the ophthalmic arteries.

EPIDEMIOLOGY

Presently, 1.4 million Americans suffer from severe visual impairments. Approximately 450,000 of these persons are considered legally blind. About half of the blind population are over 60 years of age, and 10% are school-age or younger. Approximately 70% of individuals 65 years or older have visual impairments, which prevent many of these senior citizens from performing routine activities e.g., reading and driving. About 20% of preschool and school-age children have some form or degree of visual defect; most are correctable.[10,11,12,71,72]

ETIOLOGY

The major causes of blindness can also be subdivided into prenatal and postnatal categories. Prenatal etiologic factors include (1) optic atrophy; (2) microphthalmus (1 and 2 are congenital brain defects); (3) cataracts; (4) colobamata (a developmental clefting of ocular tissue); (5) dermoid and other tumors; (6) toxoplasmosis (a parasitic infection); (7) cytomegalic inclusion disease (CID), a viral infection; (8) syphilis; (9) rubella; (10) tuberculous meningitis; (11) prematurity; and (12) development anomalies of the orbit frequently associated with syndromes. Postnatal causes include (1) trauma; (2) retrolental fibroplasia (hemorrhage of the retinal blood vessels leading to fibrosis, retinal detachment, and blindness in an infant exposed to high concentrations of oxygen during incubation); (3) hypertension; (4) diabetes mellitus; (5) leukemia; (6) polycythemia; (7) hemorrhagic disorders; (8) glaucoma; and (9) cataracts.

The leading causes of blindness in the United States are macular degeneration, retinal hemorrhages secondary to diabetes, glaucoma, and senile cataracts.[1]

MEDICAL MANAGEMENT

The prognosis of acquired vision disorders is usually better with early diagnosis and treatment. Routine eye examinations, safety glasses at worksites where eye injuries are common, and immediate medical intervention when an injury or infection arises are recommended preventive measures.

The goal of treatment is to improve sight and stop the progression of an impairment. Surgery, drugs, and corrective lenses are the standard modes of treatment available. Approximately 95% of cataracts are effectively treated by surgical procedures, which include ultrasound and lens implants. Glaucoma is usually managed by drugs, surgery, or both.

Educational programs for the blind and visually impaired have largely been designed on the basis of the age of onset of the person's disability. A child born blind learns

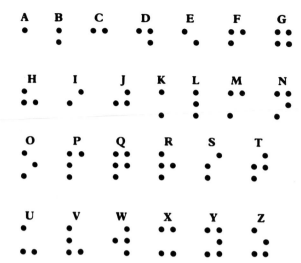

Figure 8-25. Braille. Dots are arranged in various combinations, creating patterns that represent letters of the alphabet. From Braille, Lewis, 1829, Academic American Encyclopedia. Princeton, NJ, Arete Publishing Co., 1981, Vol. 3, p. 442.

differently from an adult who acquired blindness as a result of an accident, for example. Programs usually teach visual concepts through auditory instruction, memory, and reliance on the tactile and other senses. Auditory instruction involves the use of audiocassette tapes and personalized voice-guided directives. Memory is only useful to the individual with acquired blindness because a person born blind has no repertoire of visual images from which to draw. Shape conception and recognition of the part–whole relationship is more complex and takes longer for the blind child to comprehend, unless he can identify with a significant object from his past experiences.[73] Therefore, educators must be creative and articulate when describing an object or procedure. Training in the tactile sense includes the use of Braille (a system of raised dots) for reading, writing, and typing[12] (see Fig. 8-25).[10]

OROFACIAL MANIFESTATIONS

The visually impaired tend to experience dental related anomalies at the same rate as the normal population, unless the vision disorder is associated with one or more developmental disabilities.[1] The rate of periodontal disease and trauma might be higher in the visually impaired because of inadequate oral hygiene and difficulties in ambulation, respectively.[74,75]

DENTAL AND ORAL HYGIENE TREATMENT CONSIDERATIONS

When a patient with a vision disorder is scheduled for a dental appointment, it is important for the dental health educator to determine the degree of the impairment, age at onset, existence of any other significant medical conditions, and the patient's degree of independence (if a child, the type of schooling). Over half of all blind children in the United States are mainstreamed into regular classrooms and receive supplemental services through resource rooms and itinerant teachers. Ten percent of the blind population currently uses Braille.[12]

Children with congenital blindness can have a difficult time with socialization. Many are overprotected by parents and become introverted, exhibiting stereotypic behaviors such as rocking or eye-pressing. These children can be dental management problems. A previsit to the dental office is advised. Parents or caregivers are encouraged to begin looking into and cleaning the child's mouth early. Instituting regular home care procedures is essential for emphasizing the importance of office instruction in the prevention of disease and helping the child adjust to the dental environment.

Dental health education aimed at teaching the blind is not simple. For example, conventional methods for teaching oral hygiene such as disclosing plaque, toothbrushing, and flossing, are based on visual cues. Thin accumulations of plaque can be made dramatic by the assistance of disclosing solution, but without this visual cue or memory of it, collections of plaque must be sufficient to be felt with the tongue. Outside the mouth, models of teeth coated with a sticky substance can be used to simulate plaque for the blind patient to touch.[72,76] Fabrics such as felt or burlap and raised label markers can also be used as tactile aids to support the notion of plaque, particularly when compared to silk or paper used to mimic a clean tooth surface. Toothbrushing to music or directional audiotapes are helpful guides to teach sequencing to assure that no areas of the mouth are missed.[77] As the patient practices toothbrushing in his own mouth, the dental health educator should place his hand over the patient's hand to offer guidance while describing proper technique. Flossing can be taught by pretending the spaces between the fingers on the patient's hand are the interdental spaces.[78]

The dental health educator should follow certain guidelines when caring for the visually impaired patient. They include[12,69,79]

1. Greet the patient and introduce him to the dental staff and his new surroundings by acclimating him to the layout of the waiting room, operatory, and restrooms, including placement of furniture.
2. Lead the patient by standing slightly in front of him and allowing him to hold onto a bent arm, usually near the elbow.
3. Indicate changing floor textures, turns, or obstacles in the pathway ahead.
4. Prepare the patient to be seated by removing all tray tables, lights, and chairs in his way and guiding his hands over the back, arm, and seat of the chair; allow him to seat himself.
5. Ask the patient who is accompanied by a guide dog where he would like him to stay; the corner of the operatory is advised.
6. Determine if the patient is light-sensitive, and if so, watch the placement of the unit light.
7. Avoid loud noises and announce the use of motor-driven equipment so the patient is not startled.
8. Do not speak to the patient in a loud voice as if he were deaf; speak normally and talk directly to him.
9. Be patient and verbally reassuring.
10. Describe each procedure step-by-step, incorporating the senses of taste, smell, and touch to illustrate a procedure (e.g., the smell of the rubber base, the taste of flavored polishing paste, and the feel of air on the patient's hand before the teeth are air-dried). The awareness of tactile quality can be enhanced by textures, temperatures, vibrating surfaces, and different consistencies.[74]
11. Give the partially sighted patient his glasses before beginning instruction; the glaucoma patient with poor peripheral vision requires instruction directly in front of him.
12. Changing chair positions and moving away from the patient require an explanation; speak before touching or moving the patient.

Resources for the blind patient are located in Appendix H.[10,72]

ORTHOPEDIC, CENTRAL NERVOUS SYSTEM, AND MUSCULAR DISORDERS

Disorders that affect bones, the spinal cord, or muscles can be debilitating. Although the origins of these types of ailments are different, they all exhibit deformities and motor dysfunctions that require the use of adaptive devices, body supports, and wheelchairs. Spinal cord injuries, multiple sclerosis, and muscular dystrophy have been chosen to represent this particular category of disabilities.

Spinal Cord Injuries

An individual's lifestyle changes drastically when an injury to the spinal cord results in paralysis. Paralysis occurs due to lack of blood supply to the nerve cells and pressure on the cord. Both movement and sensation are affected by paralysis. Damage to the thoracic, lumbar, or sacral vertebrae causes paraplegia. Quadriplegia results when an injury damages the cervical portion of the vertebral column.[12]

EPIDEMIOLOGY

Some 200,000 Americans are confined to wheelchairs as a result of spinal cord injuries. Approximately 10,000 new injuries occur annually in the United States. Of these, approximately 80% involve males, averaging 19 years of age.[11]

CLASSIFICATION

Spinal cord injuries are classified in two ways: (1) by the level of damage at the site on the vertebral column that corresponds to the last undamaged portion on the spinal cord and (2) by the relationship between the skeletal site of damage and the most distant intact cord segment. Cord damage can result above or below the level of bone injury.[12]

ETIOLOGY

Approximately 50% of all spinal cord injuries are caused by motorcycle or automobile accidents. Nearly 4 million people are involved in motor vehicle accidents each year. Safety belts can prevent 40 to 60% of injuries and deaths. Safety helmets can prevent up to 80% of head injuries for cyclists.[80] Occupational accidents are the second leading cause of spinal cord injuries, accounting for about 25% of them. Approximately 20% of spinal cord injuries result from sports such as diving, football, and gymnastics; the remaining 5% are accounted for by falls or violence such as gunshot wounds or stabbings.[11,81]

MEDICAL MANAGEMENT

The team approach to rehabilitation is used to manage the individual needs of each spinal cord injury patient. Coping with the shock of paralysis takes a long time for some people. Professional and family support is paramount, and psychologic counseling might be required as part of the patient's total rehabilitation program. Occupational, recreational, and physical therapists are instrumental in assisting the patient with mobility through exercise and the use of adaptive devices, socialization, and return to the workplace. Treatment for spasticity includes exercise as well as drug therapy.

If paralysis of the intercostal muscles also exists, the services of a respiratory therapist must be sought to ease breathing. Gastrointestinal disturbances can require the aid of a dietician to make dietary modifications. Bowel and bladder problems are also common and can necessitate drug therapy, the insertion of indwelling catheters, and sometimes the creation of a colostomy (a surgical opening through the abdominal wall to allow for the emptying of fecal material).[12]

OROFACIAL MANIFESTATIONS

Individuals who are paraplegic have the same dental concerns as the average person. Because their paralysis is from the waist down their disability poses no particular obstacle to the performance of oral care procedures. The hemiplegic patient, paralyzed unilaterally as the result of stroke, can experience numbness of the face on the affected side. If he avoids eating on that side and practices minimal oral hygiene, food debris will tend to collect inadvertently in the vestibule due to poor control of the oral musculature. Consequently the hemiplegic patient is more susceptible to periodontal disease. Quadriplegics have even greater difficulties establishing adequate oral hygiene practices because of their more generalized loss of voluntary function.[30]

DENTAL AND ORAL HYGIENE TREATMENT CONSIDERATIONS

A patient who has just had a spinal cord injury will require the services of the hospital dental staff for several reasons. First, such an injury can involve the immobilization of a fractured jaw. Fractures can be sim-

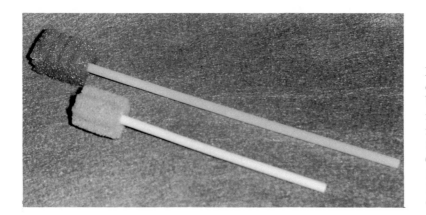

Figure 8-26. Oral sponges on a stick are ideal for swabbing the oral mucosa and removing plaque and debris from the teeth. Upper, Ora-Swab, Sage Products, Inc. 680 Industrial Drive, Cary, IL 60013. Lower, Toothette, Halbrand Inc., Willoughby, OH 44094.

ple or compound, and their treatment consists of (1) reduction (bringing together the two sides of the fracture); (2) fixation (stabilizing the fracture in the healing position with some type of apparatus); and (3) immobilization of the jaw. Uncomplicated fractures usually heal in 4 to 6 weeks. Infection poses the major complication to the patient. If feasible, an oral prophylaxis should be performed prior to wiring or placement of metal or acrylic splints.

Second, to prevent plaque accumulation and subsequent tissue irritation and infection during the treatment phase, the dental health educator should teach the patient how to clean his mouth with his jaws wired closed. Saline or chlorhexidine gluconate irrigation is often recommended, followed by fluoride rinses at bedtime. Toothbrushing

might be difficult at first due to sensitivity. A toothette (oral sponge) can be helpful initially (Fig. 8-26), followed by use of a suction toothbrush to simultaneously clean the teeth and remove oral secretions. This type of brush eliminates the fear of aspiration while performing oral care (Fig. 8-27).[69] Some patients may be able to use an interdental brush if they have adequate interproximal spacing.

Third, the dental health educator should assist the patient with his nutritional needs, teaching him how and what to eat. Adequate nutrition is necessary for healing and resisting infection. Spoon, straw (sucked through retromolar pad area or an edentulous area), or nasogastric tube (nose-to-stomach) feedings are available methods based on the extent of the patient's injury. Liquids

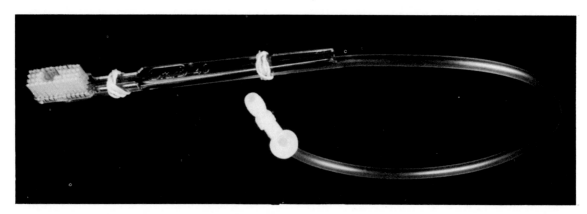

Figure 8-27. Suction toothbrush. Suction catheter tubing, attached to a suction device, is inserted through a hole in the head of a toothbrush. A suction toothbrush permits simultaneous plaque removal and evacuation of oral fluids.

(e.g., juices, milk), baby foods, and pureed table foods are advised. Liquid supplements are rich in vitamins, minerals, and calories and can be added to foods to thin them, or they can be ingested alone. Cariogenic foodstuffs must be avoided.

Fourth, when the patient's wires or splints have been removed, another oral prophylaxis is required. It is especially important to assess the lingual surfaces of the teeth. Continuing the fluoride regimen (dentifrice and mouthrinse or brush-on gel) is also suggested.[69]

Fifth, if the patient's injury has also resulted in some degree of paralysis, accomplishing his oral hygiene tasks will require a great deal of instruction and supervision by the dental staff. A task analysis that subdivides the task of toothbrushing into various components is extremely useful in determining at what point the spinal cord injury patient is experiencing difficulty, and what changes can be made to help him attain the complete behavior (Table 8-5).[12] The dental health educator can also prepare inservice programs for caregivers of dependent patients to implement at institutions for the mentally and physically disabled (Table 8-6).[82] This particular program focuses on the caregivers' ability to adequately remove plaque from their own mouths prior to performing these procedures on their clients.

C1-C4 quadriplegics are totally dependent on their caregivers for oral hygiene procedures. Many of these individuals possess normal intelligence and prefer to be as independent as possible. A dental care unit developed at the University of Mississippi was designed to eliminate the severely disabled individual's reliance on others for oral hygiene care (see Fig. 8-28).[83] Nonfoaming toothpastes (e.g., Nasadent) are recommended due to the patient's compromised respirations, cough, and gag reflex.

The sixth task of the dental health educator is the fabrication of a durable bitestick appliance that is not harmful to the occlusion for patients who rely on their mouths as important tools for performing daily functions. A variety of functional tips can be adapted to the bitestick to permit grasping objects, typing, or dialing a phone (Fig. 8-

Table 8-5. Task Analysis for Toothbrushing

The resident should
 1. Choose own toothbrush from the designated area
 2. Hold toothbrush in dominant hand
 3. Turn faucet on
 4. Wet toothbrush bristles
 5. Uncap toothpaste
 6. Spread paste on toothbrush bristles
 7. Grasp toothbrush
 8. Open mouth
 9. Place bristles against outside surface of upper left back teeth and move toothbrush in a small scrubbing motion to a count of 10
10. Place bristles against outside surface of upper left corner teeth and move toothbrush in a small scrubbing motion to a count of 10
11. Place bristles against outside surface of upper front teeth and move toothbrush in a small scrubbing motion to a count of 10
12. Place bristles against outside surface of right upper corner teeth and move toothbrush in a small scrubbing motion to a count of 10
13. Place bristles against outside surface of right upper back teeth and move toothbrush in a small scrubbing motion to a count of 10
14. Repeat steps 9–13 for inside surfaces of upper teeth
    a. Left back
    b. Left corner
    c. Front
    d. Right corner
    e. Right back
15. Repeat steps 9–13 for outside surfaces of lower teeth
16. Repeat steps 9–13 for inside surfaces of lower teeth
17. Places toothbrush on biting surfaces of left lower teeth
18. Moves toothbrush in push-pull motion across biting surfaces of left lower teeth
19. Repeat steps 17–18 for biting surfaces of right lower teeth
20. Repeat steps 17–18 for biting surfaces of right upper teeth
21. Repeat steps 17–18 for biting surfaces of left upper teeth
22. Remove brush from mouth
23. Expectorate excess dentifrice
24. Rinse mouth
25. Rinse toothbrush
26. Return brush to designated area
27. Turn off faucet
28. Recap toothpaste tube
29. Dry mouth and hands

Table 8-6. Strategy for Implementing a Dental Health Program for the Institutionalized Disabled

I. In-service training of unit personnel
  A. Pretest
     Slide-lecture presentation
     Demonstration of personal oral hygiene
  B. Evaluation of personal oral hygiene
     Demonstration of adaptive techniques for delivery of preventive dental procedures to institutionalized residents
  C. Evaluation of staff oral hygiene competency on residents at site
     Demonstration of fluoride gel application
     Post-test
  D. Graduates of training program establish similar training programs for other staff
II. Nutritional dental counseling to dietary personnel and psychologists
  A. Decrease frequency of ingestion of cariogenic foodstuffs
  B. Substitute more appropriate food tokens for behavior modification programs
III. Dental referral service for residents requiring comprehensive care

29).[84,85] This device allows the patient some degree of self-sufficiency. As is the case with any oral appliance, it is necessary to clean and soak the mouthpiece portion of the bitestick when it is not in use.

A final consideration for the dental health educator is movement of the patient confined to a wheelchair. As discussed previously, specific attachments can be connected to the wheelchair itself. When these are not available, it becomes necessary to transport the patient from the wheelchair to the dental chair. Wheelchair transfer can be accomplished by several techniques.[15,86]

1. Slide-board transfer
   a. Place wheelchair and dental chair as close together as possible; if patient is hemiplegic, position dental chair to his strong side.
   b. Adjust height of dental chair to correspond with height of wheelchair.
   c. Set brakes of wheelchair.
   d. Remove siding from the wheelchair on the side next to dental chair.
   e. Raise dental chair arm.
   f. Move footrests out of the way.
   g. Place slide board under the patient with the midpoint of the board at the junction of the wheelchair and dental chair. (The slide or transfer board is usually a beveled board 18 inches long and $\frac{3}{8}$ to $\frac{1}{2}$ inches thick.)
   h. Support wheelchair from slipping while patient transfers himself.
   i. Place patient's legs into position in the dental chair once he has completed the transfer.
2. One-person transfer
   a. Place the wheelchair at approximately a 30° angle to the dental chair to facilitate pivotal motion during the transfer.
      Repeat steps b through f for slide-board transfer.
   g. Block the patient's knee closest to the dental chair with your knees and the same foot with your foot closest to the dental chair.
   h. Have the patient place his hands around your neck while you grab him around the waist or by the belt.
   i. On the count of 3 have the patient stand, using his blocked knee as a pivot.
   j. Slowly pivot in the direction of the dental chair and let the patient down into it.
   k. Place the patient's legs and body in proper position in the chair.
3. Two-person transfer
      Repeat steps a through f for slide-board transfer.
   g. Remove top of headrest on dental chair.
   h. One person approaches the patient from behind, having the patient cross his arms if possible; place your arms under the patient's armpits and grab the *opposite* wrist of each hand.
   i. The second person is responsible for lifting and guiding the lower limbs. All lifting must be done with the legs, not the back, by bending at the knees.
   j. On the count of 3 ask the patient to pull his elbows into his body, and both persons doing the transfer lift the patient straight up. *Stop* for a second

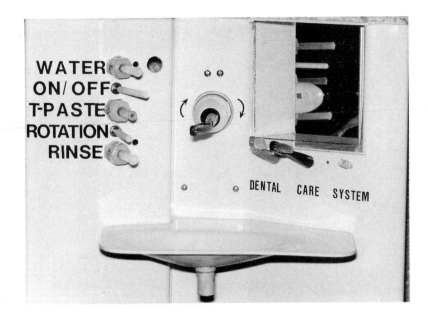

Figure 8-28. The University of Mississippi dental care system, a toothbrushing apparatus that enables the paralyzed patient to dispense toothpaste and water and brush his teeth with minimal motion. The patient selects a brush, pulls it from the holder, and installs it on the powerhead with his teeth. From Fitchie, J.G., et al.: Oral hygiene for the severely handicapped: Clinical evaluation of the University of Mississippi dental care system. Sp. Care Dent., 8:260–264, 1988.

before you move laterally to the dental chair to maximize patient position and your balance.

k. Move laterally to the dental chair, making sure to clear any obstacles, and lower the patient.

Patients should always be transferred toward their strongest side. The dental health educator can use a transfer belt to support the patient. When it is fastened around the patient's waist and gripped tightly during transfer, it provides added security if the patient begins to fall. The dental health educator should also check to see if the patient has a catheter strapped to his leg or the wheelchair. The tubing should not be twisted or bent, and the bag must be placed below the level of the patient's bladder to allow the urine to drain.

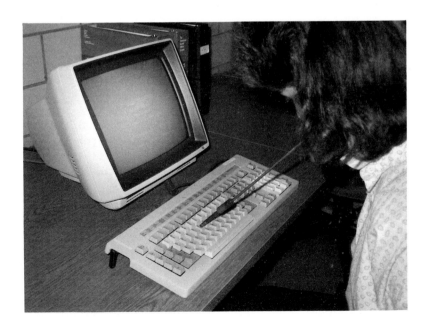

Figure 8-29. A bitestick appliance used to operate a computer; a variety of other functions are made possible for the quadriplegic patient with its use.

Multiple Sclerosis

Multiple sclerosis (MS) is a chronic degenerative disease of the white matter or myelin tissue of the central nervous system. Myelin is the fatty coating around nerve fibers, which acts as an insulator. Multiple sclerosis causes portions of the myelin sheath to be destroyed. These areas of destruction are replaced with sclerotic tissue known as plaque. Plaques accumulate until the nerve becomes permanently damaged and the conduction of nerve impulses is disrupted. MS is classified as a progressive disease, but its course can range from minimal impairment through life to rapid progression of the disease in a short time span leading to regression of neural function and death. The aggression of plaque has no particular time clock or sequence. Symptoms vary depending on the location of the lesions caused by plaques in the cerebrum, brain stem, or spinal cord.[11] Over 70% of patients experience paresthesia, which is frequently associated with the trigeminal and facial nerves. A loss of central vision also occurs in about 25% of patients. Balance abnormalities, urinary incontinence, and disruptions in thinking and behavior can also exist.[11] The course of the disease tends to oscillate between exacerbation and remission, each new attack of the disease increasing in severity. Factors which stimulate attacks include infection, stress, injury, heavy exercise or fatigue, and pregnancy.[69]

EPIDEMIOLOGY

Approximately 500,000 Americans are believed to have multiple sclerosis. The majority (95%) of individuals afflicted with multiple sclerosis are between the ages of 10 and 50 years. The mean onset is approximately 30 years of age.[11,12] Females tend to be affected more frequently than males at a ratio of 1.5:1.[87] The prevalence of MS is higher in those born and raised in the northern states.[11,12]

ETIOLOGY

There is no known cause for multiple sclerosis. Heredity, viral pathogens, and an autoimmune reaction have been implicated as possible causes, but sufficient data to support them is not currently available.[11,12]

MEDICAL MANAGEMENT

There is no cure for MS. Prednisone and adrenocortical stimulating hormone (ACTH) have demonstrated effectiveness, particularly in the relief of spastic movements and visual disturbances. When paresthesia becomes a problem, anticonvulsant drugs are prescribed. Basically the patient is told to rest and get regular exercise to maintain strength. Therapy focuses on preventing complications and potentiating residual function.[11] Psychologic and genetic counseling should not be overlooked in the comprehensive care of the MS patient.

OROFACIAL MANIFESTATIONS

The oral symptoms encountered by the MS patient are often the result of the medications prescribed. Trigeminal neuralgia is common, but it should not be assumed when the patient complains of facial pain. Advanced caries and periodontal disease can create similar pain sensations.

DENTAL AND ORAL HYGIENE TREATMENT CONSIDERATIONS

Treatment must be planned for each MS patient on the basis of his medical history findings, his dental health needs, and the degree of his disability. Short appointments might be necessary if the patient fatigues easily. Special dental considerations might not be required if the patient exhibits minimal symptoms of the disease. On the other hand, the quadriplegic patient with multiple sclerosis requires the same management considerations as outlined in the previous section on spinal cord injuries.

The dental health educator must inform the patient concerning the role infection plays in exacerbating multiple sclerosis. The patient must practice meticulous oral hygiene to reduce the risk of infection. Instruction in home care procedures should be individualized to accommodate the patient's hand strength and coordination.

Muscle weakness can compromise swallowing. The dental chair should be adjusted, a rubber dam used, and frequent evacuation employed to prevent gagging. A mouth prop might be indicated for a lengthy procedure so that the patient can maintain his mouth comfortably in the open position while permitting the operator easy access.[12]

Muscular Dystrophy

Muscular dystrophy is a conglomeration of several chronic diseases involving atrophy of the skeletal (striated) muscles. After a sufficient degree of atrophy results, the patient begins to exhibit a deformity with subsequent disability. The sequence of degeneration does not vary, but the rate of progression and the age of onset distinguish one form of the disease from another. Degeneration occurs in the following order: (1) swelling of affected muscle cells, (2) destruction of striated bands wrapped around skeletal muscles, (3) homogeneous cytoplasm, and (4) fatty deposition replacing muscle tissue.[12]

EPIDEMIOLOGY AND CLASSIFICATION

Approximately 200,000 people in the U.S. have muscular dystrophy of some type. Over 50% of muscular dystrophy patients are between 4 and 15 years of age. The three most common forms of the disease are Duchenne dystrophy, limb-girdle dystrophy, and fascioscapulohumeral dystrophy.[12,69,88]

The Duchenne type (also referred to in the past as pseudohypertrophic muscular dystrophy and juvenile dystrophy) affects about 270 out of every 1 million live male births. Males are most frequently afflicted because Duchenne dystrophy is transmitted by a sex-linked recessive factor (mothers are carriers). Duchenne dystrophy is the most debilitating form of muscular dystrophy and commonly becomes evident by the age of 3. It is characterized by weakness, which begins in the pelvis, abdomen, hip, and spine, spreads to the trunk area, and eventually involves all of the child's extremities. The child is unable to keep up with peers in regard to walking, running, and muscular coordination. As the disease progresses, falls occur frequently, a waddling gait and lumbar lordosis are noticed, the child walks on his toes, thereby enlarging the calf muscles, and he must get up from the prone position by "tripoding" or walking up his thighs with his hands (Gowers' sign). Confinement to a wheelchair usually becomes necessary. Death often results from respiratory infection or failure during mid adolescence. Congestive heart failure can exist, but it is rarely the cause of death.

Limb-girdle dystrophy is a form of muscular dystrophy that typically affects the pelvic girdle first, followed by weakness in the shoulder girdle. Limb-girdle dystrophy is inherited through an autosomal recessive trait (both parents carry the gene); therefore both male and female offspring have a 25% chance of inheriting the disease and a 50% chance of being carriers. This form of dystrophy occurs in approximately 65 out of every 1 million live births. Although most individuals are diagnosed in their twenties, the onset of this disease can occur between the first and fifth decades of life.

Fascioscapulohumeral dystrophy, as the name describes, affects the muscles of the face, shoulders, and upper arms. A general impairment of facial expressions is observed initially. The patient experiences difficulty frowning, whistling, and fully closing the eyelids and lips. This form of dystrophy is normally transmitted as an autosomal dominant trait (one parent carries the gene); each child therefore has a 50% chance of developing the disease. Symptoms usually emerge around puberty and occur in about 4 persons per 1 million live births.

ETIOLOGY

The cause of muscular dystrophy remains unknown. Researchers believe that the defect in all dystrophies might be biochemical in nature.

MEDICAL MANAGEMENT

As with most developmental disabilities, the team approach to care of the patient with muscular dystrophy is advised. Drug therapy involves treating the symptoms of the disease, but no medication has been found to arrest the progression of the disorder. To date, exercise and adaptive braces or supports are recommended to treat muscular dystrophy. Speech and oral myofunctional therapies are particularly useful for patients with fascioscapulohumeral dystrophy.

OROFACIAL MANIFESTATIONS

A loss of strength in the muscles of mastication and a diminished biting force are characteristic of all forms of muscular dystrophy, to varying degrees.[89,90] As a result, speech can be nasal and poorly articulated,[91] and foods are often eaten more slowly because the patient can only exert a maximum of 20 pounds of pressure on the molars.[92] Because the lips cannot be fully closed, mouth-breathing is common. Clinical reports also suggest a high incidence of openbite and an overexpanded maxilla in these patients.[93-98] Pseudohypertrophy of the orbicularis oris muscle gives the lips of a patient with fascioscapulohumeral muscular dystrophy a thickened or swollen appearance.[1] The occlusal disharmonies described can increase the muscular dystrophy patient's susceptibility to periodontal disease and caries.

DENTAL AND ORAL HYGIENE TREATMENT CONSIDERATIONS

In the early stages of muscular dystrophy, the approach to dental care is relatively routine. Moderate to severe impairment can result in dysfunction of the oral musculature and imbalance of the neck and trunk muscles. Securing the patient by cradling his head, using a mouth prop, repositioning the dental chair, and employing seatbelts or pillows are ideal methods for stabilization during dental treatment. Patients with chronic respiratory or cardiac problems are more comfortable in a semi-upright position. The airway should be protected by the use of a rubber dam and frequent evacuation. Foamy toothpastes and fluoride gel tray applications are contraindicated for patients experiencing respiratory congestion. Safety glasses should be provided for patients with eyelid weakness prohibiting complete closure of the eyes.

Toothbrushes and other oral hygiene implements should be adapted to the patient's range of motion and muscle strength. In addition to proper oral hygiene, the dental health educator must stress the importance of nutrition in preventing dental disease. Soft foods that are consumed because of impaired masticatory strength can be retained around the teeth and in the vestibule. To reduce the patient's risk of decay and periodontal disease, the dental health educator should recommend (1) food debris removal by employing more frequent brushing and rinsing techniques; (2) daily topical fluoride supplementation; and (3) a diet that is soft in consistency but low in fermentable carbohydrates.

If the patient's speech is so impaired that he is unintelligible, communication through written messages is suggested. The dental health educator who displays patience and understanding will ease the frustations felt by the individual with muscular dystrophy. Consequently, effective communication and treatment will ensue.

LEARNING DISABILITIES

The label learning disabled (LD) is given to children who exhibit severe difficulties learning. The federal government adopted the following definition under Public Law 94-142 in 1977:[99]

"Specific learning disability" means a disorder in one or more of the basic psychological processes involved in understanding or in using language, spoken or written, which may manifest itself in an imperfect ability to listen, think, speak, read, write, spell, or to do mathematical calculations. The term includes such conditions as perceptual handicaps, brain injury, minimal brain dysfunction, dyslexia, and developmental aphasia. The term does not include children who have learning problems which are primarily the result of visual, hearing, or motor handicaps, or mental retardation, or of environmental, cultural, or economic disadvantage.

Basically a discrepancy exists between the child's level of achievement, and his age and ability level as documented by an intelligence test and the provision of appropriate learning experiences. Signs associated with a learning disability may include

1. Disorganized work habits—messy, unsystematic
2. Inability to complete work tasks
3. Appears not to be listening to what you are saying
4. Approaches tasks impulsively
5. General air of anxiousness—knows something is wrong and can't deal with it—develops coping mechanisms—concerned with how parents feel about them
6. Peer adjustment problems, e.g., behavior disorders
7. Problems with gross and fine motor control
8. Confusion with left to right orientation
9. Confusion over instructions
10. Frustration over assignments
11. Obvious withdrawing behaviors from academic tasks or social encounters

At least 5% of all schoolchildren have learning disabilities. This disorder might be genetic or acquired and can affect the child's relationship with his peers. Future relationships and career choices can also be negatively influenced. Learning-disabled individuals tend to have a higher incidence of juvenile delinquency, drug and alcohol abuse, and divorce.[11]

The theories concerning the causes of learning disabilities are numerous, each translating into its own specific treatment program. For instance, environmental theorists believe that smog, radiation, fluoride, aerosols, fluorescent lighting, artificial food colors, or the salicylates produce educational problems such as out-of-seat behavior and inattentiveness.[100-102] The biologic model theorizes that drug therapy should be prescribed for the treatment of LD, implying that the disability has a physical cause. Researchers today generally suggest caution in regard to the use of drugs to manage learning disabilities. The contemporary approach to learning disabilities is an educational one characterized by (1) intense skill-based instruction, (2) learning in the least-restrictive environment (mainstreamed into the regular classroom if possible), and (3) a transdisciplinary approach to care.[103]

When an LD child presents for a dental appointment, the dental health educator must be patient with the child and focus his instruction on the mastery of oral hygiene skills.

A list of resources for the learning-disabled is found in Appendix I.[10]

BEHAVIOR DISORDERS

Behavior disorder (BD) is a term relevant to the society in which one lives; it is a label based on cultural norms.[104] Disordered behaviors are those that authority figures in a culture deem intolerable. Usually these adverse behaviors threaten the stability, security, or values of a society. Within the social structure, courts, schools, families, and clinics possess their own criteria for defining behavior disorders. The courts label BDs as violations of the law; schools perceive BDs as academic or social failure; clinics refer suspected BD cases to specialists; and a behavior disorder in a family violates the rules of its members and places an enormous strain on the family's well-being.

To formulate a single definition that can be used by all social agents responsible for the actions of children and adolescents is virtually impossible. It is agreed, however, that the difference between normal and disordered behavior is not the type of behavior but the rate and conditions under which the behavior in question is performed. All children throw tantrums, whine, spit, and urinate, but the situations in which disturbed children perform these acts, and the length of time and intensity with which they execute them, can separate their actions from those of normal children.[105]

Characteristics of behaviorally or emotionally disturbed schoolchildren include[106]

(1) an inability to learn which cannot be explained by intellectual, sensory or health factors, (2) an inability to build or maintain satisfactory interpersonal relationships with peers and teachers, (3) inappropriate types of behavior or feelings under normal conditions, (4) a general pervasive mood of unhappiness or depression, and (5) a tendency to develop physical symptoms, pains, or fears associated with personal or school problems.

Estimates of behavior disorder prevalence vary from 0.5 to 20% of the school population. The absence of a clear, reliable definition for a behavior-disordered person accounts for this wide range in numbers. A more reasonable estimate is 6 to 10%.[106-109] Boys appear to exhibit behavior disorders over 3 times the rate for girls.

Models such as the psychodynamic (treat underlying cause through psychotherapy), biophysical (treat with medication and genetic counseling), sociologic (work with people and events outside the student), ecologic (change the child's environment), and behavioral (set up a program to extinguish undesirable behaviors) all possess a set of viable assumptions as to why children behave as they do and how they should be treated. The eclectic approach is perhaps the most suitable for treating children with behavior disorders.

Medications e.g., methylphenidate (Ritalin) and dextroamphetamine (Dexedrine) have been prescribed for the treatment of hyperactivity. Foods containing caffeine, artificial colors (including those in toothpastes, mouthwashes, and coated/flavored medications), and foods containing natural salicylates (e.g., apples, berries, tomatoes, and pork) should be eliminated from the child's diet.

Behavior modification is effective if the child is reinforced contingent on his displaying desirable behavior or not exhibiting undesirable behavior. Many classrooms employ contingency reinforcement by dispensing tokens to students as rewards. At the end of the school week, students can redeem their tokens for prizes; the more tokens earned, the more valuable the tangible object to be purchased. Behavior modification techniques suggest that the teacher should first monitor the child's maladaptive behaviors to achieve a baseline. Later, the child can be taught to measure his own behaviors; the child is thus provided with a self-regulatory activity that gives him greater control over his own environment.[110-113]

A structured learning environment that focuses on consistency and teacher direction is paramount in the management of a child with a behavior disorder. The teacher must be an ideal role model. Clear expectations of what is expected of the child in the classroom are essential. Consistent consequences for not following the prescribed rules are to be understood by all students and enforced whenever a violation occurs. The classroom itself should have minimal distracting stimuli.

The dental health educator should structure the dental environment in the same way when the BD patient presents for an appointment. All distractions should be removed or out of the child's reach. Rules for behavior should be outlined at the beginning of the session, and parents should know the rules. These guidelines must stipulate the rewards for desired behavior and the consequences for undesirable actions. Possible consequences might include (1) time-out procedures (the dental treatment is stopped, the child is ignored and a clock is set; the child must control his inappropriate behavior by the time the alarm rings, signaling that treatment is to be resumed); and (2) the removal of an audiotape or videotape that the child is listening to or watching.

RADIOGRAPHIC TECHNIQUES FOR THE DISABLED

Radiographic evaluation of the dentition and supporting structures is an integral part of the clinical examination, and every effort should be made to secure diagnostic films. Although exposing dental radiographs is a relatively innocuous procedure, many disabled persons will not permit the dental health educator to proceed in a conventional manner. Although many of these patients lack the physical and/or mental capabilities to cooperate with the placement of an intraoral film, most will readily accept an extra oral approach.

Panoramic radiography and a 45° oblique film cassette referred to as the lateral jaw projection (Fig. 8-30) are two radiographic procedures that require minimal cooperation on the part of the patient. The reverse bitewing technique (Fig. 8-31) demands greater patient involvement, but it is ideal for the patient who has an exaggerated gag reflex but readily accepts the placement of

film intraorally. Instead of being placed lingually, the film is placed in the vestibule between the cheek and teeth and the patient closes on the bitewing tab. The emulsion side of the film faces the tube. After tilting the head to the side to be photographed, the tube is directed 0.5 inch below the angle of the mandible on the opposite side. It is important to remember that the image is reversed when viewing this film (i.e., opposite that indicated by the embossed dot on the film surface).[3,114]

OFFICE ACCESSIBILITY AND DESIGN

A disabled person might find one dental office preferable to another because of its location and accommodations for wheelchair patients. A dental office should be made physically accessible, both internally and externally, to assure a barrier-free environment for people with any kind of disabling condition.

The Rehabilitation Act of 1973, Section 504, served as the impetus for a series of laws and regulations that assured the removal of architectural barriers to permit accessibility to all persons with disabling conditions.

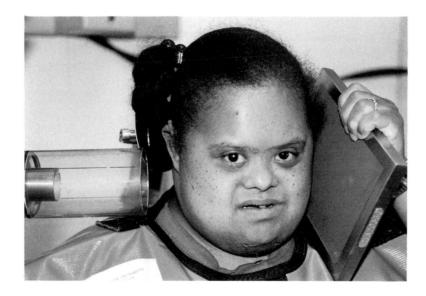

Figure 8-30. Lateral jaw projection. The film cassette is positioned with the exposure side against the skin facing the cone. The cone is aimed from the opposite side of the area being exposed. The head of the patient should be extended forward to eliminate the shadow of the cervical spine.

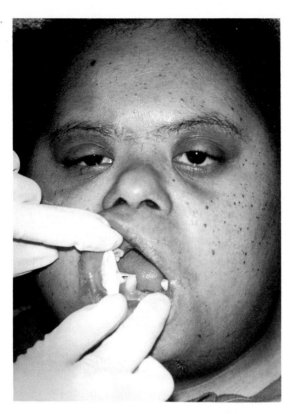

Figure 8-31. Reverse bitewing, an ideal radiographic technique for the patient who cannot or will not hold the film lingually or palatally inside the mouth.

External Considerations

Outside features designed to increase accessibility for the disabled patient include the following:[3,72,115]

Parking facilities—each handicapped-designated parking space should have a 36-inch walkway between it and the next space to allow for walkers and wheelchair manipulation. In a parking lot, a minimum of one handicapped space should be allotted for every 25 regular spaces. Each space should be paved, slip-resistant, and as close to the building entrance as possible.

Walkways—each nonskid walkway or sidewalk should be at least 36-inches in width and clear of any obstructions. Wherever a walkway joins a curb or a driveway, they should be brought to a common level.

Ramps—each ramp should have a maximum gradient or slope of 1:12, be at least 36 inches wide, and have a skid-resistant surface.

Building entrance—the door of an office building should be at least 32 inches wide, be adjusted for 10 lb of pull-pressure to open the door, and have a 5-foot-square platform centered in front of the door opening.

Wheelchair lifts—Hydraulic lifts, power-driven stairrail lifts, and elevators provide alternatives for buildings constructed with several levels.

Internal Considerations

Specifications for internal building features include the following:[3,72,115]

Corridors—all hallways should be a minimum of 48 inches wide to allow the simultaneous passage of a person in a wheelchair and an ambulatory person.

Flooring—carpets should be firm and have short pile to prevent tripping and tangles in wheelchairs. Doormats should be eliminated.

Illumination—wallcoverings that reduce glare are recommended, whereas shiny or glossy surfaces should be avoided. Daylight should be fully utilized. If the office is dependent on fluorescent lighting, pastel colors are the most soothing to the patient.

Signs—the office suite identification and elevator buttons should have raised lettering and numbers to assist the vision-impaired.

Restrooms—as with all doorways, the restroom door and stall should be at least 32 inches wide. Sinks, toilets, grab bars, and mirrors should also be installed with the wheelchair patient in mind.

Drinking fountains—the space between the floor and the base of the fountain should be 27 inches with a front pushplate control.

Telephones—no operable portion of the phone should be higher than 4 feet above the floor. An adjustable volume control for the receiver is helpful to the hearing-impaired patient.

COMMENTS

Caring for the disabled is an extremely rewarding experience for the dental health educator. Instruction is not always easy or well received, but the smallest improvements have immeasurable value. Each disability is unique and requires the dental health educator to be creative, knowledgeable, and most of all sincere. Possibly the most frightening of all barriers is the dental health educator's attitude. Many dental professionals lack confidence or fear they do not possess enough factual information for treating a person with a disability. These feelings of fear or inadequacy must be dispelled, and dental health educators must share knowledge and techniques, gain experiences, and conduct new research so that comprehensive care is available to *all* patients. Dental health educators should tap community resource groups for information concerning the particular services (e.g., health, transportation, and financial) available to their patients with disabilities (see Appendix J).[10,11]

REFERENCES

1. Nowak, A. J.: Dentistry for the Handicapped Patient. St. Louis, C.V. Mosby, 1976.
2. Miller, S. L.: Dental care for the mentally retarded: A challenge to the profession. J. Pub. Health Dent., 25:3, 1965.
3. Fenton, S. J., and DeBiase, C. B.: The handicapped patient. *In* Patient Management Skills for Dental Assistants and Hygienists. Edited by B. D. Ingersoll. Norwalk, CT, Appleton Century Crofts, 1986, pp. 136–158.
4. Stiefel, D. J.: Inclusion of a program of instruction in care of the disabled in a dental school curriculum. J. Dent. Educ., 43:262, 1979.
5. The Robert Wood Johnson Foundation. News Release, June 22, 1973.
6. American Association of Dental Schools and the National Foundation of Dentistry for the Handicapped: Curriculum guidelines for dentistry for the handicapped. J. Dent. Educ., 43:37–41, 1979.
7. American Association of Dental Schools, Section on Dental Hygiene Education: Curricular guidelines for dental hygiene care for the handicapped. J. Dent. Educ., 48:266–269, 1984.
8. Rose, T. L.: The Education of All Handicapped Children Act (PL 94–142): New responsibilities and opportunities for the school nurse. J. Sch. Health, 50:30–31, 1980.
9. Department of Health, Education and Welfare: Federal Register, 42:22678, May 4, 1977.
10. Brooks, K. S.: Being Special: A Guide to Children with Disabilities. Morgantown, WV, University Affiliated Center for Developmental Disabilities, 1983.
11. Stiefel, D. J., and Truelove, E. L.: Self-Instructional Series in Rehabilitation Dentistry: Dental Treatment of the Patient with a Disability (Modules 1–10). University of Washington School of Dentistry, Project DECOD, 1987.
12. Lange, B. M., Entwistle, B. M., and Lipson, L. F.: Dental Management of the Handicapped: Approaches for Dental Auxiliaries. Philadelphia, Lea & Febiger, 1983.
13. Neisworth, J. T., and Smith, R.: Retardation: Issues, Assessments and Intervention. New York, McGraw-Hill, 1978.
14. Voutour, J. A. C., and Voutour, M. E.: The individualized educational program (IEP)—new concept? or new label? J. Sch. Health, 50:262–263, 1980.
15. Dicks, J. L., and Dennis, E. S.: Down's syndrome and hepatitis: An evauation of carrier status. J. Am. Dent. Assoc., 114:637–638, 1987.
16. Newbrun, E.: Cariology. San Francisco, University of California Press, 1975.
17. Brown, J. P., and Schodel, D. R.: A review of controlled surveys of dental disease in handicapped persons. J. Dent. Child., 43:17–24, 1976.
18. Kahn, A. J., et al.: Defective neutrophil chemotaxis in patients with Down's syndrome. J. Perio. Res., 54:62–64, 1975.
19. Winer, R. A., and Chauncey, H. H.: Parotid saliva enzymes in Down's syndrome. J. Perio. Res., 54:62–64, 1975.
20. Kroger, J., and Day, V.: Down's syndrome: Hygienist's perspective. Dent. Hyg., 55:35–38, 1981.
21. Hall, B.: Mongolism in newborn infants. Clin. Pediatr., 5:4, 1966.
22. Shapira, J., Zilberman, Y., and Becker, A.: Lesch-Nyhan syndrome: A nonextracting approach to prevent mutilation. Sp. Care Dent., 5:210–212, 1985.
23. Fenton, S. J., et al.: ADH ad hoc committee report: The use of restraints in the delivery of dental care for the handicapped—legal, ethical, and medical considerations. Sp. Care Dent., 7:253–256, 1987.
24. OMNIA-dent USA: Lawrence Welk Drive, Escondido, CA 92026.
25. Levine, L. B.: Clinical Management of the Disabled Patient: A Working Manual for Dental Professionals. Miami, Denta Press, 1988.
26. Cerebral Palsy Facts and Figures. United Cerebral Palsy Associations, Inc., 66 E. 34th Street, New York, 1986.
27. Marks, N.: Cerebral Palsied and Learning Disabled Children. Springfield, Illinois, Charles C. Thomas, 1974.
28. Cramer, J. J., and Wright, S. A.: The bean bag chair and the pedodontic patient with cerebral palsy. Dent. Hyg., 49(4):167–168, 1975.
29. Metal Dynamics Corporation: 9324 State Road, Philadelphia, PA., 19114.
30. Boundy, S. S., and Reynolds, N. J.: Current Concepts in Dental Hygiene. St. Louis, The C.V. Mosby Company, 1977.
31. Albertson, D.: Prevention and the handicapped child. Dent. Cl. N. Am., 18(3):595–607, 1974.
32. Fox, L. A.: Preventive dentistry for the handicapped child. Ped. Cl. N. Am., 20(1):245–258, 1973.
33. Sroda, R., Plezia, R. A.: Oral hygiene devices for special patients. Sp. Care Dent., 4(6): 264–266, 1984.
34. Lancial, L. A.: Back to basics: oral hygiene for special patients. Dent. Tmwk., 1(6):230–232, 1988.
35. Hengen, M.: The role of the dental hygienist in the dental care of cerebral palsy patient. Dent. Hyg., 54(10):472–473, 1980.
36. Patriarca, J., DeBiase C., and Fenton, S. J.: You Can Prevent Dental Disease. Morgantown, West Virginia, Uni-

versity Affiliated Center for Developmental Disabilities, 1988.

37. Solomon, G., and Plum, F.: Clinical Management of Seizures. Philadelphia, W.B. Saunders, 1976.

38. Betts, T.: Epilepsy. Br. Dent. J., *143*:278, 1977.

39. Wyler, A.: Operant control of CNS activity. In Epilepsy: A Window to Brain Mechanisms. Edited by J. Lockard and A. Ward, Jr. New York, Raven Press, 1980.

40. Adams, R., Daniel, A., McCubbin, J., and Rullman, L.: Games, Sports and Exercises for the Physically Handicapped. 2nd Ed. Philadelphia, Lea and Febiger, 1982.

41. Rickens, A.: Drug Treatment of Epilepsy. Chicago, Year Book, 1976.

42. Lenard, M., and Heslin, L.: The health questionnaire in general dental practice—6. J. Irish Dent. Assoc., *17*:168–177, 1971.

43. Epilepsy Foundation of America: Basic Statistics on Epilepsies. Philadelphia, F.A. Davis, 1975.

44. U.S. Dept. of Health Education and Welfare: The Dental Implications of Epilepsy. DHEW Pub. (HSA) 78–5217, 1977.

45. Davis, R. K., Baerl, N., and Palmer, J. H.: A preliminary report on a new therapy for Dilantin gingival hyperplasia. J. Periodontol., *34*:17–22, 1963.

46. Rucker, L. M.: Prosthetic treatment for the patient with uncontrolled grand mal epileptic seizures. Sp. Care Dent., *5*:206–207, 1985.

47. Kanner, L.: Autistic disturbances of affective contact. New Child, *2*:217–250, 1943.

48. Wing, L.: The prevalence of early childhood autism: Comparisons of administrative and epidemiological studies. Psychol. Med., *6*:89–100, 1976.

49. Kamen, S. and Skier, J.: Dental management of the autistic child. Sp. Care Dent., *5*:20–23, 1985.

50. Earls, F.: Epidemiology of psychiatric disorders in children and adolescents. In Psychiatry. Vol. 3. Edited by Klerman, G. L., et al. Philadelphia, J.B. Lippincott, 1985.

51. Kopel, H. M.: The autistic child in dental practice. J. Dent. Child., *44*:302–309, 1977.

52. Hutt, C., Forrest, S., and Richer, J.: Cardiac arrhythmia and behavior in autistic children. Acta Psychiatr. Scand., *51*:361, 1975.

53. Hutt, S., et al.: A behavioral and electroencephalographic study of autistic children. J. Psychiatr. Res., *3*:181, 1965.

54. Ornitz, E. M., and Ritvo, E. R.: The syndrome of autism: A critical review. Am. J. Psych., *133*:609–621, 1976.

55. Shapira, J., et al.: Oral health status and dental needs of an autistic population of children and young adults. Sp. Care Dent., *9*:38–41, 1989.

56. Swallow, J. H.: The dental management of the autistic child. Br. Dent. J., *126*:128–131, 1969.

57. Clark, C. A., Cangelosi-Williams, P., Lee, M. A., and Morgan, L.: Dental treatment for deaf patients. Sp. Care Dent., *6*:102–108, 1986.

58. Kopra, M. A.: A brighter future for deaf people. J. Rehabil., *40*:35–38, 1974.

59. Tunes, W., and Dexter, C.: Dentistry and the hearing impaired child. J. Pedodont., *3*:321–334, 1979.

60. Nober, E. H.: Auditory processing. In Cerebral Palsy: A Developmental Disability. 3rd Ed. Edited by W. C. Cruickshank. Syracuse, Syracuse University Press, 1976.

61. Northein, J. L., and Davis, M. (Eds.): Communicative disorders in Down's syndrome. Semin. Speech Language Hearing, *1*:1–97, 1980.

62. Meadow, K. P.: Deafness and Child Development. Berkeley, University of California Press, 1980.

63. Flynn, P. T., and McGregor, D. K.: Communication disorders: An overview and practices for the dental hygienist. Dent. Hyg., *51*:455–459, 1977.

64. Miller, E., and Bentley, E. L.: Listen to the Sounds of Deafness. Silver Springs, MD, National Association of the Deaf, 1970.

65. Putnam, L.: Information needs of hearing impaired people. Health Rehabil. Lib. Serv. News J., *2*:2, 1976.

66. Riekehof, L. L.: The Joy of Signing. 2nd Ed. Springfield, MO, Gospel Publishing House, 1987.

67. Mueller, K., and Gantt, D.: Communication with the deaf patient. J. Dent. Handic., *3*:22–25, 1978.

68. O'Brien, S.: A special challenge. R.D.H., *9*:18, 20, 1989.

69. Wilkins, E. M.: Clinical Practice of the Dental Hygienist. 6th Ed. Philadelphia, Lea & Febiger, 1989.

70. Schechter-Connors, M., and Connors, W. A.: Consultants for Sign Language and Deaf Services, 9104 Babcock Blvd., Suite 5109, Pittsburgh, PA 15237.

71. Schnuth, M. L.: Dental health education for the blind. Dent. Hyg., *51*:499–501, 1977.

72. Lebowitz, E. J.: An introduction to dentistry for the blind. Dent. Clin. North Am., *18*:651–669, 1974.

73. Griffin, H. C., and Gerber, P. J.: Tactual development and its implications for the education of blind children. Ed. Vis. Handic., *13*:116–123, 1982.

74. Anaise, J.: Periodontal disease and oral hygiene in a group of blind and sighted Israeli teenagers (14–17 years of age). J. Community Dent. Oral Epidemiol., *7*:353–356, 1971.

75. Ligh, R. Z.: The visually handicapped patient in dental practice. J. Dent. Handic., *4*:38–40, 1979.

76. Winstanley, M. L.: A synopsis of the project to evaluate the use of a Braille text and tactile aids when teaching dental health to blind children. Br. Dent. J., *42*:20–23, 1983.

77. Clemens, C., and Taylor, S.: Toothbrushing to music. Dent. Hyg., *54*:125–126, 1980.

78. Ball, R. O., Zucher, S. B., and Fretwell, L. D.: Teaching preventive dentistry to patients with impaired vision. J. Dent. Handic., *4*:23–25, 1978.

79. French-Beatty, C.: Dental health for the blind. Horizons (ADHA Newsletter), *7*:1, 8, 1986.

80. Ziegler, J.: Tomorrow's check-up. Am. Health, *9*:9, 12, 1990.

81. Bromley, I.: Tetraplegia and Paraplegia. Edinburgh, Churchill Livingstone, 1981.

82. Fenton, S. J., DeBiase, C. B., and Portugal, B. V.: A strategy for implementing a dental health education program for state facilities with limited resources. Rehab. Lit., *43*:290–293, 1982.

83. Fitchie, J. G., et. al.: Oral hygiene for the severely handicapped: Clinical evaluation of the University of Mississippi dental system. Sp. Care Dent., *8*:260–264, 1988.

84. Mulligan, R.: A physiologic bitestick appliance for quadriplegics. Sp. Care Dent., *3*:24–29, 1983.

85. Cloran, A. J., Davis, W. J., and Campbell, T. M.: Special design of mouthstick device for a patient with upper extremity bilateral amputations. Sp. Care Dent., *5*:112–113, 1985.

86. Felder, R. S., Gillette, V. M., and Leseberg, K.: Wheelchair transfer techniques for the dental office. Sp. Care Dent. *8*:256–259, 1988.

87. Leibowitz, U., and Alter, M.: Multiple Sclerosis: Clues to Its Cause. New York, North-Holland, 1973.

88. Dubowitz, V.: Muscle pathology in genetic muscle disorders: Some problems in clinico-pathological correlation. In Muscle, Nerve, and Brain Degeneration. Edited by A. Kidman and J. Tomkins. Amsterdam, Excerpta Medica, 1979.

89. Hamada, T., Kawazoe, Y., and Yamada, S.: Maximum biting forces in patients with progressive muscular dystrophy. J. Dent. Handic., *3*:20–22, 1977.

90. Hamada, T., Kobayashi, M., and Kawazoe, Y.: Electromyographic activity of masticatory muscles in patients with progressive muscular dystrophy (Duchenne type): Relation between integrated electromyographic activity and biting force. Sp. Care Dent., 1:37–38, 1981.

91. Brown, J. C., and Losch, P. K.: Dental occlusion in patients with muscular dystrophy. Am. J. Orthodont. Oral Surg., 25:1040–1045, 1939.

92. Vanier, T. M.: Dystrophia myotonica in childhood. Br. Med. J., 5208:284–288, 1960.

93. Benson, H. F.: Oral manifestations of progressive muscular dystrophy. J. D. C. Dent. Soc., Summer 1977, pp. 35–41.

94. White, R., and Saekler, A.: Effects of progressive muscular dystrophy on occlusion. J. Am. Dent. Assoc., 49:4–49, 1954.

95. Ardran, G. M., Hamilton, A., and Kemp, F. H.: Enlargement of the tongue and changes in the jaws with muscular dystrophy. Clin. Radiol., 24:359–364, 1973.

96. Cohen, M. M.: Congenital, genetic, and endocrinologic influences on dental occlusion. Dent. Clin. North Am., 19:499–514, 1975.

97. Kerborg, S., Jense, B., Moller, G., and Bjork, A.: Craniofacial growth in a case of congenital muscular dystrophy: A roentgencephalometric and electromyographic investigation. Am. J. Orthodont., 74:207–215, 1978.

98. Futterman, M.: Dental anomalies associated with pseudohypertrophic muscular dystrophy. Dent. Outlook, 27:73–78, 1940.

99. Federal Register: 42(163):65083, Dec. 29, 1977.

100. Baren, M., Liebel, R., and Smith, L.: Overcoming Learning Disabilities: A Team Approach. Reston, VA, Prentice-Hall, 1978.

101. Feingold, B.: Hyperkinesis and learning disabilities linked to the ingestion of artificial food colors and flavors. J. Learning Disabil., 9:551–559, 1976.

102. Ott, J.: Influence of flurorescent lights on hyperactivity and learning disabilities. J. Learning Disabil., 9:417–422, 1976.

103. Blackhurst, A. E., and Berdine, W. H.: An Introduction to Special Education. Boston, Little Brown, 1981.

104. Burback, H. J.: Labelling: Sociological issues. In Handbook of Special Education. Edited by J. M. Kauffman, and D. P. Hallahan. Englewood Cliffs, NJ, Prentice-Hall, 1981.

105. Kauffman, J. M.: Characteristics of Children's Behavior Disorders. 2nd Ed. Columbus, Charles E. Merrill, 1981.

106. Bower, E. M.: Early identification of Emotionally Handicapped Children in School. 2nd Ed. Springfield, IL, Charles C Thomas, 1969.

107. Glidewell, J. C., and Swallow, C. S.: The prevalence of maladjustment in elementary schools. Report prepared for the Joint Commission on the Mental Health of Children, University of Chicago, July 26, 1968.

108. Graham, P. J.: Epidemiological studies. In Psychopathological Disorders of Childhood. 2nd Ed. Edited by H. C. Quay, and J. S. Werry. New York, Wiley, 1979.

109. Rutter, M., et al.: Isle of Wright studies, 1964–1974. Psychol. Med., 6:313–332, 1976.

110. Haring, N. G., Lovitt, T. C., Eaton, M. D., and Hansen, C. L.: The Fourth R: Research in the Classroom. Columbus, Charles E. Merrill, 1978.

111. Haring, N. G., and Schiefelbusch, R. L. (Eds.): Teaching Special Children. New York, McGraw-Hill, 1976.

112. Lovitt, T. C.: In Spite of My Resistance—I've Learned from Children. Columbus, Charles E. Merrill, 1977.

113. White, O. R., and Haring, N. G.: Exceptional Teaching: A Multimedia Program. Columbus, Charles E. Merrill, 1976.

114. Steinberg, A., Bramer, M., and May, B.: Simplified radiographic survey for the handicapped patient. Fortnightly Rev. Chicago Dent. Soc., 41, 1961.

115. Bill, D. J., and Weddell, J. A.: Dental office access for patients with disabling conditions. Sp. Care Dent., 6:246–252, 1986.

Chapter 9

THE MEDICALLY COMPROMISED

I believe that there are certain doors that only illness can open. There is a certain state of health that does not allow us to understand everything; and perhaps illness shuts us off from certain truths; but health shuts us off just as effectively from others, or turns us away from them so we are not concerned with them.

André Gide
The Journals of André Gide, Vol. 2

THE CHANGING DENTAL POPULATION

The patient population treated in dental practices today is somewhat different than those treated some 15 years ago. Recent strides in dentistry suggest a change in the focus of dental care from caries prevention for the child and adolescent to comprehensive care for the medically compromised and older adult.

Although only 20% of dentists in the U.S. are willing to treat patients with mentally or physically compromising conditions, an estimated 33 million people have moderate to severe medical conditions or are developmentally disabled.[1] This translates to approximately 15% of the population debilitated by cardiovascular diseases, respiratory diseases, hematologic conditions, metabolic and endocrine diseases, liver and kidney disorders, arthritis and joint prostheses, and cancer therapy complications.

Dental treatment for the patient with a systemic disease can be complicated. A thorough medical assessment of all patients prior to initiation of any form of dental therapy is mandatory. The following are some of the major reasons why the dental health educator must obtain as much information as possible regarding a patient's medical history: (1) drug interactions can occur between drugs required for dental care and those needed therapeutically for a given disease; (2) prophylactic antibiotic coverage is a necessary precaution for patients with certain conditions; (3) diseases themselves can become complicated by dental treatment, and even more important, by the lack of dental intervention; (4) a conglomerate of symptoms might suggest a particular condition to the dental health educator, therefore warranting a medical referral; and (5) a past hospitalization or record of medications currently prescribed for the patient might provide a clue to an underlying systemic disease that the patient has neglected to mention.[2]

THE HOSPITALIZED DENTAL PATIENT

The dental health educator who treats the medically compromised dental patient must be prepared to transfer these services to the hospital setting as well. Obtaining hospital privileges that permit continuity of care for the sick dental patient is both challenging and instrumental in providing the medically compromised dental patient with a sense of security.

A thorough dental prophylaxis is an essential component of preoperative care for the renal transplant, cardiovascular, or joint replacement patient preparing for surgery. Likewise, dental intervention for patients scheduled to undergo renal dialysis, head and neck radiation, or chemotherapy is generally viewed as a primary service for the prevention of infection. Dental care, which usually adds to the quality of life, can actually be responsible for prolonging life in these cases.[3]

Currently, approximately one-fifth of acute care hospitals accredited by the Joint Commission on Accreditation of Health Care Organizations have developed dental departments; over 260 general practice residency programs are available for dentists who are interested in gaining hospital-related experiences, and about 40,000 dentists are hospital staff members in at least one facility.[3]

Hospital dental departments function on three levels: service, education, and administration.[3-6] Under the service rubric, the dental health educator assumes the roles of consultant and caregiver. Dental consultations can involve initial patient screenings and consultations with physicians and other members of the health care team regarding the course of treatment for a particular patient. In the latter case, the dental health educator often acts as a resource person. Treatment, needless to say, can include any number of services. For example, clinical services might involve radiographs, treatment planning, restorative care, palliative care, oral prophylaxes, and fluoride therapy.

Health education functions might entail the coordination and presentation of hospital staff in-service oral health education programs; the coordination of continuing education programs for dental staff; the organization of educational activities for clinical externship programs or remote site opportunities for dental and dental hygiene students from area colleges; group and individualized patient education sessions for pregnant mothers, children, caregivers or guardians of persons incapable of self-care, high-risk patients (e.g., cardiovascular, renal, and leukemic), and all patients with dental prostheses requiring care and proper storage; and nutritional counseling.

Administrative duties require managerial skills. The dental health educator in the hospital setting is frequently called to serve on hospital committees, to work in team clinics, or to participate in research endeavors. Chairing a dental department within a hospital, directing a hospital externship program, and coordinating a hospital's cleft palate team clinic are examples of administrative roles. For the hospital administration, the integration of dental health into their hospital system reflects the institution's commitment to comprehensive health care and responsiveness to the health care needs of the community.

CARDIOVASCULAR DISEASE

Cardiovascular disease is the leading cause of death in the nation. The American Heart Association estimates that 63,290,000 persons in the U.S. have some degree of cardiovascular disease; many have more than one form of this disorder. The incidence of all cardiovascular diseases increases with age. According to the Framingham Heart Study, 5% of heart attacks occur in individuals under age 40, and 45% occur in individuals under age 65.[7] In addition, cardiovascular disease figures are higher among males than females, and blacks as opposed to whites (Figure 9-1[8]). It should be noted

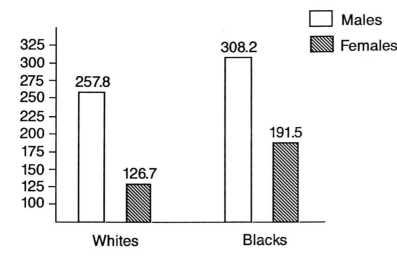

Males

Females

Figure 9-1. Age-adjusted heart disease death rates by race and sex, 1983 (rates per 100,000 population). From National Center for Health Statistics: Advance report of final mortality statistics, 1983. Monthly Statistics Report, *34*(Supp. 2), September 26, 1985.

that heart disease statistics are escalating among women.

Cardiovascular disease can be subdivided into six categories: hypertension, coronary heart disease, arrhythmia, heart valve disease, congestive heart failure, and stroke.[9] The underlying pathology for most forms of cardiovascular disease is atherosclerosis. The formation of atherosclerotic plaques is a complex process characterized by smooth muscle cell proliferation and lipid and cholesterol deposition beneath the arterial lining (subintima). Plaques gradually narrow the lumen of involved vessels and therefore compromise blood flow to organs and other areas normally supplied by the artery. Numerous risk factors have been implicated in the development of atheromatous lesions. They include high blood pressure, high blood cholesterol, cigarette smoking, diabetes, a family history of atherosclerosis, advancing age, male sex, and obesity.[10] According to a Carter Center Report, hypertension might cause 30% of all cardiovascular deaths, including 29% of coronary heart disease (CHD) deaths and 32% of deaths related to strokes. Ten percent of the nearly 1 million cardiovascular disease deaths that occur yearly have been attributed to serum cholesterol levels over 219 mg/dL, and smoking has been held responsible for 14.5% of these same deaths.[7,11]

Hypertension

Approximately 1 in every 4 dental patients has hypertension as indicated by a diastolic pressure of 90 mm Hg or greater.[12] A patient displaying a blood pressure between 140/90 and 160/95 mm Hg is described as borderline hypertensive. A diastolic reading between 95 and 104 mm Hg denotes mild hypertension; between 105 and 114 mm Hg suggests moderate hypertension; and above 115 mm Hg signifies severe high blood pressure.[13]

High blood pressure has been referred to as the silent killer because initially patients tend to be relatively asymptomatic. Early symptoms can consist of occipital headaches, vision changes, tinnitus (ringing in the ears), dizziness, weakness, and tingling of the hands and feet. Only 10% of cases can be attributed to a known cause such as renal disease, pheochromocytoma, or taking oral contraceptives. This type is referred to as secondary hypertension. The remaining 90% have essential hypertension, characterized by unknown cause. What is known is that blood pressure is elevated by an increase in blood or tissue fluid volume and a decrease in the elasticity of the larger arteries.[2,9]

Medical and Dental Management. The initial treatment for hypertension usually involves prescribing a diuretic drug that decreases intravascular fluid volume, avoiding stress and smoking, and lowering the intake of sodium. A patient who does not respond well to diuretics might require adrenergic blocking agents, vasodilators, and sedatives to control the disease.

It is important for the dental health educator to take and record a patient's blood pressure at each dental visit. Patients with undiagnosed severe hypertension can be identified and referrals made prior to starting dental treatment by routine hypertension screening practices. Because dental stress and certain dental procedures can cause an elevation in blood pressure, the dental environment can place the patient with organic disease at an even greater risk for experiencing stroke and heart attack. Significant increases in blood pressure can result from the administration of a local anesthetic containing a strong vasosuppressor or the use of epinephrine in gingival retraction cord. If a patient is being treated for hypertension, the dental health educator must request the names of the drugs taken and record them in the patient's medical history. Side effects associated with antihypertensive agents include orthostatic hypotension, syncope, depression, xerostomia, and interactions with drugs that might be prescribed by the dentist.[2,9]

Dental treatment should be postponed for the patient who has hypertension and is not being managed medically. Physician referrals should be made and dental care resumed when the patient's blood pressure has been controlled.

Coronary Heart Disease

Over 550,000 Americans die annually from heart attacks.[7] Approximately 1 in 5 males in the United States will experience symptoms related to coronary heart disease by age 60.[14] Although the incidence of coronary heart disease has been increasing over the last three decades, there is some evidence to believe that it is on the decline.[14] From 1964 to 1984, death rates for coronary heart disease dropped from 215 per 100,000 population to 129, a 40% reduction.[15]

Coronary heart disease begins with the deposition of fatty plaques in the coronary vessels. This blockage narrows the lumen of the artery and is referred to as atherosclerosis. Coronary occlusion decreases blood flow to a portion of the heart muscle (myocardial ischemia.) Both angina pectoris and myocardial infarction can manifest as a result of the heart being deprived of oxygen. Angina is characterized by chest pain of sudden onset. This pain can radiate to the chin or jaw or down the arm. Angina usually has a brief duration of 1 to 3 minutes and is a reversible process with the return of adequate coronary perfusion. Other symptoms include nausea, vomiting, palpitations, dyspnea, lightheadedness, and sweating. The damage caused by myocardial infarction, on the other hand, is irreversible. The pain associated with myocardial infarction is caused by prolonged myocardial ischemia resulting in injury to the heart muscle. The pain is similar to anginal pain but is more pronounced and can persist for hours or days.[2,9]

Medical and Dental Management. The patient with atherosclerosis and a history of angina pectoris is treated with a combination of modalities. They include a diet low in fat, cholesterol, and sodium; weight control; cessation of smoking; exercise; and drug therapy (nitroglycerine and beta blockers, e.g., propranolol, metoprolol, nadolol, and atenolol). Infarct pain is not relieved by nitrates. Victims of myocardial infarction are normally treated with oxygen, provided pain relief medications, sedated to achieve rest, treated to prevent complications such as thromboemboli and arrhythmias, treated for vascular collapse or acute pulmonary edema, and evaluated for coronary artery bypass candidacy.[9]

The number and rate of coronary bypass operations in the United States increased over 12-fold between 1970 and 1984.[16] Because more bypass patients will present to the dental office for care, the dental health educator must be apprised of any precautions that should be taken. Most coronary artery bypass patients do not require prophylactic antibiotic coverage for dental procedures after the immediate postoperative period (first 6 months); susceptibility to infection dramatically decreases 1 to 2 weeks after surgery, when the graft site has healed.[17] If in doubt regarding a patient's cardiac status, the dental health educator is advised to consult with the patient's physician.

Cardiac pain in patients with CHD can be precipitated by inadequate rest, stress, large meals, cold weather, hot humid weather, cigarette smoking, and drugs such as alcohol, amphetamines, and caffeine. Assessing the existence of pain and its causes when the patient presents for a dental appointment might help prevent cardiac complications and subsequent death.[2]

Dental patients with unstable angina or a recent history of myocardial infarction (within 6 months prior to the dental appointment) should not receive dental treatment. Patients with stable angina or who have had a heart attack over 6 months ago may receive dental treatment, but consultation with the patient's physician and following the guidelines outlined in Tables 9-1 and 9-2 are recommended.[2]

The dental health educator's role in the management of the patient with CHD should also include dietary and smoking

Table 9-1. Dental Management of Patients with Angina Pectoris

Morning appointments
Short appointments
Reduction of stress and anxiety:
  Patient should be able to express fears
  Premedication—diazepam 5 to 10 mg
  Nitrous oxide—hypoxia must be avoided
Nitroglycerin tablets available
Local anesthesia with epinephrine 1:100,000—aspirate, inject slowly; no more than 3 cartridges
Avoid use of vasopressors to control local bleeding
Avoid use of vasopressors in gingival packing material
If patient becomes fatigued or develops significant changes in pulse rate or rhythm during appointment, terminate appointment

From Little, J.W., and Falace, D. A.: Dental Management of the Medically Compromised Patient. 3rd Ed. St. Louis, C.V. Mosby, 1988, p. 162.

Table 9-2. Dental Management of Patients with History of Myocardial Infarction

Consultation with patient's physician concerning management
No routine dental care until at least 6 months after infarction
Patients on anticoagulant therapy who need deep scaling or surgical procedures:
  Check prothrombin time (coumarin) or bleeding time (aspirin)
  Have physician reduce prothrombin time to 2 times normal or less; bleeding time reduced to 1½ times normal
  Give antibiotics after surgery to minimize possibility of postoperative infection
Morning appointments
Short appointments
Reduction of stress and anxiety—premedication with diazepam
Local anesthesia with epinephrine 1:100,000—aspirate, inject slowly; no more than 3 cartridges
Avoid use of vasopressors to control local bleeding
Avoid use of vasopressors in gingival packing material
If patient becomes fatigued or develops significant changes in pulse rate or rhythm during appointment, terminate appointment

From Little, J.W., and Falace, D.A.: Dental Management of the Medically Compromised Patient. 3rd Ed. St. Louis, C.V. Mosby, 1988, p. 162.

cessation reinforcement. These patients need constant encouragement to maintain what are often drastic changes in their lifestyle. A low-cholesterol diet means a diet low in saturated fat, a fact that is often misunderstood.

Cardiac Arrhythmias

Disorders in cardiac conduction originate from the effect of the vagus nerve on the sinoatrial (SA) node. The SA node is located superior to the right atrium. This node possesses its own intrinsic rhythm, promoting the conduction of each heartbeat.[9] Disturbances in heart rhythm can arise from the atrium or ventricle. Three such irregularities might be observed by the dental health educator:

1. Sinus arrhythmia is a normal irregularity in pulse rate; it is common in children and adolescents. In a sinus arrhythmia the heart is normal but the pulse rate increases noticeably during a forced inspiration and decelerates as the patient exhales.

2. Atrial fibrillation is recognized by a completely irregular pulse. The atria do not contract as a unit, therefore adversely affecting the ventricular rhythm. Atrial fibrillation can be secondary to coronary heart disease, hyperthyroidism, or mitral stenosis.

3. Premature ventricular contractions (PVCs) exhibit a definite pause in an otherwise normal rhythm. The heart appears to have "skipped" a beat because abnormal electrical activity in the ventricle has resulted in a premature contraction. When the SA node signals the ventricles to contract to produce the next heartbeat, they cannot react because they are still in recovery. This produces a pause in the rhythm until the next SA impulse is initiated.

In addition to irregular pulse rates, patients with arrhythmias experience syncope, nausea, vomiting, confusion, dizziness, and increased perspiration.[9]

Medical and Dental Management. Treatment for arrhythmias can involve the administration of anticoagulants (to reduce the risk of emboli formation in the fibrillating atria), antiarrhythmia drugs (e.g., procainamide and quinidine), or the placement of an internal pacemaker. Pacemakers are usually installed in patients who have slow, ineffective, and irregular cardiac rhythm caused by CHD, myocardial infarction (MI), or hypertension. Pacemakers with internal leads do not require prophylactic antibiotic coverage for dental procedures.[9]

If a patient presents with tachycardia or a heart rate over 100, the dental health educator should have the patient rest and use calm reassurance. If the pulse remains over 100, no treatment should be rendered; a referral to a physician is advised.[9]

Heart Valve Disease

Valvular heart disease can be congenital (a cardiac defect present at birth) or acquired (caused by rheumatic fever or bacterial endocarditis). Congenital heart disease occurs in about 0.5% of all live births.[2] All but about 5% of the heart disease cases in children can be traced to rheumatic fever and its sequelae.[18–20] Regardless of the time of onset, the anatomy of one or more of the heart valves is abnormal, resulting in a wide variety of symptoms. Surgical closure of a defect or valvular replacement might be required.

CONGENITAL HEART DISEASE

Congenital malformations of the heart can be caused by fetal hypoxia or endocarditis, prenatal rubella, certain drugs, vitamin deficiencies, and chromosomal aberrations (e.g., Down syndrome). The types of congenital defects include[2,9]

1. *Atrial septal defects* permit the communication of blood between the two atria, causing blood flow from the left to the right atrium. This is the most common congenital cardiac defect.

2. *Ventricular septal defects* enable blood to flow between the two ventricles, also causing a left-to-right shunting of blood.

3. *Patent ductus arteriosus* is an embryonic connection between the pulmonary artery and the aorta. This defect often corrects itself by age 2.

4. *Transposition of the great vessels* is characterized by an embryonic reversal whereby the root of the aorta opens into the right ventricle and the pulmonary artery opens into the left ventricle. This defect is life-threatening.

5. *Tetralogy of Fallot* involves four malformations: pulmonary stenosis, a ventricular septal defect, a dextraposed aorta, and hypertrophy of the right ventricle.

6. *Pulmonary stenosis* involves a narrowing of the pulmonary artery that reduces pulmonary blood flow. Subsequent dilation

Table 9-3. Signs and Symptoms of Congenital Heart Disease

Dyspnea
Cyanosis
Ruddy color, polycythemia
Clubbing of fingers or toes
Murmurs
Congestive heart failure
Distention of neck veins
Enlarged liver
Ascites
Weakness
Dizziness, syncope, coma

From Little, J.W., and Falace, D.A.: Dental Management of the Medically Compromised Patient. 3rd Ed. St. Louis, C.V. Mosby, 1988, p. 116.

and hypertrophy of the right ventricle result, and heart failure eventually ensues.

7. *Coarctation of the aorta* refers to a constriction of the aorta that reduces systemic blood flow. Hypertension, cerebral hemorrhage, endarteritis (inflammation of the lining of an artery), or an aneurysm can result.

The signs and symptoms common to congenital heart defects are listed in Table 9-3.[2] Initial left-to-right blood shunting as described in defects 1 to 3 causes a recirculation of oxygenated blood to the systemic capillaries, preventing cyanosis from occurring. Initial right-to-left blood flow (defects 4 and 5) bypasses the lungs, resulting in an increased number of red blood cells being produced by the bone marrow to compensate for the decreased oxygen content of the blood (polycythemia). Some individuals with congenital heart defects experience delayed growth patterns.

ACQUIRED HEART DISEASE

A valvular defect can be acquired from a case of rheumatic fever. A sore throat involving group A streptococci can develop into rheumatic fever if untreated and if antibodies to one of the various antigens found on the bacteria are elevated. Circulating antibodies combine with the antigens, causing an allergic necrosis. The connective tissue of the heart and heart valves is extremely susceptible to this autoimmune form of destruction.[2,9] Although all four heart valves can be affected, damage to the aortic and mitral valves on the left side of the heart is most common. Murmurs can indicate a valvular defect. Rheumatic fever manifests in approximately 3% of persons with symptomatic exudative streptococcal pharyngitis.[19] Children between the ages of 5 and 15 are most commonly affected.

Bacterial endocarditis is an infection that involves the deposition of bacteria on the heart valves or the lining of the heart chambers, which have been damaged by congenital or acquired means. Prosthetic heart valves also attract blood-borne bacteria. Bacterial vegetations can detach from the valve(s), resulting in emboli with subsequent complications that include reinfection, congestive heart failure, renal disease, and stroke.[9] The infection can be sudden and acute or subacute (exhibiting a slow, quiet onset). The subacute signs include loss of appetite, weight loss, fever, and weakness.[9] The frequency of bacteremia from a variety of dental procedures, including toothbrushing, increases in the presence of periodontal or periapical disease. Transient bacteremias associated with dental manipulation are usually of short duration and are cleared from the blood stream within 10 to 30 minutes.[21–23]

Medical and Dental Management. Patients with cardiac conditions or untreated defects and patients who have undergone surgical procedures to correct a cardiac defect have varying degrees of risk for developing endocarditis (Table 9-4).[24] A thorough medical history should reveal these patients and identify questionable conditions such as (1) a history of rheumatic fever with an unknown determination of valvular disease and (2) murmurs of undiagnosed origin.[24]

Although the cardiac patient's need for prophylactic antibiotic coverage is crucial and has been addressed countless times in the literature, the role of the dental health educator in patient education cannot be overemphasized. The patient at risk for endocarditis, whether he is not a surgical candidate or is about to undergo cardiac sur-

Table 9-4. Degree of Risk for Infective Endocarditis

High risk
  Prosthetic valves
  Recent surgical repair of cardiovascular defect
  Previous infective endocarditis
Moderate risk
  Arterovenous fistulae
  Patent ductus arteriosus
  Ventricular septal defect
  Aortic valve disease
  Intravenous catheter (ventricular-jugular shunt)
  Coarctation of aorta
  Tetralogy of Fallot
  Marfan syndrome
  Mitral insufficiency
Moderate to low risk
  Mitral valve prolapse (with regurgitation)
  Tricuspid valve disease
  Pulmonary valve disease
  Pure mitral stenosis
  Idiopathic hypertrophic subaortic stenosis
  Large atrial septal defect
  Surgically corrected cardiac-valve lesion with prosthetic implant (>6 mo after operation)
Low to negligible risk (usually no antibiotic coverage indicated)
  Arteriosclerotic plaques
  Coronary sclerosis
  Small atrial septal defect
  Cardiac pacemaker
  Surgically corrected C-V lesion with no prosthetic implant (≥6 mo after operation)
  Syphilitic aortitis

From Little, J.W.: Prevention of bacterial endocarditis in dental patients. Gen. Dent., 35 5:385, 1987.

gery, needs to (1) be taught how to perform effective plaque-control procedures (which might include chlorhexidine rinses to reduce the size of the bacterial inoculum)[25]; (2) receive routine dental examinations, radiographs, oral prophylaxes, and fluoride treatments; and (3) know the antibiotic prophylactic protocol suited to him verbatim, to reduce the risk of self-inflicted or iatrogenic bacteremia. If possible, cardiac surgery should not be scheduled until the patient has had his teeth cleaned and is able to exhibit competence in personal oral hygiene care.

A standard oral care protocol for cardiac transplantation patients has not been developed. Presently, a great degree of disagreement exists nationally on appropriate dental management of the cardiac transplant patient.[26]

A prosthetic valve recipient remains at risk because his valve attaches to the heart with nonabsorbable sutures. Conversely, a Dacron patch used to cover a defect usually becomes covered by repair tissue in a relatively short period of time, reducing the patient's susceptibility to endocarditis after the first 6 months. Prophylactic antibiotics are usually not indicated once healing is complete.[2] For a complete list of the indications for prophylactic antibiotic coverage, see Table 9-5.[17,27] Prophylactic doses of antibiotics have been prescribed for patients with cardiac defects who require oral surgery or periodontal treatment since 1940.[24]

Table 9-5. Indications for Prophylactic Premedication to Prevent Infective Endocarditis

Heart Disease Risk
  Rheumatic and congenital heart disease
  Rheumatic fever and other febrile diseases that predispose to valvular damage
  Prosthetic valves and prior cardiac surgery
  Previous episode of infective endocarditis
  Other heart conditions advised by the physician
  Mitral valve prolapse with regurgitation
  Hypertrophic cardiomyopathy
Other Conditions
  Patients with a reduced capacity to resist infection associated with poor healing, immunosuppression and other conditions
  Uncontrolled, unstable diabetes
  Grossly contaminated traumatic facial injuries and compound fractures
  Anticancer chemotherapy
  Blood disease, particularly acute leukemia and agranulocytosis
  Corticosteroid or immunosuppressive therapy
  Renal transplant and hemodialysis; glomerulonephritis and other active renal disorders
  Liver and other organ transplants
  Prosthetic joints

Adapted from Shannon, S.A.: Infective endocarditis. Dent. Hyg., 59:554, 1985, which lists the following reference: Wilkins, E.M.: Clinical Practice of the Dental Hygienist. 6th Ed. Philadelphia, Lea & Febiger, 1989, pp. 85, 90.

Table 9-6. 1990 American Heart Association Recommendations for Bacterial Endocarditis Prevention

Special regimen for high-risk patients
1. Patients not allergic to ampicillin
   2 g ampicillin IM or IV, plus 1.5 mg per kg of body mass gentamycin, 30 min before procedure, followed by amoxicillin, 1.5 g, orally 6 h after initial dose
2. Patients allergic to ampicillin
   1 g vancomycin IV over the 60 min prior to the dental procedure

Standard regimen for low- to moderate-risk patients
1. Patients not allergic to amoxicillin
   3 g amoxicillin orally 1 h before procedure; then 1.5 g amoxicillin 6 h after initial dose
2. Patients unable to take oral penicillin/amoxicillin
   Erythromycin ethylsuccinate, 800 mg, or erythromycin stearate, 1 g, orally 2 h before procedure; then half the dose 6 h after initial dose

   or

   Clindamycin, 300 mg, orally 1 h before procedure and 150 mg 6 h after initial dose

Total pediatric dose should not exceed total adult dose. Consult source for initial pediatric doses.

From Dajani, A.S., et al.: Prevention of bacterial endocarditis. Recommendations by the American Heart Association. *JAMA* 264:2919–2922, 1990.

The American Heart Association dosage guidelines can be found in Table 9-6.[24,28]

Congestive Heart Failure

Congestive heart failure (CHF) usually begins with a weakening of the left ventricle due to either an increased workload or a disease of the heart muscle. Increased workload can be caused by hypertension, aortic valve disease, or anemia. The heart muscle can be damaged from infections, rheumatic fever, or infarction. If the left ventricle fails, blood cannot be forced out into the systemic circulation. An accumulation of blood in the pulmonary vessels results, referred to as pulmonary edema. Consequently the right ventricle becomes overworked to compensate for the back flow of blood from the lungs, often leading to right-sided heart failure as well.[2]

Dyspnea and fatigue are common signs of pulmonary edema. Systemic congestion usually is exhibited by distended neck veins, pitting edema in the extremities, cyanosis, and clubbing of the fingers. The prognosis of patients with CHF is relatively poor; only half of the patients with this condition live beyond 3 years.[2,9]

Medical and Dental Management. Treatment of the patient with CHF usually involves the administration of cardiac glycosides such as digitalis, which serve to increase the contractile force of the ventricle, increasing cardiac output. Diuretics are also employed when edema results in a gain in weight of over 1.4 kg in 1 week. Potassium replacement is usually necessary to prevent arrhythmias from diuretic-induced electrolyte depletion. A diet low in sodium and high in potassium (bananas and fruit juices) is recommended. Exercise is usually curtailed, and some CHF patients take sedatives to treat dyspnea.[2]

If the CHF is not under medical supervision, the dental health educator should refer the patient and delay dental care until the condition is medically controlled. Modifications to dental care for the CHF patient can include (1) minimizing procedures that can induce gagging, because individuals taking digitalis can experience nausea and vomiting; (2) seating the patient with pulmonary congestion upright throughout the appointment; (3) monitoring the patient's prothrombin time if he is being treated with an anticoagulant; (4) prescribing prophylactic antibiotics to prevent infective endocarditis; and (5) terminating the appointment if the patient begins to experience fatigue.[2]

Stroke

Stroke or cerebrovascular accident (CVA) is the third most common cause of death in the nation. Of the nearly 2 million stroke patients in the United States, 800,000 require special services and 200,000 need total care.[14] The extent of sensory and motor disability depends on the cerebral vessel involvement and the magnitude of the injury.[29] Hypertensive vascular disease, atherosclerosis, myocardial infarction, and atrial fibrillation can result in stroke.[30] Cerebral thrombosis (clot) actually accounts for 75% of the strokes in the U.S. Although less common, intracranial hemorrhage and cerebral emboli can also interrupt cerebral blood flow.[2]

Risk factors that predispose an individual to stroke include previous stroke or transient ischemic attack, hypertension, atherosclerosis, cardiac abnormalities, erythrocytosis, diabetes mellitus, elevated blood lipids, tobacco, alcohol, or drug abuse, stress, and inactivity.[31]

The warning signs of stroke consist of: (1) a sudden, temporary unilateral weakness of the face or an extremity, (2) temporary aphasia (total loss of speech) or dysarthria (a speech difficulty caused by neuromuscular weakness), (3) temporary dimness or loss of vision in one or both eyes, and (4) dizziness and an inability to walk without falling.[2,29] *Medical and Dental Management.* A patient with a history of stroke is treated prophylactically with an anticoagulant (e.g., heparin for short-term therapy and coumarin or aspirin for long-term therapy). Surgery must be required to remove a superficial hematoma or an obstruction in the neck or thorax. Lifestyle changes to reduce risk factors and rehabilitation for residual damage (e.g., speech or physical therapy) are imperative for recovery. Although many individuals improve greatly, many retain some degree of impairment.[2]

The dental health educator should identify risk factors for stroke when conducting medical history assessments and encourage patients to alter their behaviors. Patients with a history of stroke should[2,29] (1) be scheduled for short morning appointments; (2) have their blood pressure monitored; (3) not be given a vasoconstrictor in an anesthetic if possible, and epinephrine in gingival retraction cord should also be avoided; (4) have their prothrombin time (PT) monitored when being treated with coumarin (anticoagulation therapy adjusts the patient's PT to 2 to 3½ times the normal rate of 11 to 14 seconds); if a dental surgical procedure is required the anticoagulation level must be reduced to a level of 1½ to 2 times the normal PT to ensure safety; (5) have their bleeding time (normal = 1 to 6 min) checked when taking aspirin therapeutically (if abnormal consult physician); (6) be provided with modified dental care devices if necessary, designed to accommodate their particular limitations in manual dexterity; and (7) be given palliative assistance with oral problems such as food impaction related to weak oral musculature or drug-induced xerostomia.

RESPIRATORY DISEASE

Respiratory disease ranks second in prevalence to cardiovascular disease in the United States. The three major respiratory diseases discussed in this section include asthma, chronic bronchitis and emphysema, and cystic fibrosis.

Asthma

The American Lung Association estimates that as many as 6 million persons have asthma in the United States. One-third of the asthmatic population is under 17 years of age; asthma is the leading cause of chronic disease in children.[32]

The extrinsic or allergic form of asthma usually affects children prior to the age of 10; approximately half of the children with this form of asthma begin to experience wheezing by 5 years of age,[32] and most become asymptomatic by the time they reach adulthood.[33] There is generally a family history of allergies associated with the extrinsic form of asthma.[2] Bronchospasms triggered by smoke, pet hair, exercise, and climate changes can cause an antigen-antibody response. Histamine is produced, resulting in chronic airway inflammation, bronchial secretions, and edema. Consequently, the smooth muscle surrounding the airway narrows and the flow of air is obstructed.[32,34] Emotional disturbances, once believed to be a major causal factor in the development of asthma, are more often related to the hyperventilation associated with the stressful episode rather than the stress itself.[32]

In contrast, intrinsic asthma is not associated with a family history of allergy and is not triggered by a readily identifiable stimulus.[9] It is generally observed in middle-aged adults and is usually correlated with an upper respiratory infection.[35,36]

Clinically, typical asthma is characterized by dyspnea, wheezing, and coughing. A sudden attack is accompanied by tightness in the chest, persistent cough, labored respirations, and wheezing observed particularly during the expiratory phase of respiration.[2,32] Episodes are usually self-limiting, with the exception of a severe form of asthma referred to as status asthmaticus.[33] This form of asthma is considered a medical emergency because death can ensue in minutes. Status asthmaticus is refractory to routine therapy and requires hospitalization.[32] *Medical and Dental Management.* Asthmatic episodes can be prevented by avoiding specific precipitating factors that are known to induce symptoms. Drug therapy is the most widely used treatment for the asthmatic; it typically includes bronchodilating agents from the methylaxanthine, beta-adrenergic, chromone, anticholinergic, and corticosteroid categories.

The dental health educator must be attuned to the specific medical history of the asthmatic dental patient. The patient should be asked his age at onset of the condition, the frequency and severity of attacks (was hospitalization required?), the timing of the last episode, the precipitating factors responsible for triggering such attacks, and the method(s) of treatment used.

Because emotional disturbances can secondarily induce an asthmatic attack, the dental health educator should make a concerted effort to provide the patient with a stress-free dental environment. A medical history of recent steroid use can indicate the need for a supplemental dose of the steroid to prevent adrenal crisis (Table 9-7).[33] Extended steroid ingestion limits the useful-

Table 9-7. The Rule of Twos

Adrenocortical suppression should be suspected if a patient has received glucocorticosteroid therapy:
1. In a dose of 20 mg or more of cortisone or its equivalent daily
2. Via the oral or parenteral route for a continuous period of 2 weeks or longer
3. Within the last 2 years

From Malamed, S.F.: Handbook of Medical Emergencies in the Dental Office. 3rd Ed. St. Louis, C.V. Mosby, 1987, p. 124.

ness of the adrenal gland, causing it to shut down, thereby suppressing the release of corticosteroid from the gland. Stress places an increased demand on the gland to secrete corticosteroid. A nonfunctioning adrenal gland cannot respond to this rapid requirement for additional cortisol to cope with the stress, and adrenal crisis ensues. Athletes taking anabolic steroids to increase their stamina and muscle mass are also at risk for adrenal crisis under similar stressful conditions.

Proper pain-control measures are necessary. Sedative premedication, nitrous oxide, and local anesthesia can be used, but some anticholinergics such as scopolamine should be avoided. Antihistamines and narcotics should also be avoided because they can cause histamine release and respiratory depression respectively.[2] Aspirin, nonsteroidal anti-inflammatory drugs, and penicillin are contraindicated because of their allergic potential.[33] Erythromycin is not recommended for the patient taking a theophylline preparation.[37] If a patient has an inhaler, the dental health educator should keep it readily available during the appointment.

Chronic Bronchitis and Emphysema

Chronic bronchitis and emphysema affect approximately 10 million people in the United States. Chronic bronchitis is defined as a daily productive cough that persists for at least 3 months for 2 consecutive years.[9]

In chronic bronchitis the bronchial tree becomes inflamed in response to either a prolonged upper respiratory chemical and physical infection or chronic exposure to irritants, e.g., coal dust, smoke, and air pollutants. Occupational exposure to pollutants places many individuals at high risk. Families of smokers, and of course smokers themselves, are extremely susceptible to developing upper respiratory infections.

Emphysema is an abnormal condition of the pulmonary system that features both overinflation and destructive changes in the alveolar walls, resulting in a loss of lung elasticity and decreased CO_2-O_2 exchange[38] from the reduction in surface area.[9] As the alveoli lose their elasticity and tear, air spaces are created that resist air flow. Consequently, breathing becomes labored. Carbon dioxide becomes trapped in the lungs and is not easily expired, giving the patient a hyperinflated or barrel-chested appearance. In addition to dyspnea, wheezing and coughing occur. Occasionally cyanosis of the lips and fingertips results because of the reduced level of oxygen-rich blood in circulation. The workload of the heart increases as it attempts to oxygenate the tissues of the body.[2,9,34]

Chronic emphysema usually accompanies chronic bronchitis and can be associated with asthma and tuberculosis. Both chronic bronchitis and emphysema result in airway obstruction and are caused chiefly by cigarette smoking.[38] In chronic bronchitis, mucus plugs the airways early in the illness, limiting gas exchange in the lungs. In emphysema, serious damage to the anatomy of airways usually occurs in the later stages of the illness.[9]

Medical and Dental Management. Patients with chronic bronchitis should avoid irritants that induce allergic symptoms and are best treated with postural drainage of mucus and with antibiotics for bacterial infections.[34] Bronchodilators such as those used for the treatment of asthma are ineffective.

During the dental appointment, the patient should be given ample opportunity to cough. Plaque removal and antimicrobial mouthrinses to reduce the accumulation of plaque and mucus are recommended.[34]

Medical considerations for the emphysema patient include (1) a low concentration of oxygen with humidification for several minutes hourly, (2) the prescription of bronchodilators, antibiotics, expectorants, and corticosteroids, (3) postural drainage if chronic bronchitis exists concurrently, (4) breathing exercises, and (5) the consumption of 2000 to 3000 ml of fluid daily.[38] Needless to say, the patient is strongly urged to quit smoking.

Afternoon dental appointments during warm weather are recommended for the patient with emphysema. Waiting rooms with people who are smoking or have upper respiratory infections must be avoided. The patient should be seated upright during dental procedures, and rubber dams should be used cautiously if at all because of the airway obstruction that can be created when the dam is in place.

The dental health educator should also monitor the length and dosage of steroid administration, and avoid the use of narcotics, barbiturates, and high oxygen concentrations usually used with nitrous oxide, which depress respiratory function.[34]

Cystic Fibrosis

Cystic fibrosis (CF) is an inherited disorder that affects approximately 90,000 persons in the United States.[9] One out of every 20 Americans is believed to be a carrier of the CF trait. Because CF is transmitted by a mendelian autosomal recessive gene, there is a 25% chance that the child will have CF, a 50% chance the child will be a carrier, and a 25% chance the child will be neither when both parents carry the gene for CF. The incidence rate for cystic fibrosis is about 1 in 1800 live births annually.[39] Males and females are equally affected; Caucasions of European lineage are more susceptible than Orientals, blacks, or Indians.[40,41]

Cystic fibrosis was named by Dr. Guido Fanconi in 1936. He discovered that a large number of children who were dying early had experienced similar symptoms of diarrhea, retarded growth patterns, and frequent lung infections.[42] Since Fanconi's time it has been found that CF is a generalized disorder that affects the exocrine glands of the body. The exocrine glands are resonsible for the secretion of mucus, saliva, and sweat. In a person with CF, these secretions are abnormally viscous and sticky, impeding the function of the lungs and pancreas.[43]

Gastrointestinal complications are caused by viscous pancreatic juices that block the pancreatic duct, resulting in an inadequate secretion of pancreatic enzymes into the duodenum. Patients with CF experience a failure to gain weight despite increased food consumption and have frequent, bulky, foul, fatty stools due to an inability to metabolize ketone bodies.

Thick mucus secretions accumulate in the bronchi and bronchioles of the lungs of CF patients. These secretions paralyze the cilia and thus impair normal respiration and the filtering of dust and microorganisms from the lungs. The CF patient exhibits a chronic productive cough and a lowered tolerance to physical exertion.[34] Eventually, pulmonary infections, atelectasis (collapse of the air sacs), and emphysema result even with treatment. Clubbing of the fingers and toes is usually observed in more advanced disease. Diabetes, cirrhosis of the liver, male sterility, and psychologic complications also arise, particularly as these patients are able to live longer with treatment.

Cystic fibrosis patients exhibit two to five times the normal level of sodium and potassium in their perspiration. Parents sometimes notice their child tastes salty when kissed. Because of this inability to conserve electrolytes, dehydration becomes a concern for the CF patient, particularly during warm weather or while exercising.

CF patients exhibit enlarged submaxillary and sublingual salivary glands. The flow rate of the saliva is slowed and the consistency is more viscous, causing xerostomia. Such an oral environment makes wearing dental prostheses difficult. Interestingly, CF patients have less caries, plaque accumulation, and gingivitis than the average person, but their calculus deposits appear heavier. The teeth are frequently discolored from impaired oxygenation or the prolonged use of antibiotics for respiratory infections. Mouth breathing might compensate for the patient's difficulty breathing due to lung or nasal obstructions or might be acquired as a result of open-bite malocclusion.[34]

Medical and Dental Management. The dental health educator might wish to test the chemical composition of the saliva if other symptoms suggest CF during a review of a child's medical history with a parent. More realistically, the educator should advise the parents that their child should see a pediatrician or an endocrinologist to receive a "sweat test" to determine the existence of CF.

Treatment for cystic fibrosis requires a team effort. Physician, dental health educator, nurse, nutritionist, respiratory therapist, social worker, psychologist, parents, and child must work together to reduce the patient's risks. Antibiotics are prescribed to manage lung infections. Aerosol inhalants or nebulizers are used to expand the bronchial tubes and hydrate the mucus, therefore enhancing its elimination from the body. Mist tents during rest periods also promote hydration. Daily postural drainage exercises, which involve cupping, clapping, and vibrating the lungs, are compulsory for CF patients to encourage mucus drainage and expectoration.

Digestive complications are managed by reducing total fat while increasing calories and protein. The intake of salt and fluids must be adequate, particularly in the summer months, due to excessive perspiration. Inadequate metabolism caused by a reduction in the pancreatic enzymes trypsin and chymotrypsin contributes to the CF patient's poor physical growth. Pancreatic enzymes and vitamin and mineral supplements are prescribed to provide nutrients that the body cannot metabolize efficiently.

The patient with cystic fibrosis should not be scheduled during the winter months to avoid exposure to persons with colds or flu who might be sitting in the waiting room, or hot summer months, when perspiration might be extensive. Late afternoon appointments are suggested so the child does not have to miss additional school. A rubber dam should be used with caution, and the chair should be placed in a more upright position to permit uncomplicated breathing. Bleaching might be considered to treat the esthetic ramifications of intrinsic staining on the anterior teeth. Frequent prophylaxes to remove calculus and reinforce oral hygiene instructions are strongly recommended. Diet counseling from a caries standpoint might also be required for patients who consume large quantities of fermentable carbohydrates to boost their calorie intake.

The frail, underdeveloped child or adolescent with CF often suffers from self-image problems. Illness can place stress on parents and siblings, particularly if health care expenses become costly. Genetic counseling is suggested for adolescent CF patients and parents with one CF child contemplating a larger family. The major goal of cystic fibrosis research is to devise a test that identifies CF carriers.[34]

BLEEDING DISORDERS

Many bleeding disorders are iatrogenic because bleeding can result from drugs pre-scribed by physicians for heart conditions or arthritis. Two major diseases characterized by abnormal bleeding tendencies are hemophilia and leukemia. Hemophilia is discussed in detail in this section, and leukemia is outlined in the section of this chapter on cancer.

Hemophilia

Estimates suggest that hemophilia occurs in about 1 out of every 4000 live male births.[44] Hemophilia is a sex-linked hereditary bleeding disorder transmitted on a gene of the X chromosome. This blood coagulation disorder is caused by a deficiency or an inactivity of clotting factor essential for clot formation and hemostasis. A hemophiliac male cannot pass this disorder on to his sons, but all of his daughters will carry the gene for the disease; hence his daughters are carriers and have the ability to pass hemophilia on to the next generation. A woman who is a carrier has four possibilities with each subsequent pregnancy: a normal son, a normal daughter, a son with hemophilia, or a daughter who is a carrier (Fig. 9-2).[45]

There are four common types of hemophilia:[46]

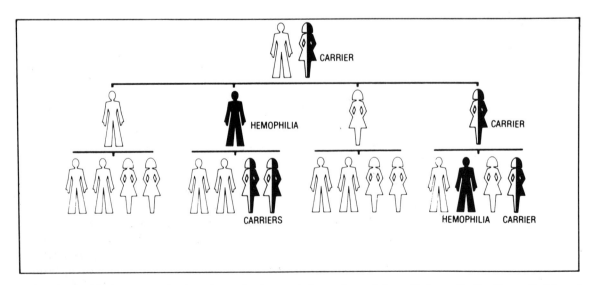

Figure 9-2. The pattern of inheritance for hemophilia. Adapted from Eckert, E. F.: Your Child and Hemophilia. Berkeley, Cutter Biological, 1983.

1. Factor VIII or antihemophilic factor deficiency refers to hemophilia A or classic hemophilia. This is the most common form of hemophilia and affects approximately 80% of all hemophiliacs.
2. Factor IX or a plasma thromboplastin component deficiency is known as hemophilia B; it is also referred to as Christmas disease. Approximately 19% of all hemophiliacs possess this form of the disease.
3. Factor XI deficiency is observed predominantly in European Jews and is also known as hemophilia C. This bleeding disorder is not as severe as factor VIII or IX deficiencies. Abnormal bleeding occurs only as a result of trauma or surgery. Less than 1% of hemophiliacs have this type of deficiency.
4. Von Willebrand disease is also a rare clotting disorder and also affects less than 1% of the hemophiliac population. This disorder is characterized by low factor VIII levels, prolonged bleeding times, and poor platelet adhesion. Von Willebrand disease occurs in both males and females.

The degree of severity of the disease depends on the level of coagulation factor present in the blood. Normal concentrations of coagulation factors range from 50 to 150%. *Severe* hemophilia refers to frequent and spontaneous bleeding into the joints (hemarthrosis) from any physical or emotional trauma. Sometimes there is no apparent cause for the bleeding. A baby with severe hemophilia can induce hemorrhage by simply crawling. Routine hemorrhage damages the joints and muscles and leads to eventual disability. A severe hemophiliac has from 0 to 2% of active clotting factor in his blood plasma. *Moderate* hemophilia consists of infrequent spontaneous hemorrhage after minor trauma. Moderate disease is likely to go undetected for a long time, perhaps until the boy begins some form of contact sport. Between 2 and 5% of the deficient factor is present. An individual with *mild* hemophilia has a factor range of 5 to 50%. Bleeding only occurs after severe injury and can go unnoticed for years. A person with mild hemophilia is able to live a fairly routine lifestyle.[47-49]

When the hemophiliac is injured, he does not bleed faster than normal, but instead bleeds longer. The deficiency in factor prevents a firm clot from forming. The soft platelet plug that does result is inadequate and eventually breaks down and bleeding begins again.

Medical and Dental Management. All forms of hemophilia require venous injections of clotting factor. Mild forms of hemophilia are treated with fresh-frozen plasma containing the factor. Severe hemophilia is managed with one of the two types of normal plasma extracts, cryoprecipitate and concentrate.[45,46] Cryoprecipitate is freeze-dried clotting factor prepared from a large number of donors, and it can be stored at room temperature for 6 months or refrigerated for up to 2 years. Concentrate is factor prepared fresh from a single blood donation and stored in the freezer.

When a bleeding episode occurs, prompt treatment is necessary to prevent deformities. With the advent of concentrate and cryoprecipitate, many hemophiliacs infuse themselves at home if a hemorrhage begins or is suspected. This enables the hemophiliac to be treated early, remain independent, and lead a more normal lifestyle. Important disadvantages of numerous infusions of blood products include the susceptibility of the individual to development of inhibitor (antibody that destroys coagulation factor) and the risk of contracting AIDS or hepatitis. Several therapeutic approaches exist to eradicate inhibitor. These include neutralization of the inhibitor by continuous infusion of massive doses of factor VIII concentrate, dilution of the inhibitor by plasmapheresis, injection of a purified porcine factor VIII called hydrate C, and bypassing the inhibitor with prothrombin complex concentrates (PCCs). Two types of activated PCCs (FEIBA and Autoplex) have been quite effective in controlling serious bleeds.[50]

Hemophiliacs who have been receiving blood products are strongly advised to obtain the hepatitis vaccine. The average hemophiliac receives 45,000 to 50,000 units of concentrate annually.[51] The testing of both donor and final product has had a major effect on the amount of the hepatitis B virus in final pooled plasma products.[46]

Treatment of the hemophiliac requires a team approach involving a hematologist, nurse, physical therapist, psychiatric social worker, rehabilitation counselor, dentist, and dental hygienist. Preventive dental care and prompt treatment of dental emergencies are vital components of the overall management of the patient's health.

Prior to performing dental treatment, the dental health educator should ascertain the type and severity of the hemophilia and the form of replacement therapy used. Although the use of concentrates makes local anesthesia less risky, infiltration and block anesthesia should be used with caution. Block anesthesia is a greater concern because of the possibility of a dissecting hematoma that could obstruct the airway. Oral premedication (intramuscular injections are contraindicated), hypnosis, and nitrous oxide analgesia are advised when appropriate.

Care must also be taken:[47,49] (1) to avoid the development of a sublingual hematoma when placing a film packet in the mouth; (2) to avoid laceration of the lip or tongue when using dental instruments; (3) to line the impression tray with wax when taking impressions; (4) to place saliva ejectors or high-speed vacuum carefully (rubber-padded ejector tips are preferable); and (5) to adapt and place orthodontic bands and other prosthetic devices in such a way as to avoid trauma to the oral tissues.

Dental procedures that cause some small degree of bleeding include subgingival scaling, the extraction of one erupted tooth, and dental restorations completed without local anesthesia.

Although quadrant scaling is preferable for the patient with moderate to severe periodontal involvement, a single scaling procedure is advised for patients requiring replacement therapy for the procedure. Ultrasonic scaling is not contraindicated but should be used with caution. Rubber-cup polishing requires careful adaptation beneath the marginal gingiva. Replacement factor is administered prior to these services

to raise the factor level in the blood to at least 30%.[46] Epsilonaminocaproic acid (Amicar) is given by mouth postoperatively and during healing to maintain the blood clot.[46] Amicar is not used postoperatively when prothrombin complex concentrates are used.[52]

More excessive bleeding can be caused by multiple extractions of teeth, the removal of impacted teeth, and periodontal surgery.[46] A 50% factor level is necessary for these dental procedures, and Amicar is given postoperatively. Local hemostatic agents, e.g., Surgicel, Avitene, and Oxycel, are impregnated with topical thrombin and sodium bicarbonate and offer additional protection in the maintenance of a clot. The patient's physician should be consulted prior to all dental procedures.

Good oral hygiene is necessary to minimize gingival bleeding. For patients exhibiting joint deformities and arthritis, toothbrush modifications are suggested to meet their dexterity needs. A hemophiliac who has never used dental floss and exhibits moderate to severe gingival inflammation should probably be instructed by the dental health educator to use dental tape first, because it is less traumatic to the tissue. Following the mastery of dental tape the patient can progress to dental floss. Fluoride supplementation might be necessary if the young hemophiliac lives in a fluoride-deficient area or appears to be prone to dental caries. A diet beneficial to the patient's oral and general health should be encouraged.

Accidents involving the mouth are not uncommon during childhood. In most cases firm pressure and the use of an oral adhesive paste are sufficient to promote hemostasis in the hemophiliac, but some cases might require local first aid, factor replacement, and play restrictions. The following safety rules should be given to children to reduce the risks of trauma:[53] do not run with objects in the mouth, chew food slowly to avoid cheek and tongue bites, do not put writing implements or other pointed objects in the mouth, and wear seat belts when riding in a car.

Analgesics containing aspirin can induce bleeding and should be avoided. Classic anti-inflammatory drugs, e.g., phenylbutazone and indomethacin, normally prescribed for joint pain, are contraindicated because they also potentiate the bleeding disorder by altering platelet function. Nonnarcotic analgesics that can be safely prescribed for pain include acetaminophen (Tylenol), pentazocine hydrochloride (Talwin), propoxyphene hydrochloride (Darvon). Narcotic analgesics include codeine, meperidine hydrochloride (Demerol), Morphine, and hydromorphone hydrochloride (Dilaudid).[49]

Hemophiliacs frequently experience hemarthroses, arthritis, and the eventual need for total joint replacement due to their disability. Infections (e.g., ear, urinary, and oral) have been known to complicate the outcome of prosthetic joint replacement surgeries. When such a procedure is indicated, it is imperative that the patient receive a dental examination so existing periodontal infections or abscessed teeth can be treated. All necessary treatment to eliminate infection must be accomplished prior to joint replacement surgery. Following the surgery, prophylactic antibiotics are required for any procedures (particularly dental) in which a bacteremia could result that would increase the risk of infection in the area of the prosthetic joint.

DIABETES

In 1982, 2.54% of the American population or about 5.77 million people in the United States were diagnosed diabetics.[54] Females appear to be affected slightly more than males. Blacks over 25 years of age have a higher prevalence of diabetes than whites, but whites in the 0 to 24 age bracket are more frequently afflicted than blacks of the same age group.[55]

Diabetes mellitus is a chronic disease complex of impaired glucose metabolism caused by a deficiency in the action of the hormone insulin. As blood glucose becomes elevated (hyperglycemia), alterations in lipid protein metabolism result, increasing the diabetic's risk of early-onset atherosclerosis, vision impairment, and kidney disease. The causes of diabetes include[2] (1) a genetic disorder of unknown transmission; (2) a primary destruction of the islets of Langerhans of the pancreas (responsible for the production of insulin) caused by inflammation, cancer, or surgery; (3) an endocrine imbalance resultant from such diseases as hyperpituitarism or hyperthyroidism; and (4) the administration of steroids.

There are two major forms of diabetes. Insulin-dependent diabetes mellitus (IDDM) occurs in approximately 10% of diabetics who depend on insulin for the prevention of ketoacidosis. IDDM, also referred to as type I or juvenile-onset diabetes, has a sudden onset and most often affects persons under 40 years of age. Type II, maturity-onset or noninsulin-dependent diabetes (NIDDM), usually has a slow onset of symptoms. It occurs predominantly in adulthood (over 40 years) and constitutes about 90% of all cases. These patients are often managed with oral hypoglycemic agents and diet modifications.

The symptoms of diabetes are found in Table 9-8.[2]

Although blood glucose levels are high, many of the body's cells are unable to metabolize the glucose because of insulin insufficiency. This results in cellular starvation—a depletion of the cells' energy level. The body interprets the situation as a low supply of glucose and responds by supplying glucose from other sources (e.g., muscle and liver glycogen and protein). As glycogen is depleted, the energy needed for muscle contraction is obtained from fatty acids. Excessive fatty acid conversion in the liver leads to ketone bodies with subsequent metabolic acidosis.[56] Acidosis is further established by increased excretion of electrolytes in the urine. Severe acidosis leads to coma if undetected or untreated. The signs of diabetic coma include[9] fruity acetone breath; cardinal symptoms of Type I diabetes; signs of dehydration; abdominal tenderness; Kussmaul breathing (rapid and deep); fever in the presence of an infection; and depressed sensorium.[9]

Medical and Dental Management. Treatment of the diabetic condition is multifa-

Table 9-8. Symptoms of Diabetes

Type I diabetes
  Cardinal symptoms—common
    Polydipsia
    Polyuria
    Polyphagia
    Weight loss
    Loss of strength
  Other symptoms
    Recurrence of bed-wetting
    Repeated skin infections
    Marked irritability
    Headache
    Drowsiness
    Malaise
    Xerostomia
Type II diabetes
  Cardinal symptoms—rare
  Common symptoms
    Weight fluctuations
    Urination at night
    Vulvar pruritus (females)
    Vision impairments
    Paresthesias
    Loss of sensation
    Impotence
    Postural hypotension

From Little, J.W., and Falace, D.A.: Dental Management of the Medically Compromised Patient. 3rd Ed. St. Louis, C.V. Mosby, 1988, p. 202.

ceted. Nearly 70% of adult diabetics are overweight. The basis for successful management of the diabetic patient involves the balance of total caloric intake with physical activity and body weight. Sometimes patients reach their ideal weight on the diabetic diet alone and their symptoms reverse. A diabetic diet to lower body weight should consist of[56] (1) 1000 calories daily, (2) a reduction in simple-sugar ingestion, (3) a decreased intake of fats and cholesterol, and (4) the regulation of food intake and exercise to the amount of insulin taken, if applicable. Patients who reach their ideal weight and still have symptoms of hyperglycemia and an elevated blood glucose level require the addition of insulin therapy to their total regimen.

Insulin preparations differ in unit dosage, onset, duration, and route of administration. Insulin is available in concentration of 100 units/ml and a variety of preparations administered alone or in combination can last from 2 to 36 h. In most cases, two-thirds of the total dose is given before breakfast and the remaining one-third before dinner. Patients become quite knowledgeable about their condition, by learning to (1) monitor their urine for glucose levels, (2) assess their need for snacks, and (3) change their insulin dosages on the basis of fluctuations in blood glucose levels related to diet, exercise, and stress. Some diabetics administer their own insulin by injection, whereas others have an insulin pump that releases continuous small dosages of insulin throughout the day. Many individuals with type II diabetes are treated with oral hypoglycemic agents because the beta cells of the pancreas are still capable of secreting some degree of endogenous insulin.

A condition known as insulin shock can occur if the level of insulin in the body is too high and consequently the level of glucose in the blood is too low. Insulin shock can result from three factors: a missed meal after an injection of insulin, excessive exercise, or an overdose of insulin. Untreated acute hypoglycemia (blood sugar ≤ 40 mg/dl) associated with insulin overdose can cause permanent brain damage, seizures, and death.[9]

Dental patients suspected of having diabetes should not be treated unless they are currently under a physician's care and are well-controlled. A patient with an estimated fasting blood glucose level of 140 mg/100 ml or above should be referred to a physician. Repeated headaches, xerostomia, paresthesia, rapidly progressive periodontal disease, and frequent periodontal abscesses can indicate a hyperglycemic condition.[2]

Controlled diabetics can be treated with relative ease. Medical history assessment should include information concerning (1) type of diabetes, (2) concomitant medical complications, (3) treatment regimen (if treated with insulin, how much, when last administered, and if a meal followed the injection), and (4) patient's monitoring of his urine and the results that particular day or evening prior to the dental appointment. The dental health educator should always keep 50% glucose, sweetened fruit juice, or candy available to manage an insulin shock episode.[2,56]

Dental appointments for diabetics should be in the morning, between breakfast and lunch. Local anesthesia injections should be limited to one, because epinephrine can raise blood glucose levels. Diabetic patients are prone to infections and take longer to heal, so caries, periodontal disease, and trauma should be prevented and antibiotics prescribed when necessary. Because erythromycin is renally excreted, penicillin is recommended. Tetracycline can be given to young diabetics after tooth development. Fungal growth can be problematic after antibiotic therapy and should be managed with nystatin. Xerostomia is also a concern and is the result of a general dehydration from electrolyte loss. The oral mucosa becomes dry and inflamed, making it difficult for the patient to wear removable prostheses. Periodic dental evaluations, meticulous oral hygiene, and daily use of a topical fluoride gel are important for reducing the risks of infection.

LIVER DISEASE

Patients with liver disease have historically posed a great concern to members of the dental profession. Protection against transmission of hepatitis B and more recently the dental management of the liver transplant candidate are issues which require consideration when addressing the effects of liver disease on the provision of dental care.

Hepatitis B

Hepatitis B, also known as serum hepatitis, is a highly contagious viral infection and approximately 11.5% of the general population have hepatitis B virus (HBV) markers.[57] Dental practitioners are believed to be at three times the risk of the overall populace. Volunteer dentists surveyed at the American Dental Association's annual ses-

sions exhibited a 27 to 37% marker prevalence from 1983 to 1985.[58]

Transmission of hepatitis B can occur through blood, saliva, semen, and bodily secretions.[59] Intraorally, the gingival sulcus has the greatest concentration potential of hepatitis B,[60,61] therefore placing the practitioner at highest risk during the performance of oral prophylaxis, periodontal surgery, or other oral surgical procedures. Only a small amount of inoculum (0.0001 ml blood) is necessary to transmit the disease. HBV is extremely difficult to destroy. It is much more stable than the AIDS virus and can live on inanimate objects and under fingernails for several days.[62]

The incubation period for HBV is between 15 and 180 days, averaging about 2 months. Viral hepatitis is characterized by degeneration and necrosis of liver cells. The liver becomes inflamed and is invaded by lymphocytes and mononuclear phagocytes.[63] Because the liver is unable to metabolize bilirubin as it normally does to aid in the emulsification of fats, bilirubin accumulates in the blood, giving the skin an amber hue (jaundice). The patient also suffers from nausea, anorexia, and malaise. Recovery is usually observed approximately 4 months after onset of jaundice. Abnormal liver function values and hepatomegaly can persist. Many cases of hepatitis are subclinical, and the patient can have the disease without any knowledge of it.[64,65]

Patients with or without jaundice can develop chronic carrier status. Hepatitis carriers are individuals who have the hepatitis B surface antigen (HB$_s$Ag) circulating in their blood indefinitely. An estimated 10% of persons with hepatitis B viral infections become carriers.[62] Although all carriers have the potential to transmit the disease to their contacts, they are not equally infectious. Infection, by direct and indirect percutaneous inoculation, absorption through mucosal surfaces, and the indirect handling of instruments or other items contaminated with their blood increases with the existence of both HB$_s$Ag and HB$_e$Ag in the blood.[66]

Medical and Dental Management. Although the frequency of transmission of hepatitis B from dental practitioner to patient is extremely low, the reverse is somewhat higher. Therefore this section emphasizes the dental health educator's role in reducing his susceptibility. The dental health educator must take a thorough medical history to ascertain the type of hepatitis, the existence of carrier status, and the treatment rendered to determine a patient's degree of infectivity if he admits to having had the disease. Potential risk groups can also be identified by their occupation, geographic origin, behaviors, and selected sexual practices.[67]

Hepatitis vaccinations are strongly recommended for dental practitioners. Heptavax-B (made from the plasma of human HBV carriers) and Recombivax HB (genetically engineered with no connection to blood or blood products) are both considered effective vaccines for achieving immunity to HBV.[62] Antibody levels should be checked periodically to ensure immunity. If the level falls below 10 SRU, a supplemental booster is indicated.

The concept of universal precautions in relation to infection control suggests that optimum barrier protection to prevent cross-contamination should be taken with all patients; all patients should be treated as if they are infectious. Gloves, eyewear, masks or faceshields, and disposable gowns are recommended. All instruments should be heat-sterilized. Handpieces should be sterilized after each use. Contaminated impressions should be rinsed and disinfected (10 min in glutaraldehyde, or 5 min in iodophor or diluted bleach for alginate) prior to being sent to the laboratory. Equipment and surfaces that are difficult to disinfect, such as hoses, light handles, and x-ray heads, should be wrapped with plastic or aluminum foil which is discarded following each patient.[68] Iodophors are best suited for hard-surface disinfection. All disposable contaminated materials should be bagged separately for each patient and discarded in one large receptacle marked "disposables." Needles and other sharp objects should be disposed of in marked puncture-proof containers.

If nonvaccinated dental personnel accidentally stick themselves with a contaminated needle or instrument and exposure to HBV occurs, the Centers for Disease Control recommend the following: (1) hepatitis B immune globulin (HBIG) injection within 24 hours, and (2) Hepatitis B vaccine intramuscularly within 1 week of exposure, the second and third doses 1 and 6 months, respectively, after the initial dose. Those exposed who have already been vaccinated should have an antibody titer done unless it has been done within the past year. If antibody levels are insufficient, one HBIG dose and an HBV booster are administered.[57,68]

Liver Transplants

Dental health educators should follow the following protocol for patients about to undergo liver transplant surgery:[70]

1. Perform a complete oral examination and radiographic survey to identify any potential sources of infection.
2. Complete all necessary restorative treatment needs.
3. Place the patient on an oral hygiene regimen and assess his progress daily. If the patient is hospitalized, an oral prophylaxis, plaque-control procedures, oral hygiene instructions, antimicrobial rinses, and daily fluoride therapy are advised to control infection, gingival bleeding, and cyclosporine-induced gingival hyperplasia. (Cyclosporine is a drug used to prevent organ rejection without producing myelosuppression.)
4. Have a complete laboratory screening done prior to performing any periodontal or oral surgical procedures. A complete blood count with differential, prothrombin time, partial thromboplastin time, and bleeding time should be obtained. If coagulopathies are noted, fresh-frozen plasma, packed red cells, platelets, or vitamin K should be considered. Local hemostatic agents (e.g., epinephrine and topical thrombin) might be indicated during oral surgical procedures.
5. Minimize the prescription of drugs primarily metabolized by the liver.

6. Administer antibiotics prophylactically 1 day prior to surgical procedures, the day of the surgery, and for 1 week after surgery.

RENAL DISEASE

Renal dialysis and kidney transplantation are the two modes of treatment most commonly employed for patients with end-stage renal disease (ESRD). Approximately 72,000 Americans are dependent on dialysis (artificial filtration of the blood), and about 8000 persons across the country have received kidney transplants. Kidney disease affects approximately 8 million people in the United States, ranking fourth among major health problems in the nation. Of the 8 million afflicted, 7.5% die annually.[9]

End-stage renal disease begins as renal insufficiency and can only be detected by slight laboratory abnormalities, such as a lowered glomerular filtration rate. As the disease progresses, functioning nephrons are damaged, limiting the kidneys' ability to perform their excretory, endocrine, and metabolic functions; this condition is referred to as uremia. Each kidney contains about 1 million nephrons. Clinical manifestations of ESRD occur when about 75% of these nephrons have been destroyed. The complications observed as a result of this loss include anemia; hypertension; dilute urine excretion; hyperkalemia, sodium depletion, and other electrolyte disturbances; an accumulation of urea (azotemia) and other waste products in the blood because of poor filtration; changes in bone formation (renal osteodystrophy), increasing the individual's susceptibility to fractures; bleeding tendencies primarily caused by a decrease in factor III (sometimes factor VIII) levels and abnormal platelet aggregation; and an increased incidence of coronary artery disease.[9,71] Patients with uremic syndrome can also demonstrate depression and muscular hyperactivity in the form of convulsions. Gastrointestinal complications, ranging from nausea and vomiting to constipation and diarrhea, are common, particularly later in the disease process. Occasionally, a whitish coating of the arms and trunk (uremic frost) occurs. This "frost" forms from residual urea crystals left on the skin after perspiration evaporates. Oral signs of renal failure include ulcerations, candidiasis (commonly in renal transplant patients), and parotitis, leaving an ammonia-like breath odor and metal taste in the mouth from urea in the saliva. The retention of pigments that would normally be excreted by the kidneys can cause hyperpigmentation of the skin and teeth if uremia was present during tooth development. Hypoplasia can also be observed, as well as osteomalacia of the mandible and loss of lamina dura.[2,9] Patients on dialysis classically have pale pink oral mucosa and increased formation of dental calculus.[9]

Medical and Dental Management. Conservative treatment for kidney disease includes drug therapy and diet alterations aimed at reducing azotemia and balancing electrolyte levels. Unfortunately, patients with ESRD cannot metabolize drugs due to their kidney impairment, and toxic levels of these drugs can accumulate.

As more nephrons become destroyed, dialysis is required. The technique requires the surgical implantation of a Teflon-Silastic shunt or an arteriovenous fistula that allows repeated access to the patient's circulation without needle punctures. The blood leaves the body from the shunt or fistula site, enters the machine where it is filtered, and returns to the patient. Heparin is administered to prevent clotting. The disadvantages of dialysis are: dependence on a machine every 2 to 3 days, 3 to 5 hours per day, increased risk of contracting hepatitis B, and the possibility of infection surrounding the fistula site.

A patient who wishes to be free from dialysis has one alternative—a kidney transplant. Kidney transplantation, although miraculous, is not without complications. The major problem is graft rejection. Despite advances in antirejection therapy, over 80% of transplant recipients experience infection.

Consultation with the renal patient's physician is essential before instituting dental care. Early stages of the disease require the monitoring of blood pressure and a hematologic profile. Antibiotics are only required if an infection is present or aggressive dental treatment is about to be rendered. Meticulous oral hygiene is also critical to infection control and paves the way for performing any other forms of dental service that might be needed. Phenacetin, acetaminophen, tetracyline, the long-term administration of penicillin VK, and other drugs that are excreted by the kidneys should be avoided or the dosage monitored to prevent retention in the kidneys.[2,9]

It is easier to manage the medically treated patient than to provide dental services to the dialysis or transplant patient. Dialysis patients with Teflon-Silastic shunts always require antibiotic premedication before dental treatment to prevent a bacterial endarteritis from a resulting bacteremia. Arteriovenous fistulae are less susceptible to infection because the devices are fabricated from a native vein or prosthetic conduit. These fistulae therefore do not always require prophylactic premedication. The dental health educator should consult with the patient's physician. With regard to impaired coagulation and hemorrhage, the day after therapy or midway between two dialysis sessions is the best time to treat the renal dialysis patient.[72]

Transplant patients should be placed on a strict oral hygiene regimen and examined thoroughly for infection and to determine susceptibility to infection. Extraction of questionable teeth is preferred over extensive reconstructive work. When severe infection exists or major dental procedures are warranted, hospitalization might be necessary. If high doses of steroids are given to reduce inflammation and subsequent infection, supplementation might be needed in the presence of stress (see Table 9-7). In addition, patients are usually placed on azathioprine (Imuran) or cyclosporine therapy. The patient on azathioprine therapy to prevent organ rejection displays the highest risk for infection because of the myelosuppression that occurs as a result of the drug. Cyclosporine's major advantage over azathioprine is that it reduces the risk of organ rejection without inhibiting the bone marrow. Prophylactic antibiotics should always be given for dental procedures to decrease the chance of bacteremia and subsequent postoperative infection at the surgical site. Transplant patients also are at increased risk for contracting hepatitis B and should be screened routinely for HB_sAg.[2]

ARTHRITIS

Arthritis is a general term used to describe a group of disorders that are characterized by inflammation of the joints, with associated pain in the joints and connective tissue. Over 37 million Americans have some form of arthritis.[73] Physicians began discussing these various forms of rheumatic disease as early as the eighteenth century. Included within the category of rheumatic disease are the following subcategories: rheumatoid arthritis, osteoarthritis, juvenile rheumatoid arthritis, ankylosing spondylitis, Sjögren syndrome, gout, scleroderma, systemic lupus erythematosus, temporal arteritis, Reiter syndrome, osteoporosis, and rheumatic fever. This section of the chapter emphasizes osteoarthritis and rheumatoid arthritis because they are the arthritic disorders most often encountered and because their symptoms and treatment are applicable to the other forms of arthritis as well.[2,9]

Osteoarthritis

Osteoarthritis is the most common form of arthritis, afflicting approximately 16 million Americans or about 50% of all arthritics.[74] Classified as a noninflammatory type of joint destruction, osteoarthritis can unilaterally affect one or more larger joints that have been damaged as a result of a congenital defect, insufficient blood supply, or disease or injury from the past.[34] Osteoarthritis usually affects younger men and older women and seems to become more painful with physical activity. Wear and tear on the larger joints that bear weight might be related to age, occupation, and strenuous exercise. The hands, feet, hips, knees, cervical and lower lumbar vertebrae, and temporomandibular joint are commonly affected by the disease.

Initially, the signs of osteoarthritis involve swelling of the cartilage covering the ends of the diseased bone. This swelling reduces the density of the cartilage, causing a cracking sound when the joint is flexed. A range of destruction occurs, from mild pitting of the cartilage to serious sloughing. If the cartilage is lost, the bone ends contact, resulting in bony spurs known as osteophytes. A dull ache is experienced which is normally relieved by immobility of the joint or rest. Stiffness in the morning, after a period of sitting, or exposure to cold and dampness is usually noted.

As the disease progresses, spurs build up and can detach, limiting the movement of that joint. As the pain becomes more constant, there is an increased likelihood that the patient will favor the joint and reduce its use.

Rheumatoid Arthritis

Rheumatoid arthritis is the second leading form of arthritis in the United States. Approximately 5 million adults and 250,000 children have this disease.[34] Two to three times more women are afflicted than men, with a peak incidence between 25 and 55 years of age.[75] Rheumatoid arthritis appears as a chronic bilateral inflammation of the peripheral joints such as the wrists and hands which can ultimately result in a crippling disability. The exact cause of rheumatoid arthritis is unknown, but three basic theories have been implicated:[9] infection (bacterial or viral), biochemical and physiologic abnormalities, and abnormal immune response.

Edema of the inner lining of the joint capsule due to an inflammation of the blood vessels supplying the synovium occurs initially. Later, the lining thickens and folds and is referred to as pannus. Swelling of the lining continues until the synovium overlaps the cartilage between the bones and

causes cartilage degeneration. The articulating bones join together as a result of this loss of cartilage. The final outcome of this fusion or ankylosis is a loss of mobility.

Rheumatoid arthritis usually affects the small joints of the hands and feet. Patients complain of tenderness, swelling, and heat. In some the temporomandibular joint is involved. Approximately one in four patients with rheumatoid arthritis also develops subcutaneous nodules at common pressure points like the elbow. Remission of the disease is experienced by about 20% of adults and 60 to 70% of children. On the other side of the spectrum, approximately 10% of rheumatoid patients experience total disability.[76]

Medical and Dental Management. The treatment of osteoarthritis depends on the stage of the disease at the time of intervention. Some patients require monitoring without treatment; others require drug therapy such as aspirin and non-steroidal anti-inflammatory drugs (NSAIDs), hot or cold compresses, and intermittent periods of rest and exercise to strengthen muscles and relieve pressure from affected joints. Walking aids or braces can be helpful. Operative procedures usually involve implantation of artificial joints. Individuals with osteoarthritis do not benefit from the use of oral steroids.[2,9,34]

Rheumatoid arthritis is treated somewhat differently from osteoarthritis. Daily management can include administration of aspirin and NSAIDs, e.g., ibuprofen and sulindac. Other anti-inflammatory and immunosuppressive drugs, e.g., gold compounds, phenylbutazone, adrenocortical steroids, methotrexate, and indomethacin, are also popular. Surgery can be performed to restore function to deformed immobile joints and can involve total replacement of a diseased joint with an artificial prosthesis.[2,9,34]

Dental management usually consists of making the patient comfortable during treatment. The waiting rooms and operatories should be climate-controlled to alleviate cold air or drafts that may cause joint stiffness. If temporomandibular joint pain is present, moist heat and anti-inflammatory agents are suggested. Mouth props are recommended to reduce patient discomfort and fatigue from keeping the mouth open for long periods of time. Lengthy appointments are not advised, but if necessary the patient should change positions frequently and support affected joints.

The dental health educator must be cognizant of the side effects of drug therapy for the patient with arthritis. A patient on prolonged steroid therapy is susceptible to adrenal crisis. An arthritic's bleeding time provides essential information when the patient has been taking aspirin therapeutically; deep scaling procedures or extractions might need to be delayed. Methotrexate, a chemotherapeutic drug occasionally prescribed for the treatment of rheumatoid arthritis, is stomatotoxic and has been known to produce oral ulcerations. Stomatitis has also been reported with the administration of gold salts.[2] Patients who have undergone prosthetic joint replacement must receive prophylactic antibiotic coverge prior to dental care.

An arthritic with compromised manual dexterity might have difficulty with plaque-control procedures. When finger joints are involved, electric toothbrushes, manual toothbrushes with enlarged handles, proxabrushes, floss holders, and irrigating devices are recommended (see Chapter 8).

CANCER

Cancer is the second leading cause of death in the United States. One in four Americans will eventually develop cancer. Of the estimated 1,040,000 new cases of cancer diagnosed in 1990, it is believed that approximately 50% will result in death.[77]

Cancer is a complex disease that includes over 100 distinct forms. All forms of the disease are characterized by the haphazard proliferation of abnormal cells. The unrestricted growth of abnormal cells results in a tumor or growth that spreads locally, invades adjacent structures regionally, or metastasizes to distant sites via the blood or lymph.

This section emphasizes the role of the dental health educator in cancer care by focusing on oral cancer and leukemia—two major types of cancer that involve disease manifestations and treatment modalities that can be detrimental to the oral cavity. Presently the treatment of cancer is accomplished through (1) surgery (total or partial excision of the tumor, which can include bone marrow transplantation); (2) radiotherapy (termination of the growth and replication of cancer cells by destroying the cell nucleus with radiation in the form of x-rays, gamma rays, or atomic particles such as electrons); (3) chemotherapy (drugs that suppress the growth and spread of malignant cells); (4) immunotherapy (drugs such as interferon that use the body's own defenses to combat cancer without overt toxicity, as is sometimes seen with radiotherapy and chemotherapy); and (5) hyperthermia (raising the body's temperature to destroy the malignant cells). Immunotherapy and hyperthermia are relatively new forms of treatment and are still viewed as experimental in many areas of the country. A combination of treatment modalities might be indicated to promote palliation and reduce the debilitation and toxicity that result when only one form of treatment is instituted.

A variety of self-help organizations are available that can assist an oncology patient in achieving complete recovery. Appendix K provides a resource list of the agencies that provide support groups, educational materials, and funding for oncology patients and their families before, during, and after therapy has been rendered.

Oral Cancer

Oral cancer accounts for about 3% of all cancers (see Chapter 7). Of the estimated 30,500 new oral cancer cases in the United States for 1990, slightly over one-third will result in death.[77] If the oral lesion is detected early when it is localized (less than 3 cm in diameter) and prompt treatment is

Table 9-9. American Cancer Society Seven Warning Signals for Cancer

Change in bowel or bladder habits
A sore that does not heal
Unusual bleeding or discharge
Thickening or lump in breast or elsewhere
Indigestion or difficulty in swallowing
Obvious change in a wart or mole
Nagging cough or hoarseness

rendered, survival rates increase significantly.

The dental health educator has an important role in screening for oral abnormalities. In addition to the professional assessment, the dental health educator must be active in teaching patients how to conduct oral self-examinations so they can be cognizant of changes in their own mouths between office visits (see Fig. 7-15). Table 9-9 lists the seven warning signals for cancer. The acronym is **CAUTION.** Patients must be made aware that all signs with the exception of the first (change in bowel or bladder habits) can be related to the head and neck area. Sores that persist beyond 2 weeks should be evaluated.

Diagnosis. As discussed in Chapter 7, oral cancers can present in a variety of ways. A diagnosis is determined by one or more of the following histologic techniques:[9] vital dyes, exfoliative cytology, biopsy-incisional (excise a portion of the lesion), and excisional (excise the entire lesion).

Toluidine blue is a vital stain that identifies tissues with higher than normal levels of DNA and RNA. When applied directly to the oral mucosa, the dye reacts metachromatically with malignant cells, thereby differentiating them from normal tissue. This test can also be helpful in demarcating specific sites that are best suited for biopsy. False positives can occur with this diagnostic method.

Exfoliative cytology can also result in false positives or negatives, but it tends to be about 90% accurate. This procedure consists of obtaining a scraping or cell smear from a lesion and placing it on a slide for microscopic examination.

Biopsy is the most reliable method (ap-proximately 99%) for detecting malignancies. A biopsy must be large enough to be representative of a tumor, but at the same time its depth and circumference must be planned in accordance with the location of the lesion, the total size of the lesion, and the suspected tumor's relationship to other critical anatomic structures.

Treatment. Selecting a treatment regimen for oral cancer depends on the following: (1) stage of the tumor (size, lymph node involvement, and presence of metastasis); (2) histology of the tumor; (3) location of the tumor; (4) grade of the tumor; (5) previous treatment rendered, if any; (6) nutritional status of the patient; and (7) psychologic, religious, and economic constraints influencing the patient's decision.

Surgery and radiotherapy alone or in combination are still the most widely used forms of therapy for the patient with a head and neck malignancy. Although chemotherapy has traditionally been used for palliation in advanced inoperable cases of head and neck cancer, it appears to be gaining some acceptance as a combination form of therapy with radiotherapy.[2]

Patients exhibiting small to moderate lesions with no evidence of regional or distant metastasis are usually treated surgically. Surgery is not recommended for bilateral metastatic nodal involvement, but it has been widely performed unilaterally as radical neck dissection. The major disadvantage of radical surgery centers around the loss of structure that accompanies the removal of the lesion. Functional and cosmetic rehabilitation is often necessary. Combining surgery with radiotherapy permits a more conservative surgical approach. If radiotherapy is performed prior to surgery, approximately 2 weeks should elapse between the two modalities to allow normal surrounding cells to repair the injury caused by the radiation.

Radiotherapy alone is usually administered via an external beam at an average dosage of 5000 to 7000 rads over a 6- to 7-week period, with 4 or 5 treatments per week. Application in small doses over a long period of time increases the injury to tumor cells while providing 2- or 3-day intervals between a treatment series to allow injured normal tissues to recover. Squamous cell carcinomas of the lip, buccal mucosa, soft palate, tongue, and floor of the mouth seem to respond well to radiotherapy.

Dental Management. Prior to surgery or radiotherapy, the oral health of the patient should be stabilized. A thorough oral examination, including radiographs and photographs, should be conducted to obtain baseline information for measuring oral complications associated with therapy and evaluating the effectiveness of oral care. Pretreatment of any existing oral disease should be accomplished. Existing prostheses should be remade or removed if they are ill-fitting, and hopeless teeth that are periodontally or periapically involved should be extracted. Recontouring of the bone following extraction is necessary to prevent infection, and healing should be largely complete (at least 2 weeks) before initiating therapy. Orthodontic appliances that are causing irritations and breaks in the mucosal integrity should be temporarily removed. Other potential sources of irritation that must be alleviated include rough, fractured cusps and overhanging restorations. Any existing carious lesions should be restored, and a thorough oral prophylaxis should be performed. Patients and their families should also be taught the proper methods for plaque removal and nutritional counseling to maintain a healthy mouth. Abrasive foods that can traumatize the oral mucosa should be avoided. Examples of such foods include toast, crackers, and potato chips. All forms of trauma (mechanical, e.g., rough foods or improper toothbrushing; chemical, e.g., spicy foods, tobacco, and alcohol; bacterial, e.g., plaque; and thermal, e.g., hot temperature beverages or foods) must be eliminated. Due to the erythema produced by the radiation (Fig. 9-3), patients should be instructed to avoid sunlight, ultraviolet rays, soaps, and lotions within the irradiated field because they can contribute to soft tissue necrosis[78] (Fig. 9-3). There is evidence that pretreatment oral disease, unrelated to the cancer, increases the patient's risk of oral complications during therapy.[79] If the salivary glands are in the

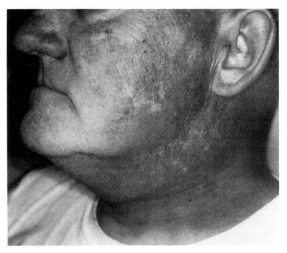

Figure 9-3. Skin erythema from exposure to therapeutic doses of radiation. Courtesy of J. E. Bouquot, D.D.S., M.S., West Virginia University.

irradiated field, the patient with retained teeth will require impressions so that custom fluoride carriers can be fabricated.

During radiotherapy, side effects can be numerous, including mucositis, xerostomia, osteoradionecrosis, hypogeusia, and trismus.

Mucositis. Mucositis emerges within 2 weeks of the onset of therapy. Mucositis refers to an inflammation and sloughing of the oral mucosa that usually persists for several weeks beyond the conclusion of treatment (Fig. 9-4). Initially the mucosa in the path

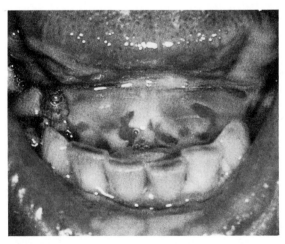

Figure 9-4. Oral mucositis in a patient receiving radiation therapy for a tumor of the head and neck. Courtesy of J. E. Bouquot, D.D.S., M.S., West Virginia University.

Table 9-10. Alcohol Content of Commercial Mouthwashes

Brand Name	Percentage Alcohol
Listerine	26.9
Scope	16.6
Signal	14.5
Cepacol	14.0
Lavoris	Second ingredient
Act	7
Listermint	6.6

of radiation appears swollen and red. It eventually becomes ulcerated and produces pain, making it difficult for the patient to speak, eat, or taste. The suggested palliative management of mucositis consists of [2,9]

1. Frequent rinsing with normal saline (0.9%) alone or in conjunction with sodium bicarbonate.
2. Avoiding commercial mouthwashes due to their high alcohol content, which produces an astringent or drying effect (Table 9-10).
3. Rinsing with or painting topical anesthetic solutions, e.g., dyclonine hydrochloride (Dyclone) and unflavored viscous lidocaine (Xylocaine), directly on ulcerated areas.
4. Coating inflamed mucosa with an unflavored, low-sodium antacid, e.g., Kaopectate and Maalox.
5. Applying topical steroids to reduce the inflammatory reaction.
6. Swabbing the oral mucosa two to three times daily with saline-soaked gauze or toothettes to remove debris, necrotic cells, and bacteria, thereby reducing the risk of infection. Sore, inflamed oral tissues are potential sources of infection.

Xerostomia. Salivary dysfunction resulting in xerostomia or dry mouth is another common sequela of irradiation of the head and neck. Xerostomia begins about the third week into therapy, and in most instances salivary flow rates never return to normal. As salivary volume decreases, the saliva becomes more viscous and tenacious and loses its buffering, lubricating, diluent, and cleansing properties. Mastication and swallowing become impaired by the combination of xerostomia and mucositis, resulting in poor nutritional intake. The patient might be unable to tolerate his dentures due to a reduced surface tension between the dry mucosa and the prosthesis and might experience an increase in candidiasis and periodontal infections as a result of a lack of self-cleansing ability.[79] The oral flora also changes in a dryer environment. Acidogenic organisms increase in quantity, thereby lowering the oral pH and increasing the patient's susceptibility to "radiation caries."[30]

The oral management of xerostomia is multidimensional and includes

1. A lifetime of daily fluoride applications (0.4% stannous or 1.0% sodium fluoride) in customized trays and over-the-counter fluoride mouthrinses is recommended to reduce the risk of caries. Radiation caries is extremely destructive and provides potential sources of infection. Decay caused by radiation-induced xerostomia typically occurs around the cervical third of the tooth (Fig. 9-5). The dental health educator must schedule the radiotherapy patient weekly to examine salivary flow and determine caries susceptibility by assessing the patient's compliance with the fluoride regimen prescribed, the oral hygiene measures delineated, and the low-fermentable carbohydrate diet recommended.
2. Artificial salivas and saliva substitutes are advised to keep the tissues lubricated. They possess a viscosity and an electrolyte composition similar to saliva and remain in the mouth longer than mere water or saline solutions. Table 9-11 lists artificial saliva preparations accepted by the American Dental Association Council of Dental Therapeutics.[81] Pilocarpine is currently being investigated for its use in stimulating salivary secretions.[79,81]
3. Perioral tissues should also be kept moist with petroleum jelly. Dry, cracked lips can permit the passage of infection.
4. Denture patients should keep their dentures out to avoid mucosal irritation. If they fit well and mucositis is not acute,

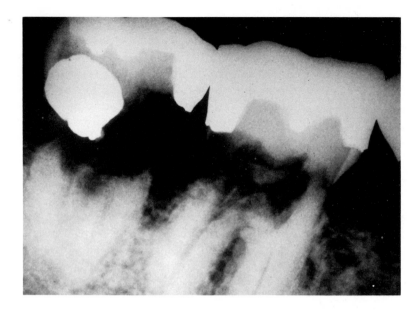

Figure 9-5. Radiograph displaying "radiation caries"—the pattern of cervical decay that can present in a patient experiencing xerostomia secondary to irradiation of the salivary glands (courtesy of J. E. Bouquot, D.D.S., M.S., West Virginia University.)

the patient may wear them briefly during eating and for visitors. Cleansing dentures is paramount in preventing Candida infection. Disposable denture cups and a chlorhexidine gluconate soak are advised to retard fungal growth.[82]

5. The patient must practice meticulous oral hygiene to decrease the risk of periodontal infection. Chlorhexidine gluconate (Peridex) rinses are also suggested to assist in the reduction of bacterial plaque.[9]

6. Bland semi-soft foods that are low in citric acid, and sucrose should be consumed. Foods should not be eaten hot. Sauces and gravies are recommended to aid the patient with chewing and swallowing.

Osteoradionecrosis. Irradiation of the oral cavity affects the vascularity of the bone, particularly the mandible.[78,83] This factor, in conjunction with exposure to trauma in any form, accounts for the development of osteoradionecrosis. Trauma to tooth-bearing areas of the jaw before or after irradiation can produce conditions that predispose to bone exposure, infection, and necrosis[80] (Fig. 9-6). Because irradiated bone loses its ability to heal, it must be protected by intact mucosa. Dry mucosa that becomes irritated and breaks down as a result of hot or abrasive foods, plaque, or ill-fitting prostheses becomes a portal of entry for secondary infection in an area where compromised bone cannot respond. The initiating injury resulting in osteoradionecrosis is frequently caused by extraction of a tooth from an irradiated mandible. Highly questionable teeth must be removed prior to radiother-

Table 9-11. Approved Artificial Salivas

Brand Name	Form	Manufacturer
Moi-Stir	Spray or swabsticks	Kingswood Laboratories, Inc. Carmel, IN
Orex	Squeeze bottle	Young Dental Company Maryland Heights, MO
Salivart	Spray	Westport Pharmaceuticals, Inc. Westport, CT
Xerolube	Spray	Scherer Laboratories, Inc. Dallas, TX

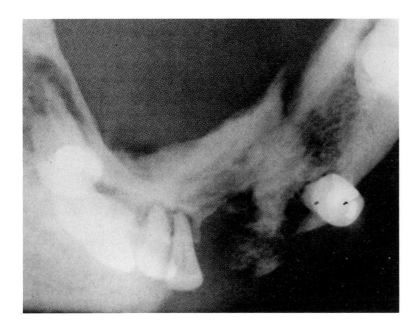

Figure 9-6. Osteoradionecrosis. A radiograph of mandibular necrosis and bony sequestration caused by a localized infection in a patient with a history of head and neck radiotherapy. Courtesy of R. Marshall, D.D.S., Lewisburg, West Virginia.

apy.[78] Patients exhibiting osteoradionecrosis usually complain of a constant aching pain at night or when masticating[80] and should be treated by oxygenating the damaged bone.[79] The dental health educator must stress to the radiotherapy patient the risk of osteoradionecrosis if oral hygiene, proper diet, and dental follow-up appointments are not strictly maintained.[83] Vulnerability to osteonecrosis seems to be at its peak within the first 2 years after radiotherapy.[84] In the event that an extraction is required after therapy, antibiotic coverage and meticulous surgical technique must be enforced.

The risk of developing osteoradionecrosis is life-long. Therefore it is imperative that patients remain on an effective recall program after radiotherapy. For the first year following therapy the patient should be seen on a monthly basis to monitor oral hygiene, fluoride compliance, diet, and the general course of recovery. Recall examinations should also focus on assessment of the head and neck for recurrent lesions. The dental health educator should constantly remind the patient of the importance of seeking professional care when the tissues become inflamed, sore, or irritated. Dentures should be checked periodically for pressure points and adjusted if an area of irritation develops.

Hypogeusia. Radiation damage to the outermost cells of the taste buds on the tongue may alter the patient's taste acuity (hypogeusia). Sweet, salty, acid, or bitter taste can be lost, depending on the location of the primary beam of radiation.[80] Bitter and acidic tastes are most commonly impaired.[85] In most patients taste is restored 1 to 4 months after treatment.[86] Nutritional foods should be prepared that are pleasing to the patient. Some authors have reported the use of zinc supplements to restore taste, but effectiveness has not been established.

Trismus. Trismus (a limited range of opening of the jaw) can be a delayed result of irradiation due to a fibrosis of the muscles of mastication and the temporomandibular joint. The patient should begin preventive exercises early in the course of radiation therapy to stretch and mobilize muscles. The patient can use a tongue blade measuring device to keep track of his range of opening.[9,78,79]

Leukemia

The estimated new cases of leukemia for 1990 is 27,800, similar to the number of oral cancer cases. The difference is in mortality rates: approximately two-thirds of all leukemics die from their disease.[77]

Leukemia is characterized by an overproduction of abnormal leukocytes. The malignant potential of the disease varies, depending on the type of white blood cell involved and the number of cells capable of dividing. In acute leukemias, large numbers of immature nonspecific leukocytes are produced. In the chronic form of the disease, leukocytes appear well-differentiated and able to mature, yet their immunologic capacity is significantly decreased. As leukemia progresses, displacement of hematopoietic tissue in the bone marrow by immature leukocytes results in diminished production of platelets, erythrocytes, and normal leukocytes.[87] Consequently, the patient can suffer from spontaneous hemorrhage, anemia, malaise, and opportunistic infections.

Chemotherapy. Antineoplastic drugs function by suppressing the growth and spread of rapidly proliferating tumor cells. Because chemotherapeutic drugs are essentially nonspecific, normal cells in various parts of the body that also display a high mitotic index are also adversely affected.[88] These drugs directly interfere with cell production, maturation, and replacement at such body sites as the mouth, digestive tract, bone marrow, hair follicles, and reproductive tract. The patient can exhibit mouth sores, nausea, alopecia (hair loss), and myelosuppression. Indirect toxicity is caused by the myelosuppressive action of the drugs, resulting in generalized immunosuppression.[89,90] This action suggests neutropenia, lymphocytopenia, and thrombocytopenia, making the patient susceptible to infection and bleeding. The systemic hematologic nature of leukemia, coupled with the comparatively large doses of antineoplastic drugs required to manage the disease, frequently results in major oral complications, which can be lethal to the compromised host.[88]

Chemotherapeutic agents that are typically known to be stomatotoxic are the antimetabolites, which include methotrexate, 5-fluorouracil, and 6-mercaptopurine. Antitumor antibiotics, hydroxyura, VP-16, and procarbazine are also responsible for the development of oral ulcerations.[79] A combined chemotherapeutic regimen, using two or more drugs with varying mechanisms of action and toxicity, is employed to (1) increase the effectiveness of the treatment, (2) distribute side effects among various organ systems, thereby increasing the patient's tolerance, and (3) decrease the chance of the patient developing resistant cancer cells.[91] Research shows that patients who develop some form of toxicity during the initial course of treatment frequently experience the same side effects during subsequent courses of treatment if the drugs or their dosages remain unchanged.[92]

Dental Management. Although many of the chemotherapy-induced oral complications are the same as those caused by radiotherapy, chemotherapeutic side effects are relatively short-term. Generally, after a cycle of chemotherapy, side effects such as bleeding or xerostomia usually resolve 2 to 3 days prior to recovery of the bone marrow. Nevertheless, side effects such as fulminating infection in an immunocompromised host can be life-threatening. Table 9-12 provides a protocol for the treatment of chemotherapy patients with an emphasis on preinduction care to establish a baseline and to attempt to prevent oral complications from arising during therapy.

The direct oral side effects of chemotherapy include mucositis, xerostomia, and ulcerations.[88] Indirect effects include infection and hemorrhage.

Mucositis. Mucositis is the most common of all chemotherapy-induced oral complications. Mucosal cells have a normal lifespan of 10 to 14 days. Although they are continuously reproducing, the rate at which these cells form is independent of their mortality.[89] After the induction of chemotherapy, mucosal cells die at a faster rate than they are produced. The sloughing of stratified squamous nonkeratinized oral epithelium leads to a loss of normal barrier function. Within 3 to 5 days after chemotherapy induction, the dental health educator can expect signs of erythematous mucositis. Ulcerative mucositis usually occurs approximately 1 week after therapy is initiated. Several measures can be used to relieve the discomfort associated with mucositis and minimize the chances of secondary infec-

Table 9-12. Oral Care Protocol for Cancer Chemotherapy Patients

Goal
　To provide the cancer patient with an asymptomatic, functioning oral environment, ultimately free
　　of infection or of other complications commonly associated with chemotherapy
Objectives
　Assess the oral status of cancer patients
　Attempt to prevent oral complications in cancer patients
　Identify existing oral complications in cancer patients
　Treat oral complications that occur
Methodology
　Patient consultation and treatment provided by a dentist and dental hygienist (if the program is
　　associated with a dental school, dental and dental hygiene faculty, general practice residents, and
　　supervised dental hygiene students may provide services)
　Research: to provide answers to questions raised in the objectives
　Education: oncology staff dental inservice teaching and an elective course for dental and dental
　　hygiene students entitled "Oral care for the cancer patient undergoing radiation or chemotherapy"
Service
　Preinduction phase (before chemotherapy)
　　Admission
　Dental consultation: assess the patient's mouth to establish a baseline for measuring changes and
　　evaluating effectiveness of oral care: orofacial soft tissue examination; examination for caries,
　　impacted teeth, and improperly fitting dental appliances; periodontal examination including
　　plaque and calculus index; amount and consistency of saliva; and previous history of oral com-
　　plications with chemotherapeutic agents
　Teach patient about oral complications associated with chemotherapy
　Oral prophylaxis
　Oral hygiene instructions:
　　Brushing with a soft toothbrush and fluoride dentifrice after meals and before bed
　　Flossing with unwaxed floss once daily
　　Oral preventive rinses twice daily
　Perform the necessary treatment to eliminate any potential pathogenic findings
　Induction phase
　(Active chemotherapy)
　　Routine oral examinations
　　Oral hygiene instructions (dependent on side effects)
　　Diet recommendations
　　Conservative dental treatment if warranted
　Remission phase
　　Oral prophylaxis
　　Oral hygiene instructions:
　　　Brushing with a soft toothbrush and a fluoride dentrifice after meals and before bed
　　　Floss with unwaxed floss once daily
　　　Oral rinsing once daily
　Elective dental treatment to be accomplished by patient's private dentist if possible

tion. If the patient has mild mucositis, brushing with a soft nylon toothbrush and 1 part hydrogen peroxide to 4 parts saline solution is recommended twice daily with equal rinses every 4 hours while awake. A suction toothbrush (Fig. 8-27) or the commercially designed Plak-Vac[93] can be used if the patient is comatose or intubated. Dentifrice is not recommended because it can cause pain or irritation. Flossing is not suggested for patients receiving chemotherapy unless they are extremely adept in the technique. If the mucositis is severe, the oral cavity should be gently cleaned with gauze dipped in a solution of 5 ml sodium bicarbonate and 500 ml saline twice a day with identical rinses every 2 hours while awake.

If the patient is unable to rinse, the dental

health educator can use a disposable enema bag or an irrigation syringe. To prevent aspiration, elevate and turn the patient's head to the side and suction any fluid or debris present. It is important for the patient with mucositis to avoid commercial mouthwashes because of the high alcohol and phenol content. Hydrogen peroxide should always be diluted and is not recommended for long-term use or in any form for the patient in whom fresh granulation tissue is forming, because it tends to break down the tissue. Recent studies show that the prophylactic use of chlorhexidine mouthrinse reduces oral soft tissue inflammation and mucositis.[82,94] Lemon glycerine swabs are contraindicated for mucositis patients. Research shows the swabs to be ineffective in removing plaque and debris from the teeth; the acidity of the swabs easily decalcifies the teeth (particularly when the patient experiences xerostomia as a side effect); and the swabs are painful to the denuded epithelium because glycerine is anhydrous, therefore drying the mucosa.[95] Minor mechanical or bacterial trauma can easily disrupt the integrity of the thin, inflamed, friable oral mucosa, resulting in ulcerations that often become the portal of entry for systemic infections. The severity of such an occurrence cannot be overemphasized be-

cause oral microbial infections in a patient who is already immunosuppressed and myelosuppressed can be fatal.

Ulcerations. Ulcerations can be deep or shallow, broad or oval. If ulcers are deep, they usually emerge with a necrotic white center encompassed by a dense red band (Fig. 9-7). Effective treatment for these ulcerations includes allowing the patient to swish with an unflavored viscous lidocaine rinse at meals, at bedtime, and before oral hygiene care. Some individuals recommend dyclonine hydrochloride (Dyclone) 0.5%, 5 to 10 ml, instead of lidocaine spray because of its longer duration and decreased cardiac toxicity. A kaolin-pectin oral rinse is advised for mild erythematous mucositis, and the addition of Benylin syrup to kaolin-pectin in a 50:50 concentration is particularly soothing for the patient with ulcerative mucositis. Kaolin-Pectin provides a protective covering over the mucosa, and Benylin acts by reducing the oral discomfort associated with the inflammation. Benadryl elixir is not recommended because as an antihistamine it causes drying of the oral mucosa and irritation is produced by the alcohol content of the drug.[91,96]

Ulcerated tissues are also highly sensitive to temperature and pressure extremes. An unpleasant odor is often emitted from the

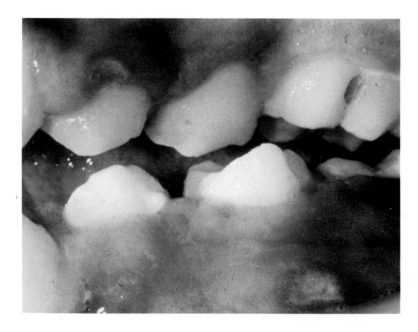

Figure 9-7. Chemotherapy-induced oral ulcerations. Courtesy of P. Hagan, D.D.S., M.S., University of Sydney Dental Hospital, Sydney, Australia.

necrotic mucous membranes, and patients have diminished taste acuity and difficulty in talking, chewing, and swallowing. Consequently their nutritional intake diminishes. Modifications in the diet to ensure comfort involve recommending a bland, semisoft diet that is low in sucrose and citric acid. Alcohol and cigarettes should be deleted as well. Foods should be served at room temperature to avoid irritation of the mouth and throat. The thinning of foods with sauces, milk, or gravy proves more acceptable for the patient with masticatory or swallowing difficulties. A straw can also make swallowing more comfortable.[97]

Disruptions in the integrity of the oral epithelium are generally imitated by equivalent alterations in the mucosal lining of the digestive tract.[92] Some dietary suggestions that might help to alleviate the side effects of nausea, vomiting, diarrhea, and constipation are the frequent consumption of small meals throughout the day to remain satiated but not full; restricted intake of fluids to 1 hour before or after eating; avoidance of sweets and fried, fatty, and highly seasoned foods; slow consumption of warm rather than hot meals; thorough mastication of foods to facilitate digestion; consumption of dry foods such as toast or crackers in the morning to prevent nausea (contraindicated if patient suffers from mucositis); ingestion of cool, clear, unsweetened beverages such as apple juice; ingestion of light meals before receiving treatment; avoidance of food preparation if the smell of food cooking causes nausea; and avoidance of lying flat for at least 2 hours after eating (though it might be helpful for the patient to rest after eating because activity slows digestion and increases discomfort).[98]

Xerostomia. Xerostomia, or dry mouth, is often caused by medications, mouth breathing, or an elevation in temperature.[96] The reduction in salivary flow alters the oral self-cleansing mechanism, yielding the accumulation of more plaque and debris. A decrease in saliva also contributes to a drop in pH of the oral cavity that encourages an acidogenic flora and predisposes the patient to dental caries. Dental disease, coupled with the fact that dry mucosa is more susceptible

to trauma, intensifies the affected area as a portal of entry for infection. Lack of saliva can also produce atrophy of the tongue papillae, resulting in the loss of taste perception previously discussed.[99]

Several artificial salivas are available for the treatment of xerostomia. Lip care must also be considered. For cracked, ulcerated, or hemorrhagic perioral tissues (not to be confused with herpetic lesions), frequent applications of surgical lubricant (Surgi-Lube or K-Y jelly) or lanolin are suggested.[96] Petroleum jelly is not advised because of the possibility of aspiration pneumonia.

Infection. Infection is one of the most serious complications of cancer chemotherapy. Antineoplastic drugs depress competent neutrophil production, prohibit the mononuclear cell function of the inflammatory reaction, and inhibit normal gamma globulin formation. A lengthy drug-induced neutropenia and lymphocytopenia compound the risk of infection. Due to the impaired immune response, opportunistic pathogens and subsequent nosocomial infections are able to colonize in the oral cavity and enter the bloodstream through a break in the mucosa. The dental health educator must practice strict infection control when examining or treating the immunosuppressed patient. Although the patient might exhibit communicable infections of concern to the dental health educator, of equal or greater concern is the exposure of the patient to pathogens when his defense mechanisms are dysfunctional.

The most common bacterial infections are the gram-negative aerobic bacilli (Pseudomonas, Klebsiella, Serratia, Enterobacter, Proteus, and Escherichia coli). The lesions are usually raised, white to yellow, moist, glistening, spreading, and nonpurulent, with a smooth-edged border seated on a painful superficial ulcerated base.[100] Broad-spectrum intravenous antibiotics are advised immediately on emergence of the lesions, particularly when the patient becomes febrile, to reduce the risk of gram-negative sepsis. Once the culture is identified a specific treatment plan can be administered.[101]

Candida infections are responsible for approximately half of all oral infections encountered by leukemics receiving chemotherapy and almost two-thirds of oral infections in solid tumor patients on chemotherapy.[102] The most frequent sites of the oral cavity to be infected by Candida include the tongue, buccal mucosa, gingiva, palate, pharynx, and the commissures of the lips. Candida lesions are characterized by white, raised, milk-curdle-like lesions that can be scraped away, leaving a red, hemorrhagic base. Antifungal agents used in the treatment of Candida consist of nystatin or clotrimazole oral suspensions, popsicles, or suppositories used as a lozenge; ketoconazole by mouth if the fungal infection becomes systemic in the immunocompromised host; and Amphotericin B intravenously for severe systemic infections. Ketoconazole tablets and IV amphotericin B should be used with caution because they are known to impair renal and liver function if used over an extended period of time.[91] The severity of Candida infections has been dramatically reduced by the use of chlorhexidine.[82,94]

The most common viral infection exhibited intra- and extraorally is herpes simplex. These lesions begin as painful vesicles that rupture, shed the virus, and become encrusted. They often cover large areas periorally and are easily spread to other body sites because of the patient's immunosuppressed status. Acyclovir (Zovirax) is considered standard treatment for oral herpetic lesions. It should be applied 6 times daily for 1 week or administered intravenously if severe debilitation ensues.[103]

Hemorrhage. Hemorrhage (disease and drug-induced) is caused by thrombocytopenia from inadequate production of megakaryocytes. Bleeding is rare in platelet counts of 50,000 cu/mm or more. Yet the chance of hemorrhage at counts below 20,000 cu/mm rises to 50%.

Bleeding usually occurs as an intermittent oozing. Fragile, soft blood clots form, break down, and reform. Often patients require platelet transfusions.[90] Hemorrhagic oral complications are seen more frequently in patients with local factors such as incorrect oral hygiene techniques causing trauma,

preexisting periodontal conditions, mobile teeth, decayed or fractured teeth or restorations, orthodontic bands or wires, or oral habits such as nailbiting, even when the patient's hematologic values are within normal limits.

To assess the oral bleeding site, one must evacuate all debris, clots, and saliva.[96] Periodontal packing or topical thrombin applied to the oozing areas is recommended for hemostasis.[87] Keeping the oral cavity as immaculate as possible will reduce the incidence of oral complications. Toothbrushing is not recommended for the patient with a platelet count below 20,000 cu/mm. Gauze squares or a toothette soaked in saline solution or other suggested preparations are quite effective and atraumatic for plaque removal.

Once chemotherapy has begun, dental treatment should be provided judiciously because the patient's platelet count alone will not ensure safety. In addition, a complete coagulation profile and a granulocyte count are necessary.[87] Parenteral antibiotic prophylaxis should be administered to the patient who has a functional granulocyte count below 2000 cu/mm.[104] With optimum conditions, oral surgery and operative dental procedures can be accomplished for the patient with a platelet count of 50,000 cu/mm. Reports show that patients can undergo oral surgery with platelet counts below 20,000 cu/mm, but transfusion therapy is required at the time of surgery.[96] During remission, routine dental procedures can be accomplished without hesitation.

Bone marrow transplantation was once considered the final treatment measure reserved solely for leukemic patients. Today it serves as an effective treatment for other cancers as well. Unfortunately, oral complications arise both before and after actual transplantation. Stomatotoxic side effects associated with chemotherapy and whole-body irradiation performed to render the bone marrow sterile, septicemia from oral microorganisms associated with periodontal or periapical infections, and graft-versus-host disease all can affect the ultimate success of the transplantation.[79] The use of a 0.12% chlorhexidine mouthrinse in oncology patients receiving bone marrow transplants was found to be effective in reducing oral soft tissue disease and oral microorganisms. Chlorhexidine also produced a significant decrease in oral mucositis and Candida infections.[82]

COMMENTS

The dental practices of the nineties are different from those of a mere decade ago. Dental diseases are no longer routine. They are influenced by a variety of acute and chronic illnesses and disabilities that claimed many lives at a relatively early age prior to advances in medical science. Many of these conditions and their treatments are reflected visually in the oral cavity.

Dental health educators must accept the responsibility for the recognition of these signs and symptoms. Prompt action can retard the disease process, relieve the patient's discomfort, and save an individual's life. It is the obligation of the dental health professional to educate patients and their families concerning the technique and importance of optimum oral care and the oral manifestations that can result from their specific disease and treatment. The dental health educator caring for the medically compromised will find that the professional challenges are numerous and the energy invested is miniscule in comparison to the rewards gained.

REFERENCES

1. McCarthy, F. M.: Essentials of Safe Dentistry for the Medically Compromised Patient. Philadelphia, W. B. Saunders, 1989.
2. Little, J. W., and Falace, D. A.: Dental Management of the Medically Compromised Patient. 3rd Ed. St. Louis, C. V. Mosby, 1988.
3. Giangrego, E. (Ed.): Dentistry in hospitals: Looking to the future. J. Am. Dent. Assoc., 115:545–551, 554–55, 1987.
4. Smith, B. W.: Dentistry in the hospital setting. Spec. Care Dent., 4:56–57, 1984.
5. DeLaney, D. F., VanOstenberg, P., and Salley, J. J.: A dental hygienist in the hospital. Dent. Hyg., 57:31–34, 36–37, 1983.
6. Poupard, J. M.: The development, function and administration of a section of dental hygiene in affiliated teaching hospital dental services. Dent. Hyg., 45:297–301, 1971.
7. American Heart Association: 1986 Heart Facts. Dallas, American Heart Association, 1985.
8. National Center for Health Statistics: Advance report of final mortality statistics, 1983. Monthly Vital Statistics Report, 34(Suppl. 2): September 26, 1985.
9. Stiefel, D. J., and Truelove, E. L.: A Self-Instructional Series in Rehabilitation Dentistry: Dental Treatment of the Patient with a Disability (Modules 1-10). University of Washington, School of Dentistry, Project DECOD, 1987.
10. U.S. Department of Health and Human Services: Disease Prevention/Health Promotion: The Facts. Palo Alto, Bull Publishing, 1988.
11. Haynes, S. G., et al.: Closing the Gap for Cardiovascular Disease: The Carter Center Health Policy Project Interim Summary. Atlanta, Carter Center of Emory University, Nov. 26–28, 1984.
12. Hancharik, S. D.: At risk: Hypertensive patients. R.D.H., 4:23–25, 30, 1984.
13. Dustan, H. P.: Pathophysiology of hypertension. In The Heart. 5th Ed. Edited by J. W. Hurst. New York, McGraw-Hill, 1983.
14. Kannel, W. B., Thom, T. J., and Hurst, J. W.: Incidence, prevalence, and mortality of cardiovascular disease. In The Heart. 6th Ed. New York, McGraw-Hill Book Co., 1986.
15. National Heart, Lung and Blood Institute: Fact Book, Fiscal Year 1985. Bethesda, MD, National Institute of Health, 1985.
16. National Center for Health Statistics. Unpublished data.
17. Shannon, S. A.: Infective endocarditis: What every dental hygienist should know. Dental Hygiene, 59:552–556, 1985.
18. Santoro, J.: Streptococcal infections and rheumatic fever. In Internal Medicine for Dentistry. Edited by L. F. Rose and D. Kaye. St. Louis, C. V. Mosby, 1983.
19. Stollerman, G. H.: Rheumatic fever. In Harrison's Principles of Internal Medicine. 10th Ed. Edited by R. G. Petersdorf et al. New York, McGraw-Hill, 1983.
20. Stollerman, G. H.: Acute rheumatic fever and its management. In The Heart. 5th Ed. Edited by J. W. Hurst. New York, McGraw-Hill, 1983.
21. Bender, I. B., Naidorf, I. J., and Garvey, G. J.: Bacterial endocarditis: A consideration for the physician and dentist. J. Am. Dent. Assoc., 109:415–420, 1984.
22. Guntheroth, W. G.: How important are dental procedures as a cause of infective endocarditis? Am. J. Cardiol., 54:797–801, 1984.
23. Jaspers, M. J., and Little, J. W.: Infective endocarditis: A review and update. Oral Surg., 57:606–615, 1984.
24. Little, J. W.: Prevention of bacterial endocarditis in dental patients. Gen. Dent., 35:382–387, 1987.
25. Garfunkel, A. A., Massot, S., and Galili, D.: Oral treatment needs for patients requiring heart surgery. Spec. Care Dent., 7:167–170, 1987.
26. Boraz, R. A., and Myers, R.: A national survey of dental protocols for the patient with a cardiac transplant. Sp. Care Dent., 10:26–29, 1990.
27. Wilkins, E. M.: Clinical Practice of the Dental Hygienist. 6th Ed. Philadelphia, Lea & Febiger, 1989.

28. Committee on Rheumatic Fever and Bacterial Endocarditis of the Council on Cardiovascular Disease in the Young of the American Heart Association: Prevention of bacterial endocarditis. Circulation, 70:1123A–1127A, 1984.

29. Kleinman, C. S., Zafran, J. N., and Zayon, G. M.: Dental care for the stroke patient. Dent. Hygiene, 54:237–239, 1980.

30. Mohr, J. P., et al.: Cerebrovascular disease. *In* Harrison's Principles of Internal Medicine. 9th Ed. Edited by K. J. Isselbacker et al. New York, McGraw-Hill, 1980.

31. Toole, J. F., et al.: Vascular diseases. *In* Merritt's Textbook of Neurology. 8th Ed. Edited by L. P. Rowland. Philadelphia, Lea & Febiger, 1989.

32. Mungo, R. P., Kopel, H. M., and Church, J. A.: Pediatric dentistry and the child with asthma. Sp. Care Dent., 6:270–273, 1986.

33. Malamed, S. F.: Handbook of Medical Emergencies in the Dental Office. 3rd Ed. St. Louis, C. V. Mosby, 1987.

34. Lange, B. M., Entwistle, B. M., and Lipson, L. F.: Dental Management of the Handicapped: Approaches for Dental Auxiliaries. Philadelphia, Lea & Febiger, 1983.

35. McFadden, E. R., Jr., and Austen, K. F.: Asthma. *In* Harrison's Principles of Internal Medicine. 9th Ed. Edited by K. J. Isselbacher et al. New York, McGraw-Hill, 1980.

36. Weiss, E. B.: Bronchial asthma. Clin. Symp., 27:3–72, 1975.

37. Walker, J., and Hendeles, L.: The interaction of erythromycin and theophylline in the asthmatic dental patient. J. Am. Dent. Assoc., 99:995–996, 1979.

38. Glanze, W. D., Anderson, K. N., and Anderson, L. E. (Eds.): Mosby's Medical Nursing and Allied Health Dictionary. 3rd Ed. St. Louis, C. V. Mosby, 1990.

39. Professional Education Committee, Cystic Fibrosis Foundation: Guidelines for Health Personnel—Cystic Fibrosis. Rockville, MD, Cystic Fibrosis Foundation, 1980.

40. Anderson, C.: Pancreatic disease in childhood. *In* The Exocrine Pancreas. Edited by J. Howat and H. Sarles. Philadelphia, W. B. Saunders, 1979.

41. Schaap, T., and Cohen, M.: A proposed model for the inheritance of cystic fibrosis. *In* Cystic Fibrosis: Projections into the Future. Edited by J. Mangos and J. Talamo. New York, Stratton Intercontinental Medical Book Corp., 1973.

42. Gardner, L. J.: Endocrine and Genetic Diseases of Childhood. Philadelphia, W. B. Saunders, 1969.

43. Anfenson, M.: The school-age child with cystic fibrosis. J. Sch. Health, 50:26–28, 1980.

44. The National Hemophilia Foundation: What You Should Know About Hemophilia. New York, World Federation of Hemophilia, and the National Health Council.

45. Eckert, E. F.: Your Child and Hemophilia. Berkeley, Cutter Biological, 1983.

46. Mitchell, P. F., et al.: Hemophilia in the dental patient. West Va. Dent. J., 55:18, 20–21, 1980.

47. Powell, D., and Bartle, J.: The hemophiliac: Prevention is the key. Dent. Hyg., 48:214–219, 1974.

48. Saunders, S. D.: The management perspective in the treatment of hemophilia. Dent. Hyg., 56:32–39, 1982.

49. Evans, B. E. (Ed.): Dental Care in Hemophilia. Berkeley, Cutter Biological, 1977.

50. Lusher, J. M.: Living With Inhibitors. Berkeley, Cutter Biological, 1983.

51. Hilgartner, M. W.: Managing the child with hemophilia. Pediatr. Annals, 8:68, June 1979.

52. Nowak, A. J.: Dentistry for the Handicapped. St. Louis, C. V. Mosby, 1976.

53. Ridley, K.: Preventive Dentistry and Hemophilia. Ann Arbor, Hemophilia Foundation of Michigan.

54. National Center for Health Statistics: Current Estimates from the National Health Interview Survey, U.S., 1982. Vital and Health Statistics. Series 10, (150). DHHS Pub. NO. (PHS) 85-1578. Washington, DC, U.S. Govt. Printing Office, 1985.

55. Harris, M. I.: Diabetes in America. National Diabetes Data Group (Ed.) NIH Pub. No. 85-1468. Bethesda, MD, National Institutes of Health, 1985.

56. Rothwell, B. R., and Richard, E. L.: Diabetes mellitus: Medical and dental considerations. Sp. Care Dent., 4:58–65, 1984.

57. Centers for Disease Control: Update on hepatitis B prevention. MMWR, 36:353, 1987.

58. Siew, C., et al.: Survey of hepatitis B exposure and vaccination in volunteer dentists. J. Am. Dent. Assoc., 114:457, 1987.

59. Scully, C.: Hepatitis B: An update in relation to dentistry. Br. Dent. J., 159:321, 1985.

60. Huer, G., Kaminski, R., and Smith, A.: A protocol for the treatment of hepatitis patients. J. Dent. Educ., 49:596, 1985.

61. Sampson, E.: Hepatitis B protection of patient, dentist, and staff. Proceedings of a symposium on hepatitis B: Risk, prevention and the vaccine. 123rd ADA Annual Session, pp. 16–20, 1982.

62. Maseman, D. C.: Hepatitis: Types, protection, and legal ramifications. Semin. Dent. Hyg., 1:1–5, 1989.

63. Golden, A.: Pathology: Understanding Human Disease. Baltimore, MD, Williams & Wilkins, 1982.

64. Hoofnagle, J. H.: Type B hepatitis: Virology, serology, and clinical course. Semin. Liver Dis., 1:7, 1981.

65. Cottone, J. A.: Hepatitis B virus infection in the dental profession. J. Am. Dent. Assoc., 110:617, 1985.

66. Brown, B. S.,: Viral hepatitis B perspectives: Past and present. Dent. Hyg., 55:22–28, 1981.

67. Longnecker, S. A., and Odom, J. G.: Hepatitis B treatment in dental hygiene education programs: Clinic protocols. Dent. Hyg., 62:250–254, 1988.

68. Centers for Disease Control: Recommended infection-control practices for dentistry. MMWR, 35:237, 1986.

69. Centers for Disease Control: Recommendations for protection against viral hepatitis. MMWR, 34:313, 1985.

70. Lindhout, J. A., and Parrish, A. E.: Protocol for the dental management of the liver transplant candidate. University of Michigan Medical Center, unofficial publication.

71. Brenner, B. M., and Lazarus, J. M.: Chronic renal failure. *In* Harrison's Principles of Internal Medicine. 9th Ed. Edited by K. J. Isselbacher et al. New York, McGraw-Hill, 1980.

72. Levy, H. M.: Dental considerations for the patient receiving dialysis for renal failure. Sp. Care Dent., 8:34–36, 1988.

73. National Institute of Arthritis, Diabetes, and Digestive Diseases: Arthritis, Rheumatic Diseases, and Related Disorders. DHHS Pub. No. (NIH) 85-1983. Bethesda, MD, National Institutes of Health, 1985.

74. National Arthritis Data Work Group: Prevalence of Rheumatic Diseases and Osteoporosis. Bethesda, MD, National Institute of Arthritis and Metabolic Diseases, unpublished document, April 17, 1986.

75. Zvaifler, N. I.: Rheumatoid arthritis: A clinical perspective. *In* Epidemiology of the Rheumatic Diseases. Edited by R. C. Lawrence and L. E. Shulman. New York, Gower Medical, 1984.

76. Gilliland, B. C., and Mannik, M.: Rheumatoid arthritis. *In* Harrison's Principles of Internal Medicine. 9th Ed.

Edited by K. J. Isselbacher et al. New York, McGraw-Hill, 1980.

77. Silverberg, E., Boring, C. C., and Squires, T. S.: Cancer Statistics, 1990. Ca. J. Clin., 40:9–28, 1990.

78. Engelmeier, R. L.: A dental protocol for patients receiving radiation therapy for a cancer of the head and neck. Sp. Care Dent., 7:54–58, 1987.

79. National Institutes of Health: NIH consensus development conference statement: Oral complications of cancer therapies: Diagnosis, prevention, and treatment. J. Am. Dent. Assoc., 119:179–183, 1989.

80. Jones, J. A., and Lang, W. P.: Nutrition during treatment of head and neck cancer. Sp. Care Dent., 6:165–169, 1986.

81. Gilpin, J.: Xerostomia. Dent. Hyg., 63:111–114, 1989.

82. Ferretti, G. A., et al.: Chlorhexidine for prophylaxis against oral infections and associated complications in patients receiving bone marrow transplants. J. Am. Dent. Assoc., 114:461–467, 1987.

83. Fattore, L. D., Strauss, R., and Bruno, J.: The management of periodontal disease in patients who have received radiation therapy for head and neck cancer. Sp. Care Dent., 7:120–123, 1987.

84. Dreizen, S., et al.: Oral complications of cancer radiotherapy. Postgrad. Med., 61:85–92, 1977.

85. Donaldson, S. S.: Nutritional consequences of radiotherapy. Cancer Res., 37:2407–2413, 1977.

86. Conger, A. D.: Loss and recovery of taste acuity in patients irradiated to the oral cavity. Radiat. Res., 53:338–347, 1973.

87. Carl, W., and Schaaf, N. G.: Dental care for the cancer patient. J. Surg. Oncol., 6:305, 1974.

88. DeBiase, C. B., and Komives, B. K.: An oral care protocol for leukemic patients with chemotherapy-induced oral complications. Sp. Care Dent., 3:207–213, 1983.

89. Ostchega, Y.: Preventing and treating cancer chemotherapy's oral complications. Nursing 80, 10:47–52, 1980.

90. Dreizen, S.: Stomatotoxic manifestations of cancer chemotherapy. J. Prosthet. Dent., 40:650–651, 1978.

91. Naylor, G. D., and Terezhalmy, G. T.: Oral complications of cancer chemotherapy: Prevention and management. Sp. Care Dent., 8:150–156, 1988.

92. Dreizen, S., McCredie, K. B., and Keating, M. J.: Chemotherapy-induced oral mucositis in adult leukemia. Postgrad. Med., 69:103, 1981.

93. Plak-Vac Oral Evacuator Brush. Trademark Corporation, 1053 Headquarters Park, Fenton, MO, 63026-2033.

94. McGraw, W. T., and Belch, A.: Oral complications of acute leukemia: Prophylactic impact of a chlorhexidine mouth rinse regimen. Oral Surg. Oral Med. Oral Pathol., 60:275–280, 1985.

95. Daeffler, R.: Oral hygiene measures for patients with cancer. Ca. Nursing, 3:352, 1980.

96. Toth, B. B., and Hoar, R. E.: Oral/dental care for the pediatric oncology patient. Ca. Bull., 34:66–69, 1982.

97. Donaldson, S. S., and Lenon, R. A.: Alterations of nutritional status: Impact of chemotherapy and radiation therapy. Cancer, 43:2036–2049, 1979.

98. U.S. Department of Health and Human Services: Chemotherapy and You: A Guide to Self-Help During Treatment. Bethesda, MD, National Institutes of Health, Publ. No. 81-1136, 1980.

99. Miller, S. E.: Dental management of the patient with xerostomia. Dent. Hyg., 55:42–43, 1981.

100. Dreizen, S., Bodey, G. P., and Rodriguez, V.: Oral complications of cancer chemotherapy. Postgrad. Med. 58:80, 1975.

101. Dreizen, S., Bodey, G. P., and Brown, L. R.: Opportunistic gram-negative bacillary infections in leukemia: Oral manifestations during myelosuppression. Postgrad. Med., 55:133–139, 1974.

102. Fattore, L. D., Baer, R., and Olsen, L.: The role of the general dentist in the treatment and management of oral complications of chemotherapy. Gen. Dent., 35:374–377, 1987.

103. Redding, S. W.: Oral complications of cancer chemotherapy. Texas Dent. J., 103:18–20, 1986.

104. Williams, L. T., Peterson, D. E., and Overholser, C. D.: Leukemia and dental treatment. Dent. Hyg., 55:31, 1981.

Chapter 10

DENTAL HEALTH EDUCATION FOR THE ELDERLY

Older people are neglected and left to get along as best they can. . . . If it is important to give the human animal a good start in life, it is just as important to see that he makes a good finish. We should be as much interested in actual fulfillment as in setting the stage for the realization of possibilities.

George E. Lawton
New Goals for Old Age

DEMOGRAPHICS

Older adults (age 65 years and above) currently comprise about 13% (31.8 million) of the U.S. population. By the year 2050, the older adult category of Americans is expected to reach a projected 68.5 million or 22.8% of the total population (Table 10-1).[1] The growth in numbers of persons over 85 years of age is probably the most significant of the demographic changes and the trend is expected to accelerate dramatically over the next sixty years; this segment of the older adult population alone increased 28% during the 1980s. This long-range shift in demographics appears to be primarily due to major advances in medical research and the baby boom generation reaching maturity.[2]

Women outnumber men in the over-65 age group by a ratio of about 3 to 2.[1] Although the average life expectancy for U.S. males is 71.5 years, the average 65-year-old man will live another 14.6 years. Females have an average life expectancy of 78.3 years

but can generally expect to live to about 87 years of age.[1,3] Approximately 92% of the U.S. population over 65 years of age is white.[4]

In general, older adults are less educated than the other adult population groups, but this is changing to some degree. Data indicate an increase in average years of school completed from 8.7 in 1970 to 11.4 in 1984. The median income of older adult males is $10,450; females average $6020. Twenty-one percent of older persons are considered poor or near poor (below 125% of the poverty level). The majority (75%) of Americans retire from the work force by age 65.[5]

About 20% of the older adult population group spend some time in a nursing home or an extended-care facility; about 5% of this age group reside permanently in nursing homes at any given time. For individuals over 85 years (the "fragile elderly"), the percentage living in long-term-care facilities is about 25%. As a result of the emergence of Medicare and Medicaid in 1966, the use of extended-care facilities by persons in the 65-plus age group has doubled. Usage of these facilities is expected to continue to

Table 10-1. Projected Growth of U.S. Elderly Population by Age Group for 1985–2050
(in thousands)

Year	U.S.Population (All Ages)	U.S. Elderly Population by Age Group (Percent of Total Population in Parentheses)					
		65–69	70–74	75–79	80–84	85 and over	Total 65 and over
1985	238,649	9227 (3.9)	7635 (3.2)	5534 (2.3)	3482 (1.5)	2794 (1.2)	28,672 (12.1)
1990	249,731	10,006 (4.1)	8048 (3.3)	6224 (2.6)	4060 (1.7)	3461 (1.4)	31,799 (13.1)
1995	259,631	9757 (3.8)	8766 (3.4)	6607 (2.5)	4621 (1.8)	4255 (1.6)	34,006 (13.1)
2000	268,267	9491 (3.5)	8752 (3.3)	7282 (2.7)	4936 (1.9)	4622 (1.7)	35,083 (13.1)
2025	298,252	19,257 (6.4)	15,420 (5.2)	11,378 (3.8)	6647 (2.2)	7014 (2.4)	59,716 (20.0)
2050	299,848	17,325 (5.8)	14,265 (4.7)	12,042 (4.0)	9614 (3.2)	15,286 (5.1)	68,532 (22.8)

Adapted from Projections of Population of the US 1982–2050: Current Population Reports: Population Estimates and Projections Series P-25 No. 922, Washington, DC, October 1982, and 1988–2080, P-25 No. 1018, Jan, 1989.

rise because of the major increases in numbers of the elderly nationwide.[6]

Older people usually have many medical problems. Deaths from heart disease, although declining overall, escalate steadily with increasing age. For persons between the ages of 65 and 69 the mortality rate related to cardiac disorders is about 49%; it is 64% for the 80-to-84 age group. Cancer is the only major cause of death that has actually increased, because of an increase in lung cancer among women who smoke cigarettes.[7]

DENTAL NEEDS

The changing demographic profile for older adults will affect the future of dental practice. Little emphasis was placed on dental care for the elderly prior to the last decade. As the number of older Americans increases in proportion to the total population, this once-neglected group will become a major segment of the dental practice.

Older Americans have significant oral health problems that require attention. The most recent NIDR survey of adult oral health (see Chapter 3) indicates that 41% of older adults are completely edentulous (a 20% decline in 28 years), 66% of seniors have evidence of root caries, 47% experience gingival bleeding on probing, and 95% of the dentate seniors have attachment loss, and 34% have attachment loss of 6 mm or more in at least one area.[8] In addition, the risk for oral cancer increases with age; 90% of oral carcinoma patients are 45 years of age or older.[9] Because older people are retaining all or part of their natural dentition for longer periods of time, the dental needs of the elderly will shift from the previous emphasis on removable prostheses in an edentulous mouth to periodontal treatment to maintain the health and function of the remaining teeth, particularly if implants are being considered. The restoration of teeth damaged by root caries and recurrent decay is also an integral part of geriatric dental care.[6]

Geriatric dentistry refers to dental care for older patients, many of whom possess a physical, psychological, or social condition that compromises the delivery and prognosis of that care.[10] About 90% of the elderly have one or more chronic diseases. Although the majority of older persons are active, about 17% depend on others for major activities such as bathing, dressing, and eating.[11] In order for the dental health educator to provide appropriate care, he must be prepared to approach the patient's treatment in a comprehensive manner. A number of medical conditions (e.g., cardiovascular disease, stroke, cancer, arthritis, vision and hearing disorders, postural instability, and incontinence) affect the 65-plus age group, and treatments of these conditions frequently alter the health of the oral cavity. Psychological and sociological disturbances (e.g., dementia, sleep disturbances) that prohibit the individual's successful assimilation into the home or community also require the special attention of the dental staff. The dental health educator must devote additional time to these patients. Caring communication and sensitivity to their problems can enhance the treatment outcome.[6]

Barriers to Care. Several barriers affect the demand for dental care among the elderly. It has been reported that only 40% of the age-65-plus population have visited the dentist within the past year; this corresponds to a 55% utilization rate for dentate seniors and only 13% for the edentate older adult group. This is the lowest rate of dental visits for any age group.[8]

Unfortunately for many elderly persons, cost makes dental care prohibitive. Increasing age often leads to increasing health care needs and a loss of economic independence. When the average income of the older adult is only about $8000, dental care is not a priority. Social Security is the major source of income for over a third of the over-65 population. Medicare does not cover dental services, and most older adults do not carry dental insurance. This means that approximately 95% of dental care must be paid for by the patients themselves.[2]

Physical inaccessibility of services is another major barrier related to low utilization of dental services among the elderly. Many older seniors find themselves without transportation when they give up driving because of poor health or the high cost of maintaining a vehicle. The expense of cab fare, the obligation to ask others for assistance, and inaccessibility of public transportation discourage many elderly persons from scheduling dental appointments. Older persons who have physical disabilities can have difficulty finding convenient offices that are also accessible to the handicapped. Narrow doorways and long flights of stairs can make elderly persons reluctant to seek care.[12]

The most disconcerting of all barriers involves the lack of dental awareness and misconceptions held by the elderly. The individual's self-perceived need and dental health beliefs influence his dental utilization behavior as much as his dentate status.[13] Many, young and old, believe that tooth loss and poor oral health are the inevitable prices one pays for aging, and that dental care is no longer needed once dentures are acquired. The elderly have low expectations regarding the outcome of care and are not familiar with the need for soft-tissue examinations even when they are edentulous. This self-stereotyping behavior, referred to as "ageism,"[14] is an attitudinal behavior that the dental health educator must gradually dispel through empathy and the dissemination of information. The elderly must be made aware that dental care is a right and responsibility of all persons regardless of their age.

Ageist beliefs further manifest in the elderly by their concerns over bothering a busy dentist with their problems, which they believe are inconsequential and not operational at their stage in life.[13,14] Having limited or no prior contact with a dental professional also decreases the likelihood that an older adult will seek care.[13] Individuals 75 years and over grew up in an era in which dental care was more disease-oriented; people sought treatment only when they were in pain. Currently the younger, "new" elderly (ages 65 to 74 years) in the United States, who are better educated and dentate, are more likely to have experienced dental care in a more preventive environment during their 30s or 40s;[14] this preventive attitude appears to have increased the dental-care-seeking behavior of this age group.[15] Their offspring and future generations will consequently be affected by these changes in concepts and practices.

Ageist beliefs can also be found among dental professionals. Many dental health educators have negative feelings about aging and prefer not to treat the elderly. In a study conducted to assess dentists' attitudes toward older adults, it was found that almost half of all Ohio dentists felt that elderly patients were the least satisfying of all age groups.[16] A survey of dentists in the state of Washington proved these professionals to be essentially uninformed about the aging process.[17] Negativism among dentists was also reported to exist toward older adults in regard to their oral hygiene status.[16,18] The awareness of dental professionals must be increased by educating them about the physiology of aging and the pathology of disease, oral problems experienced by seniors, methods of communication with older patients, and the impact that care of the elderly will have on their dental practices. In addition to knowledge of the medical/dental physiologic and pathologic changes in the elderly, sensitivity and attentiveness to the patient's psychosocial needs and attitudes are also essential.[14] The dental health educator should examine his own attitudes and beliefs before delivering patient care to ensure mutual satisfaction. Practitioners with unresolved prejudices should not treat the elderly.

Other impediments to the utilization of dental services by the elderly include fear of treatment and illness.[111] Low dental care utilization can be considered a form of neglect when infirm elders are isolated or mistreated by family members responsible for providing care. Physical assaults, verbal abuse, neglect, and financial exploitation are forms of elder abuse (see Chapter 5).

AGING AND DISEASE

The aging process has no exact starting time. Aging is essentially the continuation of maturation, which leads to deterioration and an eventual loss of function of an organ or group of organs.[19] The numbers of cells and their ability to proliferate decrease, causing tissue dehydration, atrophy, fibrosis, diminished elasticity, and poor repair.[20] Death is the end result.

Changes in the body over time vary from one person to another. Many times it is difficult to discern changes that occur as physiologic manifestations of aging from those that are disease-induced. Some physiologic changes actually increase the likelihood of disease. The dental health educator must be aware of the marked variability of physiologic and pathologic changes among the elderly, the multiplicity of these problems in one individual, and the frequency of atypical disease presentation. Adequate medical histories and communication with other health professionals cannot be overemphasized.[21]

Physiologic Changes

Aging decreases the reserve capacity of most organs and organ systems, resulting in a reduced ability to respond to stress[6] and an increased susceptibility to disease. Some of the normal physiologic changes encountered with age include[6,20,21] (1) decrease in bone mass, (2) drop in basal metabolism, (3) dysfunction in the regulatory mechanisms that coordinate several organ systems such as the mechanism that regulates heart rate and respiration during exercise, (4) reduction in lung capacity, (5) decrease in circulation and cardiac output, (6) loss of muscle mass and strength, (7) steady decline in brain volume, producing a slowed response rate, (8) decrease in gastrointestinal secretions and motility, (9) progressive loss of immunologic responsiveness, increasing an individual's susceptibility to infection and decreasing his healing capacity, (10) lowered level of sex hormone activity, (11) steady decline in kidney function, (12) reduction in sensory acuity, and (13) modification in appearance, e.g., hair loss, graying of hair, reduction in height, and loss of skin elasticity resulting in wrinkles. Tooth loss is not a part of the natural aging process. It is caused by extensive caries or periodontal disease.

Pathologic Changes

Chronic diseases tend to increase with advancing age. Statistics reveal that over 80% of all cancers occur in persons over 55 years of age.[22] Although such maladies as cancer, cardiovascular disease, arthritis, osteoporosis, diabetes, dementia, parkinsonism, and vision and hearing impairments are considered to be concomitant with aging, they are pathologic processes that vary in onset and severity among the elderly population. Those chronic diseases not discussed in Chapter 8 are addressed in detail in this section.

OSTEOPOROSIS

Osteoporosis is characterized by a reduced density of bone tissue, predisposing an individual to bony fractures. This condition affects about 1 in 4 women over the age of 60.[23] Only about 10 to 15% of males develop osteoporosis because of the increased density of their bone structure and larger frame. Typically, thin, small-framed Caucasion women are more susceptible to osteoporosis than heavier persons. Women who (1) have a family history of osteoporosis, (2) have had their ovaries removed at an early age, causing hormonal disturbances, (3) live a sedentary lifestyle, (4) have had a diet low in calcium and high in sodium, and (5) have been heavy users of alcohol, caffeine, or cigarettes are at higher risk of developing osteoporosis.[20] Conditions and medications that also increase the risk of osteoporosis include thyroid disorders, renal problems, long-term steroid therapy, and excessive use of antacids containing magnesium or aluminum.[6]

A reduction in bone mass is normal with age, but unfortunately with osteoporosis this decrease in bone density becomes much more advanced. Over a 20- to 30-year period, increasing sharply after menopause as a result of estrogen depletion, women can lose up to 40% of their skeletal mass.[6] Osteoporosis therefore has an insidious onset and can go unnoticed until a fracture of the spine, hip, or wrist occurs, causing pain and disability.[23] Osteoporotic bone becomes brittle, and the simple act of stepping off a curb can cause a fracture.[6]

Persons with osteoporosis can exhibit a loss of height, curvature of the spine, or a humpback appearance in progressive cases when the vertebrae fracture and collapse.[23] Residual ridge resorption of the mandible has been observed.[24]

The goal for young women should be the prevention of osteoporosis through a diet high in calcium; adequate amounts of vitamin D or short-term exposure to sunlight to enhance calcium metabolism; exercise; and avoidance of caffeine, smoking, alcohol, high-protein diets that encourage the loss of calcium through the urine, and foods and soft drinks with high phosphorus content that inhibit calcium absorption. Calcium is best absorbed when a diet with a 1:1 calcium-to-phosphorus ratio is consumed. Americans unfortunately intake about 4 times as much phosphorus as calcium in such foods as meats, eggs, and soda.[6,20,23]

Treatment for patients who already have osteoporosis includes calcium supplements, a diet high in calcium, sodium fluoride to increase bone density, a prescribed vitamin D supplement (high doses of vitamin D can be toxic and should not exceed 400 IU per day), and estrogen therapy to slow the rate of bone loss. Calcium and vitamin D also slow the degeneration process, but only exercise can stimulate the formation of new bone. Activity and exercise must be prescribed with caution to avoid fractures and accidental falls. Accidents, including falls, are the 5th leading cause of death among the elderly. Muscle-strengthening exercises are the most beneficial.[23] Severe involvement of the spinal column might require an orthopedic support or analgesic for the pain.[20] The osteoporotic dental patient with dowager's hump might also require frequent repositioning during a dental appointment.

DEMENTIA

Disease can present atypically in the older adult. For instance, infection in the form of an abscessed tooth or cystitis can manifest as confusion. Hypothyroidism can present as cardiac failure or dementia, and a person with hyperthyroidism can appear apathetic, depressed, and somewhat demented. Therefore to regard dementia as simply as a sign of old age could be fatal to the patient.[21]

True dementia, or a pathologic decrease in mental functioning, is a syndrome rather than a single disease entity. The syndrome is characterized by a short attention span, minimal memory of the very recent past, decreased immediate retention, a tendency to become confused or disoriented, unconscious or conscious fabrication of events when a lapse in memory prevents the completion of a thought, a propensity for misidentifying people or relationships, unstable emotions, strange sleep patterns, and panic or agitation when confused.[21]

Normal forgetfulness or inattention does not denote dementia. In fact, true dementia is relatively uncommon, affecting only about 5% of Americans aged 65 to 79 years and 22% of the elderly population 80 years or older.[25]

Table 10-2. Causes of Dementia

Reversible Dementias	Irreversible Dementias
Depression	Alzheimer disease
Hypothyroidism	Multi-infarct
Hyperthyroidism	dementia
Cushing syndrome	Creutzfeldt-Jakob
Hypopituitarism	disease
Neurosyphilis	Dementia pugilistica
Sensory deprivation	Pick disease
states (such as	Parkinsonism
blindness or	Huntington disease
deafness)	Brain tumor
Lifelong alcoholism	
Deficiency states	
(such as vitamin	
B_{12}, folic acid, or	
niacin)	
Normal-pressure	
hydrocephalus	
Brain tumor	
Drug intoxication	
Cardiovascular	
accident	
Tuberculosis	
Subdural hematoma	

From Neissen, L.C., and Jones, J.A.: Alzheimer's disease: A guide for dental professionals. Spec. Care Dent., 6:7, 1986.

ALZHEIMER DISEASE

In 1906, Alois Alzheimer described the clinical course of a disease that involved progressive memory loss and disorientation in a 51-year old female and resulted in a severe dementia and death within 2 years.[26] He histologically analyzed the patient's brain tissue and found a generalized atrophy with clumping and distortion of the neurofibrils.[27] This condition was later termed Alzheimer disease.

Currently, Alzheimer disease is the most common cause of dementia. Probably because of their relative longevity, females tend to be afflicted two to three times more frequently than males. It affects almost 10% of persons over 65 and 47% of those over 85 years of age. These figures account for nearly 4 million persons nationwide. An estimated 14 million older adults are expected to have Alzheimer disease by the year 2050. It is the fourth leading cause of death among adults in the United States.[23] The second leading cause of dementia is multi-infarct or arteriosclerotic dementia, which comprises 25% of dementia cases. The remainder of persons with cognitive deficits have reversible forms of dementia (see Table 10-2).[28]

The common disturbances noted in Alzheimer disease are usually categorized into three or four overlapping stages (Table 10-3).[29] Although the sequence is progressive, it can vary from patient to patient and the decline can extend for 15 years or more.[30]

An estimated 10 to 30% of Alzheimer patients have the type that is inherited.[23] It is believed the people who have parents or siblings with Alzheimer disease are four to five time more likely to develop the disease than those with no family history of the disease.[31] Research has revealed the trisomy of chromosome 21 in some Alzheimer disease patients, linking Alzheimer disease with Down syndrome.[32]

Because patients with Alzheimer disease can be aggressive or uncooperative, tran-

Table 10-3. Common Impairments Associated
with Alzheimer Disease

Early Stage
  Forgetfulness
  Personality changes
  Employment performance difficulty
  Social withdrawal
  Apathy
  Errors in judgment
  Inattentiveness
  Personal hygiene neglect
Middle Stage
  Disorientation
  Loss of coordination
  Restlessness and anxiety
  Language difficulty
  Sleep pattern disturbance
  Progressive memory loss
  Catastrophic reactions
  Pacing
Advanced Stage
  Profound comprehension difficulty
  Gait disturbances
  Bladder and bowel incontinence
  Hyperoralia
  Inability to recognize family members
  Seizures
  Aggression
  Lack of insight into deficits
Terminal Stage
  Physical immobility
  Contractures
  Dysphagia
  Emaciation
  Mutism
  Pathological reflexes
  Unawareness of environment
  Total helplessness

From Fabiszewski, K.J.: Caring for the Alzheimer's
patient. Gerodontology, 6:53, 1987.

quilizers and antipsychotic drugs have been employed to effectively manage behavior. Side effects of the prolonged use of these drugs include[30,33] (1) tardive dyskinesia (a central nervous system disorder characterized by involuntary movements of the trunk and limbs, and facial distortions, e.g., grimacing, sucking, and chewing movements, protruding of the tongue, and lip-smacking); (2) akathisia (a condition of continual movement while standing or sitting); and (3) xerostomia. Secondary oral problems related to xerostomia include caries, inflammation, ulceration, and shrinkage of the mucosa. For Alzheimer patients taking phenytoin, gingival hyperplasia can be a concern.

It is important for the dental health educator to obtain a thorough medical history of patients with Alzheimer disease and determine their disease stage. Because neglect for personal hygiene occurs during the initial stage of Alzheimer disease, dental intervention should begin early.[30] Communication and preventive care instructions must be modified on the basis of the individual's level of impairment. Speech must be slow and clear. Short words and simple sentences should be used. Nonverbal communication by the dental health educator should involve direct eye contact with the patient as he moves (even if he is wandering in the opposite direction), and deliberate facial expressions, particularly if the patient is hearing-impaired.[34] Distracting noises in the office should be kept to a minimum to enhance effective communication. Mouth props and restraining devices might be necessary to stabilize the patient. The dental health educator should work quickly, and if a radiographic survey is needed, the complete set should be taken over a series of appointments unless the patient is highly cooperative.[35]

PARKINSONISM

Specific structural pathologic changes of the brain can also be observed in patients with parkinsonism. In parkinsonism there is a deficiency in the neurotransmitters dopamine and norepinephrine and an overproduction of cholinergic neurotransmitter substance. Treatment therefore involves drug therapy with L-dopa and anticholinergic agents.[21] Parkinsonism disease is not reversible. It normally affects persons by the sixth or seventh decades of life. Males are afflicted twice as often as females. Currently, about 1 million people in the United States have this disease.[36]

Described by James Parkinson in 1817, this disease remains the most common of the extrapyramidal disorders. The disease possesses three cardinal signs:[37] bradykinesia (slow movements); tremors at rest; and rigidity, usually of the neck and trunk. Loss of dexterity, muscle weakness, pain and cramps, impaired speech, psychiatric disturbances, and paresthesia occur with less frequency. Tremors are rhythmic and can subside with voluntary movement. When the fingers are involved the patient might exhibit a behavior that simulates pill rolling or bread-crumbling.[38] Other symptoms include a shuffling gait with flexed arms and knees and a forward tilt of the body. Facial hypomimia also exists. This masklike appearance results from rigidity of the facial muscles and an overall delay in responsiveness. Excessive drooling can occur because of the patient's dysphagia or difficulty swallowing.[39]

Many parkinsonism patients have normal intellects, but approximately one-third experience dementia.[40] Depression is also a significant finding of parkinsonism, but the dental health educator should explore the patient's mental state further with other health professionals before reacting, because facial rigidity and speech alterations can mimic depression or dementia.

Dental management involves (1) palliative treatment of anticholinergic-induced xerostomia, (2) prevention and treatment of xerostomia-induced caries and periodontal disease, (3) maintenance of prostheses that do not fit well because of poor muscle function and xerostomia (the tongue movements can dislodge the mandibular prosthesis, and the rigidity of the face can prevent retention of the maxillary prosthesis; dry tissues do not cushion a denture, causing mucosal irritation), and (4) counseling on nutritious foods that can be swallowed easily. Because parkinsonism is a disability of muscle control, restraining devices, mouth props, and adaptive oral hygiene aids are usually recommended. The dental health educator should also make an effort to communicate with the patient concerning his oral health status, unless severe dementia exists.[41]

DRUG THERAPY IN THE ELDERLY

Nearly one-third of all medications, both prescription and over-the-counter, are taken by the elderly. This figure represents a major shift in the treatment of chronic disease with drugs. Such a phenomenon affects dental practice. The dental health educator must be prepared to treat elderly patients on multiple drug regimens that are either prescribed by a physician or self-prescribed.[42]

Drugs most commonly used by the elderly include analgesics, cardiac glycosides, diuretics, hypnotics, oral hypoglycemics, and sedatives.[43] Increasing age, multiple medical problems, and complicated drug therapies result in the development of adverse side effects seven times more frequently in the elderly than in any other age group.[44] These side effects are more severe in the elderly, and they take longer to recuperate. Adverse drug reactions also occur more frequently in women, most likely the result of their longevity.[42]

Alerations in drug action in the elderly are related to the effects of aging on the distribution, metabolism, and excretion of drugs. With increasing age, a lower dosage of drugs should be considered because of the following factors: (1) reduction in total body water, (2) decrease in blood flow to various organs and a diminished cardiac output, (3) decrease in albumin levels, and (4) reduction in renal function.[42]

Another concern is noncompliance, which can lead to death or a severe adverse reaction. Approximately half of all outpatients fail to take the medications that have been prescribed.[45] The elderly frequently forget to take their medicine, take the wrong dosage, take their medicines at the wrong time, or forget which pills require food or drink with them to prolong the effects of the drug or decrease gastrointestinal distress. Many are confused about drugs prescribed "as needed" and take them routinely or not at all. In addition, many elderly persons misuse over-the-counter preparations such as laxatives, antacids, and analgesics.[46] In a drug opinion survey of the elderly, about 60% of respondents indicated that they would stop taking a prescribed drug if they didn't feel it was working.[47] Antihypertensive drugs are commonly discontinued by patients because of the silent nature of the disease.

A thorough medical history with a complete listing of a patient's drugs is advised prior to dental treatment. The dental health educator should ask all elderly patients to bring their medications to their initial dental appointment.

ORAL PROBLEMS OF THE ELDERLY

Oral complications in the elderly can be attributed to changes that occur as a result of the aging process, disease, or medications prescribed to treat one or more chronic conditions. Many of the oral manifestations discussed in this chapter are not found exclusively in the elderly population and are related to disabilities and diseases addressed elsewhere in this text.

XEROSTOMIA

Saliva lubricates the oral mucosa, decreases abrasion, and facilitates speech and mastication. Because xerostomia is related to certain systemic diseases, medications, and irradiation (Table 10-4), the dental health educator should be able to anticipate dry mouth as a side effect, educate his patients accordingly, and offer palliative forms of treatment when it cannot be prevented.[48] At least 400 drugs are known to induce xerostomia[20] (Table 10-5).[48]

The clinical signs and symptoms of xerostomia include dry, smooth, shiny, inflamed oral mucosa, chapped lips and commissures that crack and bleed; denture sores and poor denture retention, if applicable; a burning sensation of the tongue caused by glossitis (inflammation of the tongue) or glossodynia (painful tongue); difficulty swallowing because of the lack of lubrication and a burning sensation also noted in the throat; difficulty speaking and sleeping; dental caries; heavy plaque accumulation due to a decrease in the oral self-cleansing mechanism; tooth sensitivity; alterations in taste and smell; Candida infections; and chronic sialadenitis.[20,48]

Table 10-4. Causes of Xerostomia

Factors affecting the salivary center
  Emotions: fear, excitement, depression, stress
  Neurosis: endogenous depression
  Organic disease: brain tumor
  Drugs such as levodopa, morphine
Factors affecting the automatic outflow pathway
  Encephalitis
  Brain tumors
  Accidents, e.g., cerebrovascular accidents
  Neurosurgical operations
  Medications
Factors affecting salivary gland function
  Sjögren's syndrome
  Obstruction and infection (sialoliths)
  Tumors
  Aplasia
  Excision
  Irradiation
Factors affecting fluid or electrolyte balance
  Dehydration (vomiting, diarrhea, sweating, hemorrhage)
  Diabetes
  Cardiac failure
  Uremia
  Edema
  Hypertension
  Thyroid disease
  Folic acid dysfunction
  Hormone dysfunction
  Parkinsonism
  Anemia
  Drugs (diuretics)

From Gilpin, J.L.: Xerostomia: A review for dental hygienists. J. Am. Dent. Hyg. Assoc., 63:112, 1989.

Management of xerostomia is covered in detail in Chapter 9.

CANDIDIASIS

Numerous factors predispose an individual to oral candidiasis (Table 10-6).[49] Fungal infections can be observed in older adult patients with poorly maintained, ill-fitting dentures. The Candida infection secondarily infects traumatized tissues and appears as painless, erythematous mucosa underlying the denture base (denture stomatitis). Chronic atrophic candidiasis is usually encountered on the maxillary arch[50] (Fig. 10-1).

Perleche or angular cheilitis (cracked

Table 10-5. Xerostomia-Causing Drugs

Analgesic mixtures	Decongestants
Anticholinergics	Diuretics
Anticonvulsants	Expectorants
Antidepressants	Muscle relaxants
Antiemetics	Neuroleptics
Antihistamines	Psychotropic drugs:
Antihypertensives	CNS depressants
Antiparkinsonians	Dibenzoxazepine
Antipruritics	derivatives
Antispasmodics	Phenothiazine
Appetite suppressants	derivatives
Cold medications	MAO inhibitors
	Tranquilizers—
	major and minor
	Sedatives
	Sympathomimetics

From Dental Hygiene News: Redi-reference insert, 3, Spring 1990.

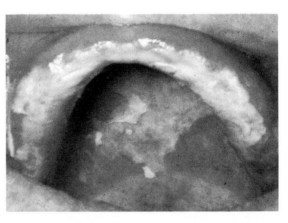

Figure 10-1. An erythematous mucosal reaction under a denture base results in development of candidiasis. Courtesy of J. E. Bouquot, D.D.S., M.S., West Virginia University.

painful commissures of the lips) can also be associated with a Candida infection. Fungal growth in the area is sometimes secondary to a decrease in vertical dimension created by improperly fitting dentures that have caused an overclosure of the arches. The

corners of the mouth become creased, allowing moisture to collect in the folds of tissue, particularly if the patient drools, thereby providing an ideal medium for the fungus to grow (Fig. 10-2). B-complex deficiencies have also been implicated as a cause of this condition.[49-51]

The treatment of candidiasis is discussed in detail in Chapter 9.

DENTURE IRRITATION

Denture irritation can manifest in several ways. The mucosa can appear inflamed, ul-

Table 10-6. Predisposing Factors in Oral Candidiasis

Systemic
  Use of broad-spectrum antibiotics
  Xerostomia
    Pharmacologically induced
    Diabetes mellitus
    Head and neck radiation
  Chronic disease processes
  Malnutrition and avitaminosis
  Immunosuppression
    Chemotherapy
    Corticosteroids
  Neoplasia
Local
  Use of dentures or partial dentures
    Overnight wear
  Ill-fitting dentures
    Lack of stability or retention
    Inadequate lip support
    Inadequate vertical dimension of occlusion
  Poor prosthesis hygiene
    Use of nonprescription reliners
    Inability to clean dentures as a result of decline in vision or digital dexterity

From Thomas, J.E., and Lloyd, P.M.: Oral candidiasis in the elderly. Spec. Care Dent., 5:222, 1985.

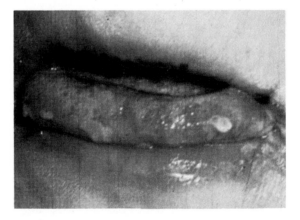

Figure 10-2. Angular cheilitis. Painful, infissured lesions at the commissures of the lips secondarily infected with Candida. Courtesy of J. E. Bouquot, D.D.S., M.S., West Virginia University.

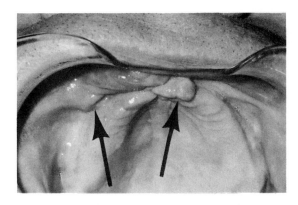

Figure 10-3 Epulis fissuratum. Folds of tissue from chronic denture irritation that have enlarged and become ulcerated. Courtesy of J. E. Bouquot, D.D.S., M.S., West Virginia University.

cerated, secondarily infected with Candida, papillomatous, hyperplastic, or keratotic. If the patient does not complain of discomfort, other signs that can indicate denture sores include difficulty chewing, holding or rubbing the mandible, and constantly taking dentures out. Denture-induced mucosal irritation can be treated by having the dentures relined or remade, reducing the site on the denture causing the irritation, leaving the dentures out of the mouth to rest the tissues for a designated period of time daily, and using a topical over-the-counter preparation such as Orabase for the treatment of ulcerations (see Table 6-2).

Epulis fissuratum is a lesion found primarily in the maxillary anterior segment, adjacent to the labial flanges of a denture. It is also caused by an ill-fitting prosthesis, and it usually results when shrinkage of the underlying ridge occurs with subsequent overextension of the denture flange as the base loses its foundation. Early epuli consist of small folds of tissue. If the source of irritation continues, the folds can enlarge and become ulcerated (Fig. 10-3). The treatment usually consists of surgical removal and an adjustment or fabrication of a new denture, depending on the severity of the problem.[51]

VARICOSITIES

Oral varicosities, particularly in the sublingual area, are a common finding in the elderly. The causes are many, but varicosities are usually due to capillary fragility associated with aging, a loss of elasticity in the venous wall, or a blockage of venous flow.[51]

Petechiae or purpurae of the oral mucosa can be indicative of more than the mere aging process. Certain conditions or drugs can initiate bleeding by interfering with platelet numbers or function.[52]

TASTE PERCEPTION

Dysgeusia or altered taste sensation due to a loss of taste buds is not necessarily the result of the aging process, as was once believed. In fact, although the elderly do experience some loss of taste sensitivity, no substantial decline in the number of taste buds occurs with advancing age.[6,50] When a change in taste is noted, it usually manifests as an increase in the thresholds for salty and sweet, due to an occlusion of the taste buds on the tongue, partially as a result of hyperkeratinization of the aging epithelium.[53] Poor oral hygiene, disease, smoking, xerostomia, malnutrition, neurologic deficiencies, olfactory complications, social living conditions (which limit the elderly person's participation in food preparation and reduce his food choices), and medications (e.g., chlorhexidine, cardiac glycosides, and some cancer chemotherapeutic agents) appear to be more influential in creating taste disturbances.[6,50,52] Because receptors on the palate are most responsive to bitter and sour tastes, patients who wear complete maxillary dentures seem to lose a great deal of their sensitivity to these tastes.[54]

Alterations in the sense of smell also seem to occur in later years. Usually older adults complain about a decreased ability to detect or identify odors. Because the odor of foods contributes to their palatability, deficits in smell and taste tend to go hand-in-hand and can ultimately result in poor nutrition because of the lack of enjoyment derived from eating and a tendency to choose unhealthful, highly seasoned, fatty, fried foods to perceive some sense of taste.[6,55]

Fissuring of the dorsal surface of the

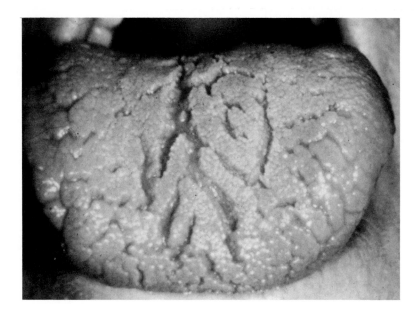

Figure 10-4. Fissured tongue.

tongue is common in the elderly (Fig. 10-4). These furrows enhance the retention of plaque and food debris. The patient notices a bad taste in his mouth that is not associated with eating, and halitosis results. Brushing the tongue is recommended to increase taste sensation. If an individual experiences an unpleasant taste when chewing, it can be due to a discharge of crevicular fluid from a diseased sulcus.[55] The dental health educator should assess the patient's periodontal status and review proper oral hygiene practices with him.

ATROPHIC GLOSSITIS

A tongue that is bald, red, and painful can indicate a nutritional deficiency. Nutritional anemias associated with vitamin B_{12}, folic acid, or iron manifest predominantly in the elderly, producing this oral side effect. Characteristically there is atrophy of the filiform papillae, giving the tongue a smooth appearance. Adequate nourishment is essential for recovery, but there might be an underlying cause such as a malabsorption syndrome, chronic alcoholism, or long-term drug use (e.g., anticonvulsant therapy triggering a folic acid deficiency).[50]

BONY ALTERATIONS

Some bone remodeling occurs in the older adult. Periodontal disease and osteoporosis actually accelerate alveolar bone loss. After tooth extraction, the bony trabeculae surrounding the socket decrease in number and thickness, thereby increasing the porosity of the bone. Tooth loss and drifting teeth also affect the patient's appearance. Hollow cheeks, a collapsed bite, and a protrusive mandible are characteristic of the edentulous patient. With the absence of teeth, the alveolar process no longer serves its primary function of tooth support, and consequently it is resorbed. Bone can be lost to such an extent that the maxillary and mandibular ridges can approach flatness, making retention of a prosthesis extremely difficult. This decrease in vertical dimension also results in diminished muscular power during mastication. Many must therefore rely on a semisoft or soft diet.[6,54]

Temporomandibular joint disorders in the elderly are primarily encountered by those who have degenerative joint disease. A limited opening, crepitus, pain, trismus, or swelling tend to occur unilaterally in the patient with osteoarthritis and bilaterally in the individual afflicted with rheumatoid arthritis.[6]

DENTAL AND PERIODONTAL CHANGES

The elderly can exhibit changes in the teeth and periodontium as a consequence of poor habits and aging. These changes include[20] (1) intrinsic staining from large dental restorations or long-term exposure to nicotine, coffee, tea, or occupational materials, e.g., dyes and coal; (2) attrition from years of wear associating with eating, bruxism, or occupational factors; (3) mechanical abrasion from use of a hard toothbrush, using a scrubbing, horizontal motion, with an abrasive dentifrice; (4) narrowing pulp chambers and canals and increased deposition of secondary dentin; (5) root caries caused by gingival recession, poor oral hygiene, and ingestion of fermentable carbohydrates; and (6) an accelerated rate of periodontal disease due to periods of oral hygiene abstinence or neglect.[11]

ORAL CANCER

One of the factors most strongly linked with oral carcinomas is age. As a person ages the cells undergo metabolic changes, the body is exposed to carcinogens in the food and the environment, immunologic function becomes altered, and cumulative contact with microorganisms over the years might be carcinogenic.[56,57] (See Chapters 7 and 9 for further details on the incidence, causes, and treatment of oral cancer.)

DENTAL AND ORAL HYGIENE TREATMENT CONSIDERATIONS

The goal of treatment for the elderly patient should be to preserve and restore the oral cavity to a state of optimal health and function. A thorough medical history must be performed to assess any problems that could compromise the treatment process or final outcome. Oral hygiene instruction and treatment plan information must be presented to the patient gradually. The treatment plan should be (1) explained clearly, at the patient's level of understanding; (2) realistic (never attempt to change life-long habits in the elderly—just those that are the most threatening to the patient's well-being); and (3) within the desires, expectations, and economic realm of the patient. The dental health educator should be sympathetic to the patient's needs, but not patronizing. The patient should be actively involved in his diagnosis and treatment options, so that he is equipped to render an informed decision regarding his care. The information presented in the treatment plan should also be in writing, and informed consent must be obtained from the patient. If the patient has been declared legally incompetent, signature by his committee or a designated family member with power of attorney is advisable before proceeding (see Chapter 12).

Although some older adults and those with Alzheimer disease lack interest in their personal appearance and neglect their oral hygiene, the vast majority of the younger elderly, aged 65 to 74 years, are still very much interested in esthetics and lead socially active lives. Rehabilitation of the edentulous patient no longer needs to be limited to the selection and arrangement of teeth. The dental health educator must address his patients' psychological concerns about how they look and want to look, and attempt to preserve their self-esteem. Implants and new denture fabrication techniques can assist in improving lip support, retention of the prosthesis, mastication, and facial contour.[58] Unsightly lesions caused by erosion, abrasion, or cervical caries can be restored esthetically with bonded resin materials. Essentially, the dental health educator should offer the geriatric patient the same treatment plan options he offers his younger patients, making adaptations in treatment procedures as deemed necessary[59] (Table 10-7).[20]

Toothbrushing, adjunct plaque-control

Table 10-7. Adaptations in Treatment Procedures for the Gerodontic Patient

Appointment Factors	Characteristic of the Gerodontic Patient	Suggested Procedure Effect During an Appointment
Medical history review	Many forms of chronic diseases	Poor medical prognosis can limit the extent of total treatment
	Variety of medications used	Need for antibiotic premedication for decreased immune response
Appointment planning	Low stress tolerance	Morning appointments
	Tires more easily than younger patient	Shorter appointments
		Need for frequent maintenance appointments to provide high-level preventive care
		Appreciation of the real effort patient has made to get there
	Slower voluntary responses	Do not rush
	Sensitivity about shortcomings of lack of motor control	Do not make the patient feel old by obvious physical assistance
	Lowered intolerance to extremes of heat and cold; less body cooling through perspiration	Adjust room temperature. Cover with blanket
	Impaired hearing; difficulty in hearing when there are distractions	Speak clearly and slowly; provide written memorandum of date and time of each appointment
		Eliminate background noises and music
Instrumentation	Loss of elasticity of lips and oral mucosa	Difficulty in retraction can provide patient discomfort
	Slowing of voluntary responses	Do not demand quick response to request for change of position of head, rinsing
	Cannot adjust to sudden muscular demands	
	Pulp recession: variable pain threshold	Ask patient before administering anesthesia; the patient might not need it
	Reduction in growth and repair processes	Provide as little trauma to gingiva as possible during instrumentation
	Decreased resistance to infection	Suggest postoperative care procedures to promote healing
	Healing slowed	
	Discomfort in the supine position	Some patients prefer to sit upright during care; pillows and blankets can be used to increase comfort
	Inability to recover readily from stresses and strains	At completion of appointment, straighten chair back slowly and let patient sit up for a time before dismissing; assist out of chair
	Unsteadiness; tendency to postural hypotension	

From Wilkins, E.M.: Clinical Practice of the Dental Hygienist. 6th Ed. Philadelphia, Lea & Febiger, 1989, p. 567.

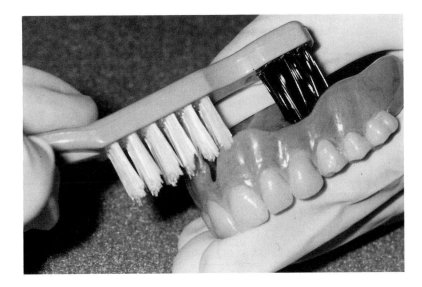

Figure 10-5. Use of the denture brush. Bacterial plaque and debris are removed from the inner impression surface with the small dark-tufted brush, and outer surface of the prosthesis is cleaned with the larger regular-bristled brush. The prosthesis should be handled carefully, preferably over a towellined sink to avoid accidental breakage.

procedures, and methods for maintaining appliances must be reviewed gradually and on a regular basis with the elderly or the caregivers of the elderly residing in an extended-care facility. If the older adult takes an *active* part in his oral hygiene, *motivation* will follow; two essential components to effective learning. Toothbrush modifications, floss holders, and other adaptive adjuncts discussed in Chapter 8 can be useful for the geriatric patient with impaired motor function; an interproximal brush might be preferred over flossing. Fluoride dentifrices, artificial salivas, and fluoride gels are advantageous to the patient with xerostomia or root caries. Mental impairment or weak oral musculature might contraindicate the use of fluoride mouthrinses. Commercial denture cleansers, household hypochlorite, or white vinegar solutions are recommended for cleaning removable prostheses. A hypochlorite solution should not be used on removable partial dentures with metal clasps. After immersion, a denture brush should be used to brush both the inner and outer surfaces of the prosthesis (Fig. 10-5). The patient should also be taught to brush the oral tissues gently with a soft toothbrush and examine the tissues for inconsistencies in size, shape, texture, or color while the dentures are soaking.

NUTRITION AND AGING

A study conducted by the U.S. Department of Agriculture Human Nutrition Research Center on Aging at Tufts University revealed that tooth loss is one of the best predictors of inadequate nutrition in the elderly. Other factors which were found to contribute to poor nutrition include low income, loneliness, poor cooking facilities, poor physical health, lack of nutritional knowledge, and a low level of interest in eating properly.[60] Nutritionally related medical conditions include diabetes, obesity, cardiovascular disease, osteoporosis, and cancer. Unless treated, each of these conditions can shorten the elderly person's life.

A major problem of many older persons is a limited ability to digest and absorb foods. Faulty dentition can make chewing difficult and decrease the individual's intake of fibrous foods. A low-fiber diet coupled with diminished intestinal muscle tone reduces motility and results in constipation.

Digestion, absorption, and utilization of nutrients are also impaired to some degree with aging because of a reduction of secretion of gastric enzymes and atrophy of the alimentary mucosa.[53] Many elderly persons suffer from heartburn, gastric distress, and flatulence after consuming foods that are rich, spicy, high in caffeine, or bulky (e.g., beans, cabbage, broccoli, and brussels sprouts).

Over 5 million elderly Americans live alone and prepare their own meals. Loneliness and apathy are two significant social factors related to malnutrition among members of this age group.[53] Eating alone is depressing for individuals who were accustomed to preparing meals and eating with a family. Mealtime is considered a time for socialization, and when that opportunity is taken away, cooking and eating become a drudgery rather than a pleasure. People who eat alone are less concerned about preparing a well-balanced, varied, and visually appealing meal. Extended-care facilities for the aged strive to make mealtime a social event by having common dining rooms, provide healthy foods prepared in a manner suited to the individuals' tastes and ability to chew, and attempt to ensure that meals are not missed by planning and scheduling mealtimes.

Overeating is common among the lonely elderly. When work and family are no longer a part of their lives, many cannot cope and turn to food for gratification. Excessive food consumption can also produce drowsiness, enabling the elderly to sleep and thus avoid their unpleasant surroundings.[53]

A diminished taste acuity for salt and sweet flavors can induce the excessive salting or sweetening of foods to enhance taste. Purchasing bakery items instead of meats, dairy products, fruits, and vegetables at the grocery store is a common behavior, because the taste of bakery items is pleasing and they do not require preparation.

Modifying food habits is not easy for any age group, but it is particularly difficult for the elderly. Gradual, consistent nutrition education is only part of the answer; the remainder lies in finding a motivator for the patient so he has a desire to eat properly and regularly. Older adults for example, might find senior-citizen lunches or regular bus trips enjoyable. As the digestive process slows with age, less food is needed. Large, heavy meals impair absorption, often cause indigestion, and disturb sleep when eaten

at the end of the day. Therefore light, small, frequent meals are advised, with training in those foods that constitute healthy snacks. In-between-meal sucking on candies because of xerostomia or a bad taste in the mouth must be explored. The dental health educator must first find the source of the dryness or bad taste and recommend reasonable alternatives; sugarless candy can be one option.

COMMUNICATING WITH THE ELDERLY

Interacting with an elderly patient might require modifications in communication technique if the patient has a vision or hearing deficit or cognitive disturbances that alter his ability to comprehend and retain new information.

These physiologic changes do not occur suddenly when one turns 65 years of age; they are gradual processes. The most common physical change is that of hearing loss; it affects approximately 30% of persons over 65 years of age living in the community and 99% of the elderly residing in extended-care facilities or nursing homes.[61] Often hearing loss can be identified when an elderly person turns one ear toward a person speaking, seems inattentive or aloof, requests information to be repeated, fails to follow directions, speaks loudly, responds with irrelevant statements, or avoids communication with others.[62] People who mistake these characteristics for unresponsiveness or confusion cause the hearing-disabled older adult to feel ostracized, powerless, and frustrated.[23]

To ensure effective communication with the elderly in the dental office, the following measures are suggested: structure the environment to eliminate outside noises; speak in a slow-paced, normal tone of voice, directly facing the patient; repeat instructions and write down important points; use gestures and visual aids to reinforce verbal instructions; and do not conlude from mere "yes" or "no" responses that the patient understands.[63]

Visual acuity is indirectly proportional to age. The dental health educator should always remember to return a patient's glasses to him prior to giving instructions. It is also helpful to suggest to the patient that he wear his glasses at home while performing oral hygiene procedures because most elderly are farsighted due to a loss of accommodation. Light-to-dark perception is similarly affected beyond 40 years of age. The patient should be advised to perform his home care in front of a well-illuminated mirror. When providing the patient with written materials, the dental health educator should compensate by using bold, large print. The operatory or consultation room where instruction is presented should also have adequate lighting.

Memory loss and poor retention can be disconcerting to both parties when one is trying to provide health-related instruction. Studies have shown that the deficit noted in cognitive learning and memory is more a problem of speed than any other factor. Older adults need more time to learn new information and more time to respond to questions.[64] Postoperative or home care instructions should be written out for the patient because spoken information is often forgotten or misunderstood. See Table 10-8

for communication techniques to counteract specific cognitive changes that can occur in the geriatric patient.

Patience is extremely important when communicating with the elderly. The dental health educator should (1) show patients respect by granting them the time to finish their thoughts, (2) avoid finishing sentences for them, and (3) be cognizant of nonverbal signals that could offend them.[65] The elderly need to feel a sense of personal achievement, whether knitting a scarf or flossing their teeth. The dental health educator should assist elderly patients in gaining a sense of accomplishment by commending them for their successes, however small.[20] Infantile nuances in communication with the elderly must be avoided. Older adults should be addressed by their title unless requested otherwise by the patients themselves. Baby talk or plural questions such as "How are we today" are contraindicated. If a caregiver or family member accompanies a patient, both should be addressed. The dental health educator should never speak solely to the caregiver as if the patient were not present.[66] A reassuring touch on the hand or shoulder can often convey more caring and sincerity to the patient than words.[65] The success of most dental treatments for the elderly depends to a great extent on the quality of communication be-

Table 10-8. Communication Problems of the Gerodontic Patient and Techniques for Addressing Them

Characteristic of the Gerodontic Patient	Suggested Communication Technique
Slowing of voluntary responses	Make suggestions gradually, over a series of appointments
Slowing of speed of thought associations	
Difficulty in timing sequential events; skills become separate movements, similar to a child	Do not demand learning a completely new procedure; adapt procedure already used
Least comfortable when must respond quickly to demanding sequential stimuli	Guide patient's demonstration of toothbrushing to prevent embarrassment
Rate of learning changed, ability to learn not changed	Do not expect perfection; go slowly, anticipate difficulties, give cues, clues
Changes in speed of vocalization	Distinguish between slowness of learning and inability to learn
Memory shortened, due mainly to lack of attention, lack of interest, or selection of what patient wants to remember	Use motivating factors carefully. Provide written instructions; spoken instructions might be forgotten or misunderstood

Adapted from Wilkins, E.M.: Clinical Practice of the Dental Hygienist. 6th Ed. Philadelphia, Lea & Febiger, 1989, p. 569.

tween the dental health educator and patient—how comfortable the patient feels, mentally, physically, and socially, in the dental office.

NURSING HOME CARE

The nursing home population, in general, has a multitude of medical problems: failing intellectual capacity (decreased memory and attention span, inability to make decisions), physical instability or immobility, and incontinence. The average institutionalized elderly person has six pathologic conditions, almost twice as many as the average older adult living in the community.[67]

Every individual in a nursing home is in need of some form of dental care. Because persons in extended-care facilities are medically compromised, their medical problems usually take priority or the patient himself has no desire to undergo dental care. Dental utilization statistics among nursing home residents are similar to those of noninstitutionalized older adults. A survey of nursing home patients disclosed that 70.3% were edentulous; of those residents who had some or all of their teeth (29.7%), most believed they were in good or fair condition. Approximately 40% of the dentate instutionalized had visited the dentist in the past year; only 19% of the edentate group had done so. Half of those who had received dental care were transported to a private office; the remaining half were seen in the facility. Of those elderly who had not received dental care, visiting dentists found that 82.5% of these persons required some form of dental treatment. Even though most patients (71%) could have their dental treatment accomplished in the dental chair, many elderly either needed bedside care or could not be treated at all due to physical or mental disabilities.[68]

The greatest dental need of nursing home patients is oral prophylaxis. Daily oral health is frequently neglected. Many investigators have commented on the difficulty they experience when attempting to do a clinical oral examination to quantify dental disease in this population group. Moderate to heavy deposits of calculus, plaque, and debris interfere with the assessment process.[11]

Although strides are being made in geriatric dental care, the needs of nursing home residents remain unmet to a large extent due to their poor physical health, their poor manual dexterity, the disinterest they display in oral health, their financial limitations, the lack of dental treatment facilities at nursing homes, the facilities' inability to supply transportation to and from private dental offices or clinics, the absence of agreements or contracts with local dentists or dental schools to provide services, the negative attitude of dentists about caring for the elderly, and a lack of knowledge, skill, and interest among nursing home staff to provide adequate oral care to their residents.[69,70] This dilemma has been addressed in several ways: (1) oral in-service training programs for nursing home staff, particularly nurses aides, enable a large population of institutionalized elderly to receive daily oral care, denture identification and cleaning, etc., when a shortage of dental health professionals exists[71,72] (see Table 8-6 and Fig. 10-6); (2) mobile dental systems, consisting of dentally equipped vehicles, transport dental health teams to extended-care facilities in a particular region or state;[73,74] (3) portable dental equipment provides on-site dental care to bedridden patients;[75] and (4) dental consultants for extended care facilities, as mandated by the federal govenment in 1974, provide in-service training for nursing staff, devise individualized oral hygiene programs based on patients' needs, recommend policies for emergency care, and help patients find dental care if they so desire.[76]

On February 2, 1990, the federal government issued new requirements for the 15,000 nursing homes in the U.S. that receive Medicare and Medicaid funding.[77] These rules stipulate routine and emergency dental care for all residents. As described above, before this time, the dental consultant merely provided education or assisted with dental referrals. Effective Oc-

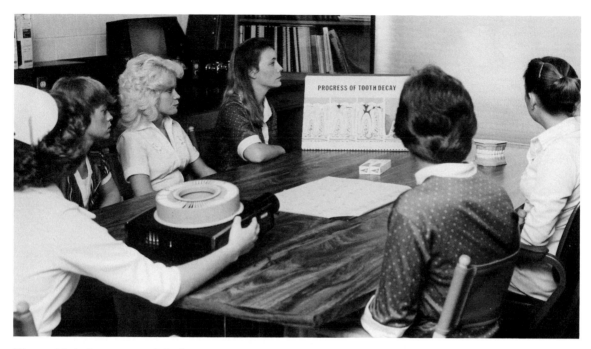

Figure 10-6. In-service slide-lecture presentation on dental disease and prevention for nursing home staff. This is the first instructional step in development of a daily oral health program for older adult residents.

tober 1, 1990, facilities became directly responsible for the dental care needs of their residents by providing (1) comprehensive assessments of their residents' needs, which include dental conditions, conducted by "appropriate health professionals," and (2) referrals to dentists for residents whose dentures have been lost or damaged. Each facility must have an agreement with a dentist to deliver dental services and make referrals. If necessary, assistance with appointment scheduling and transportation to and from the dental office must also be provided.[77]

Hospice Care. Oral management of medically compromised elderly persons can require extension of care to other interdisciplinary settings such as hospice. Hospice can be defined as a specialized program of care, providing medical, psychologic, and social care, through a multidisciplinary team approach, to terminally ill persons and their families.[78] The goals of hospice care programs are to assist terminally ill patients in living the remainder of their lives to the full-

est, surrounded by loved ones, free of pain yet alert and able to participate in activities surrounding them.

Palliative hospice care can be provided in one of three formats:[79]

1. An inpatient unit, which can be either a freestanding building such as an AIDS hospice or a palliative care ward in a hospital.
2. A home-care program, through which visiting nurses and other health professionals provide patient care at home. Family services, including support groups and bereavement follow-up, are also provided.
3. A consultation service as needed for patients requiring intermittent care for pain control, mouth sores, and other problems.

In the course of providing palliative care for the terminal patient, the dental health educator must remain in constant contact with other members of the health care team to ensure the patient's comfort and maintain his sense of dignity.

COMMENTS

The elderly represent an extremely heterogeneous group. Older adults, particularly those in nontraditional settings, provide a unique challenge to the dental health educator. Dentists and dental hygienists are the "appropriate health professionals" to conduct oral evaluations, provide in-service programs, and deliver direct patient instruction and care. Certainly, as the older adult population grows, their impact on the practice of dentistry will become increasingly dramatic. Education of the dental health educator in care of the elderly is as important as the actual patient education process. Both groups must dispel negative attitudes and increase their knowledge base regarding oral health and aging.[80] The informed dental health educator has been afforded the unique opportunity of being able to provide the older adult with factual information and services capable of producing a generation of elderly persons who are able to enjoy optimum oral health and increased self-esteem through a positive image of themselves during the later years. It is imperative that the dental health educator consult the older adult in identifying his needs to ensure the development of meaningful dental experiences worthy of promoting positive changes in behavior.

In the 1930s, dentistry for children was frowned upon, and many practitioners refused to accept children as patients although their needs were great and their numbers were many. Therefore neglected caries resulted in widespread tooth loss.[81] In the 1950s a preventive philosophy emerged. Children were viewed as the key to the curtailment of dental disease, and pediatric dentistry gained acceptance as a dental speciality. History is repeating itself as geriatric dentistry achieves professional and public recognition. The goal is to provide the older

adult with oral health care benefits equivalent to those extended to the young.[14]

For support services and resource groups for the elderly, see Appendix L.

REFERENCES

1. U.S. Bureau of the Census: Current Population Reports: Population Estimates and Projections, 1989. Washington, DC, U.S. Government Printing Office, Series P-25, No. 1018, 1989.
2. Miranda, J. E., Miranda, F. J., and Caldwell, J. K.: Bracing for the baby boomers. R.D.H., 7:26–28, 41, 1987.
3. National Center for Health Statistics: Vital Statistics of the United States. Vol. II. Mortality, Part A. Washington, DC, U.S. Government Printing Office, 1986.
4. Simmons Market Research Bureau, 1983.
5. American Association of Retired Persons: A Profile of Older Americans. Washington, DC, American Association of Retired Persons, 1985.
6. Steifel, D. J., and Truelove, E. L.: A Self-Instructional Series in Rehabilitation Dentistry: Dental Treatment of the Patient with a Disability (Modules 1–10). University of Washington School of Dentistry, Project DECOD, 1987–1988.
7. National Center for Health Statistics: Aging in the eighties, age 65 years and over and living alone: Contacts with family, friends, and neighbors. Preliminary Data, January–June 1984.
8. U.S. Department of Health and Human Services: Oral Health of United States Adults. Bethesda, National Institute of Dental Research, NIH Pub. No. 87-2868, 1987.
9. Strom, T. (Ed.): Access: meeting the needs of special patients. J. Am. Dent. Assoc., 116:319–327, 1988.
10. Ettinger, R. L., and Beck, J. D.: Geriatric dental curriculum and the needs of the elderly. Spec. Care Dent., 4:207–213, 1984.
11. Jong, A. W.: Community Dental Health. 2nd Ed. St. Louis, C. V. Mosby, 1988.
12. King, L.: Geriatrics: The changing face of oral health care. Access, Newsmagazine of ADHA, 3:6–9, 1989.
13. Wilson, A. A., and Branch, L. G.: Factors affecting dental utilization of elders aged 75 years or older. J. Dent. Educ., 50:673–677, 1986.
14. Gilbert, G. H.: "Ageism" in dental care delivery. J. Am. Dent. Assoc., 118:545–548, 1989.
15. Ettinger, R. L., and Beck, J. D.: The new elderly: What can the dental profession expect? Spec. Care Dent., 2:62–69, 1982.
16. Strayer, M. S., DiAngelis, A. J., and Loupe, M. J.: Dentists' knowledge of aging in relation to perceived elderly patient behavior. Geriodontics, 2:223–227, 1986.
17. Kiyak, H. A., et al.: Dentists' attitudes toward and knowledge of the elderly. J. Dent. Educ., 46(5):266–273, 1982.
18. Beck, J. D., et al.: Oral health status: Impact on dental student attitudes toward the aged. Gerontol., 19:580–585, 1979.
19. Blandford, G.: Normal aging versus disease. A symposium: Clinical Geriatric Dentistry, 1986. Spec. Care Dent., 7:7–44, 1987.

20. Wilkins, E. M.: Clinical Practice of the Dental Hygienist. 6th Ed. Philadelphia, Lea & Febiger, 1989.

21. Long, C.: General health considerations. *In* Oral Health and Aging. Edited by A. F. Tryon. Massachusetts, PSG Publishing, 1986, pp. 81–104.

22. Silverberg, E.: Cancer statistics, 1989. Ca. J. Clin., *39*:9–25, 1989.

23. U.S. Department of Health and Human Services, Public Health Service: National Institute on Aging. Age Pages. Bethesda, National Institutes of Health, 1986.

24. Kribbs, P. J., Smith, D. E., and Chesnut, C. H.: Oral findings in osteoporosis. Part II. Relationship between residual ridge and alveolar bone resorption and generalized skeletal osteopenia. J. Prosthet. Dent., *50*:719, 1983.

25. Gershon, S., and Herman, S.: The differential diagnosis of dementia. J. Am. Geriatr. Soc., *30*:585–665, 1982.

26. Alzheimer, A.: Veber eine ergenartige Erhranhung der Hirnrinde. Col. Nervenheilk Psychiat., *18*:177, 1907. Referenced in Wells, C. E. (Ed.): Dementia. 2nd Ed. Philadelphia, F. A. Davis, 1987.

27. State of Maryland: Task force on Alzheimer's disease and related disorders—interim report. Baltimore, MD, 1985.

28. Besdine, R. W.: Dementia. *In* Health and Disease in Old Age. Edited by R. W. Besdine and J. W. Rowe. Boston, Little Brown, 1982.

29. Fabiszewski, K. J.: Caring for the Alzheimer's patient. Gerontology, *6*:53, 1987.

30. Niessen, L. C., and Jones, J. A.: Alzheimer's disease: A guide for dental professionals. Spec. Care Dent., *6*:6–12, 1986.

31. Greer, M.: Dementia: A major disease of aging. Geriatrics, *37*:101–107, 1982.

32. Heston, L. L., and Mastri, A. R.: The genetics of Alzheimer's disease associations with hematologic malignancy and Down's syndrome. Arch. Gen. Psychiatry *34*:976, 1977.

33. Baker, K., and Ettinger, R.: Intraoral effects of drugs in elderly patients. Gerodontics, *1*:111, 1985.

34. Bartol, M.: Nonverbal communication in patients with Alzheimer's disease. J. Gerontol. Nurs., *5*:21, 1979.

35. McClain, D. L.: Dental hygiene care for the Alzheimer's patient. J. Am. Dent. Hyg. Assoc., *61*:500–503, 1987.

36. Wyngaarden, J. B., and Smith, L. H., Jr. (Eds.): Cecil Textbook of Medicine. 17th Ed. Philadelphia, W. B. Saunders, 1985.

37. Rowland, P. (Ed.): Merritt's Textbook of Neurology. 8th Ed. Philadelphia, Lea & Febiger, 1989.

38. Holm-Pedersen, P., and Loe, H. (Eds.): Geriatric Dentistry: A Textbook of Oral Gerontology. Copenhagen, Munksgaard, 1986.

39. Nowak, A. J.: Dentistry for the Handicapped. St. Louis, C. V. Mosby, 1976.

40. Loranger, A. W., et al.: Intellectual impairment in Parkinson syndrome. Brain, *95*:405–412, 1972.

41. Jolly, D. E., et al.: Parkinson's disease: A review and recommendations for dental management. Sp. Care Dent., *9*:74–78, 1989.

42. Lamy, P. P., Overholser, C. D., and Lamy, M. L.: Therapeutic effects. *In* Oral Health and Aging. Edited by A. F. Tryon. Massachusetts, PSG Publishing, 1986, pp. 105–138.

43. Hollister, L.: General principles of treating the elderly with drugs. *In* Clinical Pharmacology and the Aged Patient. Edited by L. F. Jarvk et al. Los Angeles, Raven Press, 1981.

44. Hurwitz, N.: Predisposing factors in adverse reactions to drugs. Br. Med. J., *1*:536–539, 1969.

45. Gambert, S. R.: Drugs and the elderly. Spec. Care Dent., *4*:102–103, 1984.

46. Stewart, R. B.: Drug use in the elderly. *In* Therapeutics

47. Gebhardt, M. W., Governali, J. F., and Hart, E. J.: Drug related behavior, knowledge, and misconceptions among a selected group of senior citizens. J. Drug Educ., *8*:85–92, 1978.

48. Gilpin, J. L.: Xerostomia: A review for dental hygienists. J. Am. Dent. Hyg. Assoc., *63*:111–114, 1989.

49. Thomas, J. E., and Lloyd, P. M.: Oral candidiasis in the elderly. Spec. Care Dent., *5*:222–225, 1985.

50. Thomas, J. E.: Oral care. *In* Therapeutics in the Elderly. Edited by J. C. Delafuente and R. B. Stewart. Baltimore, Williams & Wilkins, 1988, pp. 210–222.

51. Alexander, W. N.: Oral lesions in the elderly. *In* Oral Health and Aging. Edited by A. F. Tryon. Massachusetts, PSG Publishing, 1986, pp. 207–226.

52. Felder, R. S., Millar, S. B., and Henry, R. H.: Oral manifestations of drug therapy. Spec. Care Dent., *8*:119–124, 1988.

53. Nizel, A. E., and Papas, A. S.: Nutrition in Clinical Dentistry. 3rd Ed. Philadelphia, W. B. Saunders, 1989.

54. Davidoff, A., Winkler, S., and Lee, M. H. M.: Dentistry for the Special Patient: The Aged, Chronically Ill and Handicapped. Philadelphia, W. B. Saunders, 1972.

55. Weiffenbach, J. M.: Taste and smell perception in aging. Gerontology, *3*:137–146, 1984.

56. Silverman, S.: Geriatrics and associated oral problems. Spec. Care Dent., *7*:11, 1987.

57. Hill, M. W., and Rowe, D. J.: Influence of aging on oral cancer. J. Am. Dent. Hyg. Assoc., *56*:26–30, 1982.

58. Murrell, G. A.: Esthetics and the edentulous patient. J. Am. Dent. Assoc., *117*:57E–63E, 1988.

59. Koelbl, J. J.: Restorative dental procedures for the older adult. *In* Oral Health Care for the Older Adult. Edited by S. Epstein and H. H. Chauncey. Suppl., Spec. Care Dent. No date.

60. Papas, A. S., and Hefferren, J. H.: Nutrition and the preventive needs of older adults. Spec. Care Dent., *7*:13–14, 1987.

61. Public Health Service: Prevalence of chronic conditions and impairments. National Health Survey, PHS pub. No. 10000, ser. 12, 8, Washington, DC. Department of Health Education and Welfare, 1979.

62. Mauer, J.: Auditory impairment and aging. *In* Working with the Impaired Elderly. Edited by B. Jacobs. Washington, DC, National Council on the Aging, 1976.

63. Sonies, B. C.: Communicative disorders in the elderly. *In* Oral Health and Aging. Edited by A. F. Tryon. Massachusetts, PSG Publishing, 1986, pp. 139–157.

64. Kimberlin, C. L.: Communicating with the elderly. *In* Therapeutics in the Elderly. Edited by J. C. Delafuente and R. B. Stewart. Baltimore, Williams & Wilkins, 1988, pp. 37–49.

65. Geboy, M. J., and Muzzio, T. C.: The geriatric patient. *In* Communication and Behavior Management in Dentistry. Edited by M. J. Geboy. Baltimore, Williams & Wilkins, 1985, pp. 117–138.

66. Dolinsky, E. H., and Dolinsky, H. B.: Infantilization of elderly patients by health care providers. Spec. Care Dent., *4*:150–153, 1984.

67. Rowe, J. W.: Health care of the elderly. New Engl. J. Med., *312*:827, 1985.

68. Council on Dental Health and Health Planning: Oral health status of Vermont nursing home residents. J. Am. Dent. Assoc., *104*:68, 1982.

69. Empey, G., Kiyak, A., and Milgrom, P.: Oral health in nursing homes. Spec. Care Dent., *3*:65–67, 1983.

70. Napierski, G., and Danner, M.: Oral hygiene for the eden-

tulous total care patient. Spec. Care Dent., 2:257–259, 1982.

71. O'Loughlin, J. M.: A comprehensive oral care plan for nursing homes. Spec. Care Dent., 5:14–17, 1985.

72. Herriman, G., and Kerschbaum, W.: Oral hygiene care and education needs in long-term care facilities of Michigan. J. Am. Dent. Hyg. Assoc., 64:174, 196–198, 1990.

73. American Dental Association, Council on Dental Health and Health Planning: Portable Dentistry Information. Chicago, American Dental Association, 1982.

74. Bronny, A. T.: Mobile dental practice: Financial considerations. Spec. Care Dent., 9:160–164, 1989.

75. Berkey, D. B.: Improving dental access for the nursing home resident: Portable dentistry interventions. Gerodontics, 3:265–268, 1987.

76. Shaver, R. O.: Dentistry for the Homebound, Institution-alized, and Elderly. Lakewood, CO, Portable Dentistry Publishers, 1982.

77. Saunders, M. J., Reynolds, W., and Gannoe, K.: Setting and enforcing standards for oral health care in the long-term care facility. Workshop 3 of the 1st Annual National Conference on Special Care Issues in Dentistry—Part 2, Chicago, 1989. Spec. Care Dent., 9:167–168, 1989.

78. National Hospice Organization: Newsletter of the NHO, 2:1, 1979.

79. MacDonald, N.: The hospice movement: An oncologist's viewpoint. Ca. J. Clin., 34:178–182, 1984.

80. Waldman, H. B.: The dental profession and the elderly: A favorable opportunity. Spec. Care Dent., 4:9–12, 1984.

81. Blau, Z. S.: Socioeconomic variations in dental status and behavior of today's elderly. Spec. Care Dent., 9:244–247, 1989.

Chapter 11

DEVELOPMENT OF DENTAL HEALTH EDUCATION PROGRAMS

I know no safer depository of the ultimate powers of society but the people themselves; and if we think them not enlightened enough to exercise their control with a wholesome discretion, the remedy is not to take it from them, but to inform their discretion by education.

Thomas Jefferson

THE PLANNING PROCESS

Dental health educators are frequently called on to assist health agencies or organizations in the development of dental health education programs for communities, organizations, and corporations. Patient education or an individualized oral health education program in the private dental office involves a one-to-one assessment of an individual's needs and characteristics. Program planning, on the other hand, requires an understanding and analysis of an entire group as well as the individuals who comprise the group, (e.g., the local Alcoholics Anonymous) or a total health care delivery system in a geographic area (e.g., maternal and infant health care programs in a particular state).[1]

Program development is defined as the process by which a series of activities are selected and planned to achieve the goals necessary to solve the problems of a particular group.[2,3] In health education the prob-lems to solve are usually mental or physical, and the activities involve health instruction, delivery of care, and active participation in health-related activities that influence and reinforce changes in health behavior.[4]

Effective planning requires communication, cooperation, and coordination between those persons receiving services and those persons delivering services. The health educator must anticipate what will be needed during the course of the program to attain the desired goal for a specific group.

STEPS FOR PROGRAM DEVELOPMENT

Reaching a defined goal requires specific steps:[5] identification of the target population, assessment of needs, design of a specific program, implementation of the program, and evaluation of the program. There are no secret formulas in program development. It requires long, hard work in staff training and group assessment, and constant monitoring and refining.[6]

Identify the Target Population

Usually a program planner is requested when a problem is suspected within a community or group. For example, a company might contact a program planner due to a high level of absenteeism among employees. If a concrete problem has not been perceived, the dental health educator can take the initiative and approach an institution or organization with a desire to focus attention on a suspected need. For example, a dental health educator in a nonfluoridated community might like to assess the dental status of all second-graders in a school district because he suspects a high rate of decay.

Every community has high-risk groups that appear to be more prone to health problems. These groups include the elderly, the very young, the disabled, and the economically disadvantaged (particularly migrant workers and immigrants).[7]

A target population refers to a portion of a community, usually a high-risk group, that has been identified as a focus for concern and needs identification; they are the people for whom health education programs are designed and implemented. Once the target population has been defined, program planners and professionals providing service can differentiate program participants from nonparticipants. Identification of a target population emphasizes a group or groups of people who share similar needs and characteristics, thereby enhancing the cost-effectiveness of the program.[5]

Conduct a Needs Assessment

Needs assessment is the foundation not only for effective program planning but also for successful program development.[7]

When a target group has been identified, the dental health educator should conduct a needs assessment to identify the specific needs of that group. The health educator must be extremely aware that the needs thus defined are needs perceived by the target group. A common mistake of program planners is to design a program on the basis of how they perceive the need rather than how the participants themselves view their problem.

Before surveying needs or collecting data, the dental health educator should stop and think about the task at hand. It is important to first get familiar with a variety of surveys and consult with persons in agencies such as the state and local departments of health who have expertise in surveying technique. It is also advisable for the dental health educator to consult a statistician regarding sampling, records, data analysis, and presentation of findings. A pilot survey (an initial survey given to a similar group to obtain feedback relative to the survey's design, clarity, and content)[8] is essential to ensure development of a final survey that is simple and valid (i.e., that it measures what it was intended to).[8]

COLLECT DATA

The dental health educator must collect the facts to determine the extent or severity of the dental health care needs in a community. An accurate needs assessment must be thorough and include information from (1) a review of local, state, and national public health statistics so the target group can be compared to equivalent groups across the country; (2) a survey of the community's values and attitudes related to oral health and utilization of dental services; (3) an oral inspection survey, if feasible, using a standard dental index to determine the actual dental status of the group (see Dental Health Services section of this chapter); and (4) a survey of existing community resources (facilities, equipment, and manpower) that might be needed to implement the program plan. Table 11-1 describes a variety of methods for surveying community needs.

Table 11-1. Methods for Surveying Community Needs: Advantages, Disadvantages, and Suggested Uses

Pretest	Disadvantages (*continued*)
Advantages	Individuals answering might not respond to all questions
Can be anonymously taken	Might require translation into different languages
Method of evaluating an individual's knowledge or understanding	Suggested Uses
Can vary in length	Acquire information on opinions or attitudes
Specifically developed with a specific theme, e.g., understanding of preventive practices	Provide demographic data or medical or dental history
Same or similar test can be used later for evaluation	Observation
Easy to tabulate	Advantages
Disadvantages	Helpful in observing lifestyle, environment, actual behaviors
Threatening—individual might be admitting lack of knowledge	Observations can be recorded using a checklist, rating scale, or evaluation form
Might not get total cooperation	Developed for a particular activity
Poorly written or developed questions are unreliable	Disadvantages
Involves time in preparation, pilot testing if necessary, printing, and tabulation	Time-consuming
Limited to those who can read	Limited in the situations it can be used for
Suggested uses	Can introduce observer bias
For educators, administrators, parent groups, health professionals, and similar groups in which educational programs are being assessed	Suggested Uses
Questionnaire	Acquire information on attitudes, opinions, or behaviors
Advantages	Find out daily routine oral hygiene practices, dietary practices
Personally administered or mailed	Demographic data
Can be open-ended or closed format	Dental Index
Nonthreatening; anonymous responses	Advantages
Specifically developed for particular information	Designed for specific oral conditions
Easy administration—can require minimum personnel	Indicates disease patterns
Disadvantages	Efficient
Same as pretest	Provides comparison with similar groups
Questions can be misinterpreted	Can be used as an evaluation tool
If mailed, can be costly; return rate might be poor	Indexes have been developed to evaluate caries
Individuals answering might not be representative of the community	Indexes have not been developed for certain oral conditions
	Suggested Uses
	Large numbers of individuals or samples or groups

Adapted from Kostiw, U., Stephenson, M. M., and Zarkowski, P.: The Dental Health Consultant in Community Based Programs. Chicago, American Dental Hygienists' Association, 1982.

ANALYZE DATA

The data collected from outside sources, the needs survey, and the community profile must be carefully scrutinized by the dental health educator to ensure that accurate and appropriate results are concluded. Organizing, tabulating, and interpreting data comprise the sequence of events for analysis. Data analysis can vary in complexity based on the survey instruments and the statistical tests used to interpret the findings.[7] Once the needs are verified, all subsequent activities in the health education program planning process should focus on designing a program oriented to the specific target group with these identified needs.[5]

Design the Program

After a target population has been identified and their needs have been surveyed and analyzed, the dental health educator is ready to institute the methodology, which consists of prioritizing needs into specific program goals and objectives and defining strategies to accomplish these program objectives.

DEFINE GOALS AND SUPPORTING OBJECTIVES

The target population must assist the dental health educator in prioritizing their dental health needs. If their needs are many, several programs might be required to satisfy them. Assistance from a health advisory committee comprised of consumers, health professionals, and community leaders might be warranted to determine which needs should be addressed.[9]

Once the needs have been ranked in importance, a goal can be developed to meet each need. Goals are broad-based, generalized statements describing desired behavioral changes that must occur to alleviate the needs that have been identified. Because of their breadth and generality, goals tend to be timeless and require specific program objective to support their intentions. Goals provide direction in designing instructional objectives.[7,10]

Objectives are precise, short-term statements describing outcomes that build cumulatively to a goal.[10] Objectives should be written as target-group-oriented behaviors that are realistically attainable and meaningful to the population identified. They should include a time frame, a specified direction of change that is both clear and measurable, and a particular content area in which behaviors are being sought.[5,10] Goals

and objectives are solutions to the needs of a target population; they propose ways to reduce a health problem. The development of objectives helps determine the program activities that will take place. Program activities describe how the objectives will be accomplished. Program activity descriptions include three components: what is going to be done, who will be doing it, and when it will be done.[1] Activities are strategies for bringing about desired results. The number and extent of these activities is determined by program length, number and capabilities of personnel, availability of equipment needed, and sources of funding. Personnel, equipment, facilities, and funding are resources. Limitations in these areas can pose constraints and must be effectively managed by alternate strategies to ensure the success of the program. If projected costs (which should include all potential expenditures) exceed budgetary appropriations, program goals and objectives might need to be modified.[7]

The following example illustrates a problem and a need statement, a goal, and related objectives and activities that might be developed to address it:

Problem
  Migrant workers in a southern Texas oil refinery have an unusually high rate of absenteeism from pain associated with their teeth and lower jaws.

Need
  All migrant workers in southern Texas oil refineries need immediate and continuing dental care.

Goal
  All migrant workers employed in southern Texas oil refineries should receive basic dental care under their employers' health care policies.

Objectives
  1. Within the first year, dental screenings will be completed for 25% of the migrant workers employed in southern Texas oil refineries.
  2. Emergency dental care will be provided for these employees, as

deemed appropriate by the dental health educator.

3. One family member per worker will be required to attend dental prevention sessions.

Activities

1. On January 15, 10 dental hygienists will be hired in association with the five local health departments to screen migrant employees of southern Texas oil refineries for dental problems.

2. A dentist will provide emergency services one Wednesday evening per week at the local health department in Galveston.

3. Once monthly, a hygienist will travel to each southern town where an oil refinery exists and provide a preventive dental education program on caries, periodontal disease, fluoride, proper diet, and oral hygiene for families of these workers at the town hall. One family member must attend in order for the employee to continue receiving dental benefits.

DEFINE STRATEGIES TO ACCOMPLISH EACH OBJECTIVE

Once goals and objectives have been written by the dental health educator and approved by the appropriate parties, (e.g., the target group, the advisory committee, and involved health professionals), a timetable strategy is suggested. Timetables are charts that depict the dates by which particular objectives should be achieved. Objectives appear on the chart in the order in which they need to be met. As each objective is met, it is crossed off the timetable, providing visual reinforcement.

A second strategy consists of making arrangements, prior to program implementation, for all required resources needed to meet the objectives of the program.[7] Materials, media, and equipment should be purchased or reserved as far in advance as possible to guarantee their availability and delivery.

Personnel serving in the capacity of professional speakers and health care providers need to be contacted early to eliminate possible scheduling conflicts. It is also important for the program planner to choose personnel who are knowledgeable about teaching methods and criterion-referenced teaching (teaching by objectives). Those personnel performing clinical roles must be calibrated to enhance inter-rater reliability. Facilities must be adequate and accessible to all facets of the population served.

Last, grants, contract acquisitions and creative attempts at fund-raising might be necessary to obtain support dollars from the private, federal, state, or local sectors or third-party insurance carriers to meet the objectives delineated. Much money is available through grants and contracts from government agencies and private foundations.[4] Fund-raising through mailings or door-to-door canvassing is also plausible when a worthwhile project cannot be completed unless additional resources are provided.[11]

Program promotion is a third strategy for getting a program off the ground. Visible programs are more likely than obscure ones to be successful in obtaining participation and administrative support.[11] A particular program can be outstanding, but if consumers are unaware of it, attendance will be low. Whatever it is that makes a program special or different should be featured in the publicity of the program. Not only must dental health educators market programs that suit the needs and preferences of the target population, they must also design publicity programs for that population.[4] The publicity program for promoting a smokeless tobacco cessation program for adolescents would be quite different from one to promote an in-service nursing program for caregivers of the elderly. Public service announcements on television and the radio, newsletter and newspaper advertisements, and notices in specialized publications should be planned well in advance of program implementation to create an interest and peak anticipation.

Implement Program

The realization of the planning phase of a program is its implementation. When a plan is put into operation, all of the assumptions regarding resources, cooperation of personnel, and accessibility of the target group are tested. Unfortunately, not all assumptions made during the planning stages will be correct.[5] Teamwork is essential if the implementation stage is to be a success.[1] Checkpoints should be set at various points throughout the program so all responsible parties can provide feedback and review the objectives.[7]

Making program changes during implementation is not uncommon and does not mean that the program plan was prepared unsatisfactorily or is flawed. Modifying objectives and rearranging the timetable for completion of these tasks should be based on the feedback the dental health educator receives during the initial implementation of the program. If adjustments are made, they should be documented and the original program plan should be revised in preparation for program evaluation.

Evaluate Program

One of the main reasons for conducting an evaluation is to develop a new program or improve an old one. Therefore, once a program has been implemented, it must be monitored continually. A program's triumphs are determined by how well personnel are doing their jobs, how well equipment functions, how adequate funding and facilities are, and essentially how well program goals have been met by each of the objectives delineated.[1]

Evaluation is a means of providing accountability.[7] All persons involved in the planning process and implementation stage are responsible for their assigned duties. A proper approach to accountability must also assess the impact objectives from cognitive, affective, and psychomotor domains[12] have on the program participants. Although affective objectives are intangible and frequently difficult to measure, they provide insight into the humanistic benefits, if any, that might be derived from a program.[13]

Informal and formal methods for evaluation are both important. Observation is an example of an informal method of assessment. A post-test is a formal evaluation tool that can be used to assess changes in knowledge, attitudes, or behavior during the course of a program, if a pretest has been conducted to obtain baseline data.

Evaluation should be a nonthreatening experience. Program planners should be creative, flexible, and eager to evaluate progress and eliminate stagnation in their programs. Because evaluation is an ongoing process, feedback should be obtained routinely and actions to remedy concerns should be conducted in a timely fashion. Such an evaluation is referred to as formative because it provides continuous feedback to program directors and enables them to make modifications that will enhance the program. The focus of *formative evaluation* is on early program assessment. The development of a goal consensus, assessment of participant reactions to the services provided by the program, and a needs assessment of the target group conducted early in the planning stages are examples of formative evaluation. Conversely, *summative evaluation* emphasizes the end product or outcome—the degree to which goals and objectives have been met. Fiscal year assessments and course evaluations distributed after a final examination are examples of summative evaluation. A summative report is extremely important to funding agencies and is used to determine the viability of the program. Summative evaluation studies require a more sophisticated research design, which in turn requires more time, effort, and resources, than formative assessments. Evaluators must be cognizant of the temptation to assess only those areas of the program that appear to be successful; an evaluation must be comprehensive to be helpful to the total process.[11]

DENTAL HEALTH SERVICES

The three phases of a dental health education program include dental health instruction, dental health services, and dental treatment (which encompasses preventive procedures). All phases of the dental health education program are interdependent.[14] In order for one phase to be effective it must overlap others. For example, an oral cancer screening is never accomplished without some degree of preventive education. Dental instruction and dental treatment and prevention have been widely discussed throughout this text. Since the focus of this chapter is on program development, the service component is emphasized.

Dental health service programs are largely based on the needs of the group participants. Typical dental services at a school, convalescent home, or institution for the mentally retarded include dental inspections, follow-up referrals, emergency care, evaluation, and in-service training. For example, a dental health educator can plan a caries screening of schoolchildren or prepare a teacher in-service program on implementing a fluoride rinse program. Dental services are not simply ends in themselves; they require follow-up counseling and procedures.

Dental Inspections

The dental inspection should be conducted for diagnostic or assessment purposes (depending on the level of sophistication) and as a basis for educational discussions. There are four types of dental inspections: (1) complete—an entire office examination including diet counseling and radiographs; (2) limited—a recall assessment with a mouth mirror, explorer, adequate illumination, and radiographs, if indicated; (3) inspection—a basic assessment using a mouth mirror, explorer, and adequate illumination; and (4) screening—a cursory examination using only a tongue depressor and available illumination. The terms screening and inspection are often used synonymously.[14]

Inspections are advantageous because they can (1) serve as the basis for oral hygiene instructions, (2) provide an opportunity for establishing a rapport between the patient and the dental health educator, (3)

serve as motivational strategies, (4) be a fact-finding experience for the patient, parent, teacher, physician, and dental health educator, (5) provide baseline data for the evaluation of a dental health program that has been instituted, and (6) provide information as to the status of the dental needs of an individual or a target group.[14]

Some of the disadvantages of dental inspections can include (1) if a lower-level inspection is relied on as an examination the need for complete dental assessment might not be perceived; (2) inspections are of no value unless follow-up is initiated; and (3) if a child is receiving a lower-level inspection in school, the parents are not present to be informed of their child's problems and might remain unaware of the importance of follow-up.[14] Figure 11-1 is a sample screening form that could be used during screenings at various settings to reaffirm a patient's needs in writing and to inform parents or significant others about the dental status of an individual for whose care they are responsible. It also encourages follow-up at all treatment need classifications (I–IV), as stipulated by the American Dental Association. Ideally, inspections should be rechecked within a reasonable time period for individuals displaying poor oral hygiene or other dental treatment needs, e.g., restorations, extractions, and appliances.

In-Service Education

The dental health educator is an outstanding resource person for performing in-service education. Teachers, physicians, nurses, pharmacists, dieticians, social workers, and other professionals responsible for rendering care or seeing that care is provided need to keep up to date with dental health issues pertinent to their fields. Although prevention should be emphasized throughout, oral side effects related to drug therapy and their palliative management, for instance, might be of greater interest to physicians, nurses, and pharmacists; dieticians might be more interested in feeding appliances for infants with oral clefts; teachers might wish to discuss a protocol for

Department of Dental Hygiene

Medical Center
Morgantown, West Virginia
26506

West Virginia
University

ORAL SCREENING EVALUATION

_____ 1. **No treatment necessary at this time, as related to the type of inspection given.**

_____ 2. **Treatment needed, but not urgent at this time.**

_____ 3. **Conditions requiring early treatment.**

_____ 4. **Emergency treatment necessary.**

ALL RECOMMENDATIONS INCLUDE A VISIT TO YOUR DENTIST FOR AN ORAL EXAMINATION AND PREVENTIVE ORAL HYGIENE CARE.

Equal Opportunity / Affirmative Action Institution

Figure 11-1. Oral screening evaluation form.

management of traumatic oral injuries on the playground; and social workers might prefer to address those insurance carriers that provide dental coverage for their clients.

Whatever the dental health topic(s), a series of in-service programs is perhaps the best means of enriching a group, because issues can be discussed in depth and two or more sessions allow for an atmosphere of exchange. Additional sessions also enable participants to relate pertinent experiences that they have had since the last meeting. One-meeting approaches are more limiting. Regardless of the approach, the dental health educator should never attempt an in-service program unless he has first assessed the needs of the participants. In-service sessions are usually rated more highly if a variety of teaching methods is employed and if learning activities are provided that enable the participants to get more involved in the program.[10]

INSTRUCTIONAL MEDIA

Media should always be a part of instruction. To be effective, media must be both pertinent to the subject matter being addressed and an adjunct to instruction; media cannot replace a teacher or assume the actual task of teaching.[14,15]

When selecting a type of medium for instruction, one should consider certain questions:[14] (1) Is the material presented at an opportune time in the program? (2) Is the material presented at the participants' level of understanding? (3) Is the size of the participant group conducive to the instructional medium chosen? (4) Is there sufficient time to thoroughly cover the medium presented? (5) If equipment is needed, is it available and is the dental health educator acquainted with the method of operation? and (6) Is the environment (e.g., lighting, seating, room temperature) acceptable for the medium chosen?

Instructional materials, media, and equipment can take several forms. The simplest and most direct means of communicating an idea or a concept is usually the most desirable.[16] This section of the chapter considers visual and audiovisual instructional media options that can be extremely useful during various stages of the dental health education program process.

Table Clinics

A table clinic is a presentation of a specific topic that combines oral communication with a table top display. The topic of presentation may be previously documented or original research, or a technique, service, or trend in dental hygiene, dentistry, or related field.[17,18] Through preparation and presentation of a table clinic, the dental health educator expands his knowledge of a specific subject. It is not uncommon for the table clinician to use the information gained from this experience in the development of other research or publications. Table clinics can also act as mini refresher courses by providing pertinent information to observers. In a short amount of time, an observer can listen to several clinics and gain information on topics that would normally take days to research.

The initial step in planning a table clinic is to decide on a topic of interest that relates to the audience to which it is to be presented. The topic should be timely and one that can be adequately covered in the allotted time. The American Dental Hygienists' Association[17] specifies a time limit of 7 to 10 minutes, and the American Dental Association[18] specifies a 5- to 7-minute presentation. If the table clinician has no specific topic in mind, purusing current dental journals or the Index to Dental Literature might lead to discovery of an interesting topic.

Guidelines of the American Dental Hygienists' Association suggest that topics for table clinics fall into one of six categories:[17]

public and community health, private practice or clinical procedures, basic or dental science, research (documentation or original), alternative career opportunities, and foreign or international health care systems.

Once the presenter decides on a topic, he must review the literature for previously documented information on the subject. Keeping in mind the allotted time for the presentation, the clinician should then write objectives for the clinic. The objectives usually range in number from three to six.

After the subject is researched, an outline of the presentation should be written. This should include an introduction, body (presentation of facts), and a conclusion. If the table clinic involves original research, the outline should conform to a typical research format: introduction and review of literature, methods and materials, results, and conclusions.

Throughout the table clinic, advertising of a product is prohibited.[17,18] Brand names must be omitted, and products should just be described. Drugs should be identified only by their generic names.

The table top display needs to be attractive, colorful, and communicative. All displays must be confined to a table top that measures 2' × 6" or 3' × 6". Poster boards or flip charts should be no more than 3' high.[18] A display might consist of one to three poster-type boards, flip charts, slide projectors and small screens, rear-projection screens, audioviewers (self-contained screen and projectors) (the audio section must not be used), inanimate models, or combinations of these.

Models or audioviewers can be placed on the table in front of or beside the display panels, or they can be part of the actual panel display. An opening large enough to accommodate the audioviewer screen can be cut in the display board, or a model placed in front of a blank area of the board so that either is an integral part of the display. Whatever arrangement is decided on, the clutter should be kept to a minimum so as to present a neat and easily comprehensible table top display.

The layout of the poster-type display

should be easily understood and esthetically pleasing and should include the title, text, and an element that makes the visual image the center of attention (Fig. 11-2). This center of interest might be created with pictures, graphs, or even the title. Oftentimes a catchy title is the primary attention-getter. Whether it is catchy or not, it should carry the main theme of the clinic.

Once the content of the display is decided on, the arrangement of the layout must be determined.[15,16,19] By sketching scale diagrams of the display, one can determine the appropriate balance and configuration of its elements. Remember that the eye normally reads from left to right and top to bottom.

The title should be bolder and larger and can be a different color from the rest of the text of the display. Because table clinic displays are normally viewed from 3′ to 5′, 2″ letters for the title, 1″ letters for subtitles, and ½″ to ¾″ letters for the text are sufficient sizes.

Drawings and pictures should be bold and simple but should not distract the viewer's attention to exclude the other elements.[16] If any are used, they should be labeled or coded in the text. They can be attached to the display board with special glues, rubber cement, or Velcro. Color, texture, and moving parts can add excitement to the display.

The text of the display should be limited to subtitles and listings of words or phrases. Sentences should be avoided. A series of arrows or dashes between words or phrases is effective in directing the viewer through a sequence.

Table top displays of two to three hinged panels work well for table clinics. Three types of boards can be used: poster board (thin, flexible, and multicolored), mat board (heavier and multicolored), and Foamcore (foam-type material sandwiched between layers of white presentation paper to form a lightweight, durable board). Because of its rigidity and stability, Foamcore is preferable; and, although it is available only in white, color can be added by spray painting or attaching colored mat board. The individual panels can be hinged with wide tape, Velcro strips, or preformed plastic hinges.

The lettering of the table top display should be legible from 3′ to 5′ and should present an overall clean and neat appearance. Various styles, sizes, and colors of dry-transfer and precut vinyl letters are available. Lettering can also be produced with a computer and then printed with a laser printer. Neat hand lettering can be used for emphasis. Letters should be spaced optically by making spaces look equal, regardless of measured distances between them.[19]

A handout or brochure containing a sum-

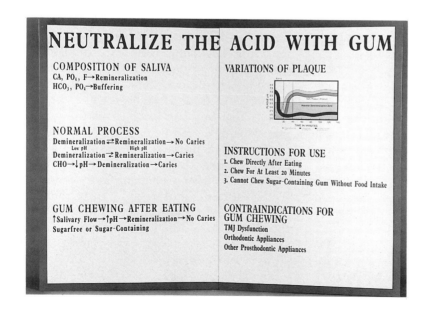

Figure 11-2. Table clinic display.

mary of the table clinic is conducive to a good table. This should include a title page (title, presenter, affiliation, and date), body (objectives, introduction, text, and conclusions), and bibliography and acknowledgments (Fig. 11-3). This handout is simply an overview of the table clinic and should not be lengthy or written as a research paper.

The parts of the table clinic are tied together by the oral presentation of the dental health educator. The dental health educator should first state the title and objectives of the clinic and then proceed with the body or text. While speaking, the table clinicians should utilize the display by pointing to key sections so that the audience can easily follow along.

Knowledge of the subject is a must; the subject can be described with ease if the clinician has thoroughly researched it. Annoying mannerisms, such as rocking back and forth, saying "you know," and playing with a pointer or note cards should be avoided. Note cards, if used, should be small and discrete. The presenter should use eye contact and create rapport with the audience.

Preparation and presentation of a table clinic can be a gratifying experience if the dental health educator chooses the topic well and allows sufficient time to research and prepare the clinic. A table clinic is an excellent means of providing information on a subject to colleagues at professional meetings.

Exhibits

Relaying information to consumers about new techniques in dental care can be accomplished by an informal type of table clinic or exhibit. Health fairs, conducted mainly in shopping malls in towns and cities across the country, display less-formal tabletop programs and screening clinics (e.g., cholesterol or blood pressure) sponsored by a variety of health care agencies and professionals in private practice.

Health fair exhibits should visualize the positive side of dental health and should offer some free samples such as toothbrushes, floss, balloons with a preventive message, and stickers to attract consumers. The presenters should be dressed profes-

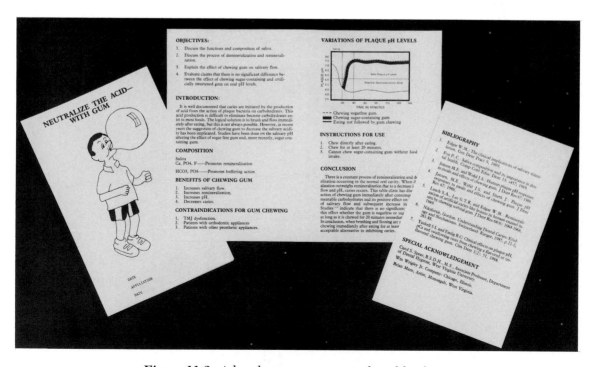

Figure 11-3. A brochure summarizing the table clinic.

sionally and should remain at the booth at all times to discuss their topic and answer any questions that might be asked. The enthusiasm displayed by the dental health educator will be communicated to those who stop by the booth and will increase their interest in the information offered.[20]

Children's Dental-Health-Month Fairs

For over 40 years, February has marked a national monthlong observance of children's dental health. Activities include dental health screenings, health fairs, and contests. Many states conduct events such as puppet shows for special audiences, gain mass media exposure through radio and television public service announcements, and stimulate new program activities[21] (Fig. 11-4).

To assist state and local dental societies in developing National Children's Dental Health Month programs and publicizing the event, the American Dental Association has created a comprehensive planning kit.[22]

Health fairs have proven to be a valuable educational tool for children, particularly if teachers, trained by dental health educators,

prepare the students concerning prevention prior to the fair; students participate in events rather than just listen; and students have the opportunity to observe various dental procedures in a nonthreatening environment (e.g., demonstrations of radiographs, sealants, fluoride applications).[23]

Bulletin Boards and Teaching Displays

Bulletin boards and teaching displays (chalkboards, felt boards, charts, posters, and models) are among the least expensive of the visual instruction resources. They function by:[16] stimulating interest and motivation, saving time, encouraging thought, providing a simplified view or summary, assisting the user or creator in learning to communicate ideas visually, and providing an attractive addition to an office or classroom.

Preparation of visual displays should begin early. As in the table clinic process, a theme must be decided on and a plan sketched out before construction begins. Simplicity and clarity emphasizing the main idea of the display, proper placement pattern, balance, effective use of pictures or illustrations, vibrant compatible colors, vary-

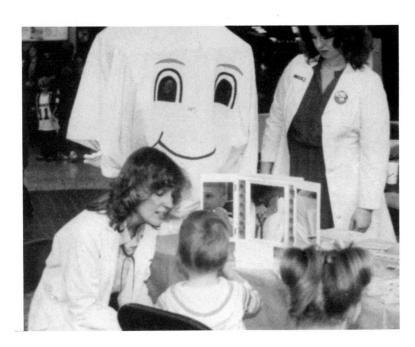

Figure 11-4. Children's Dental Health Month activities.

ing shapes and sizes, and legible, professional-looking lettering are essential.

BULLETIN BOARDS

The main purpose of a bulletin board is to gain the attention of the viewer so that he will want to stop, look, and learn. One central idea with simple supporting material is advised so that the message is comprehensible in a short period of time. Word play and familiar themes or characters can be a suitable approach to getting the message across (Fig. 11-5). Bulletin boards should be changed periodically to avoid saturation of an old theme and enable the representation of new and interesting ideas. Dental health educators should use bulletin boards as motivational tools for increasing interest in dental health; the power of suggestion can be a strong force in changing behaviors.[14]

CHALKBOARDS

Most training centers still have chalkboards; they are one of the oldest instructional aids available. Skill and some degree of artistic talent are needed to use a chalkboard effectively (Table 11-2).[15] Chalkboards should be used primarily for displaying symbols, words, and numbers.[14] Going to the board to solve an arithmetic problem is a prime example. Metallic boards will gradually replace chalkboards. Felt markers are used for writing on these boards, and sponge erasers are used to remove the ink.

FELT OR CLOTH BOARDS

Hard boards covered by felt or cloth are useful because materials can be placed, rearranged, or removed at will. This feature enhances small group involvement and is ideal for the young learner. They are convenient to use, easily transported, and can be prepared ahead of time. Felt illustrations adhere directly to the felt board (Fig. 11-6). If the board is cloth, Velcro strips are first glued to the back of the pictures to be placed on the board, enabling them to adhere to the cloth.

CHARTS, POSTERS, AND MODELS

Charts, posters, and models, like most visual displays, are designed to be self-instructional; they do not require the assistance of another person to interpret the information.

Charts and posters can be created by

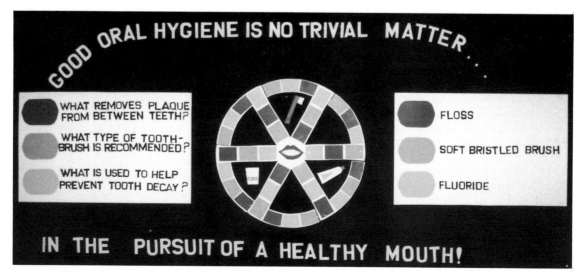

Figure 11-5. Bulletin board utilizing a familiar board game theme to attract the viewer's attention.

using pictures from magazines, original drawings, or clipboard pictures. Clipbooks are commercially available sourcebooks for obtaining black-and-white line drawings of a wide variety of subjects. Another type of ready-made artwork is dry-transfer art, which is sold as illustration, number, and letter forms printed on the underside of an acetate sheet. The picture is transferred to the working surface with a burnishing tool.[19]

Line, bar, and circle graphs are ideal techniques for visualizing statistical data. Flow charts and diagrams are also helpful in summarizing a complex concept by depicting the flow of a process, thereby connecting parts into a working relationship (Fig. 11-7). Flip charts are handy devices for presenting information in a sequence.

Models are tactile, three-dimensional learning media. They can supplement wall charts and are ideal for anatomy courses. Removable parts allow the learner to view the

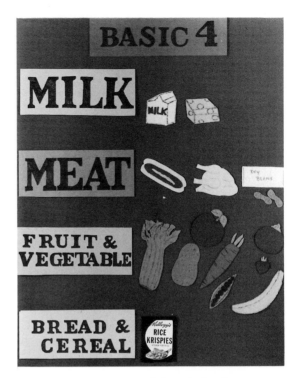

Figure 11-6. Felt board display.

anatomic structures internally as well as externally.[16]

Projected Visual Media

Sheets of transparent acetate material can be prepared ahead by drawing or writing on them with felt-tip markers. When placed on an overhead projector the light passes through them and projects the image onto a screen. This medium can facilitate discussion sessions; the educator can illustrate as he speaks and receives feedback from participants. The user must write legibly and large enough to project adequately and should avoid putting too much information onto one transparency sheet.[15]

Slides are the most commonly used still-projection medium, and they are effective in most instructional situations. Slides can be produced to match the unique design of a presentation describing a program or technique. Slides from various presentations can be mixed and matched to create new pre-

Table 11-2. Correct Techniques for Using a Chalkboard

1. Print, unless your writing is especially easy to read
2. Verify that your words are large enough to be seen easily from the back of the room
3. Use colored chalk to separate ideas or add emphasis
4. Do not try to talk and write at the same time. When you write on the board stop talking and concentrate on what you are writing
5. Maintain eye contact with the class, not with the board. Avoid looking at the board during discussion, but use a long pointer instead so that you can stand aside, using peripheral vision to see the board
6. Write short sentences or phrases, but avoid abbreviations; students taking notes will have difficulty later in deciphering your shorthand
7. Hold the chalk like a knife and pretend you are slicing tomatoes on the kitchen counter. Use firm downward strokes, and rotate the chalk as you use it so that lines will be uniform as the chalk wears

From Simonson, M. R., and Volker, R. P.: Media Planning and Production. Columbus, Charles E. Merrill, 1984.

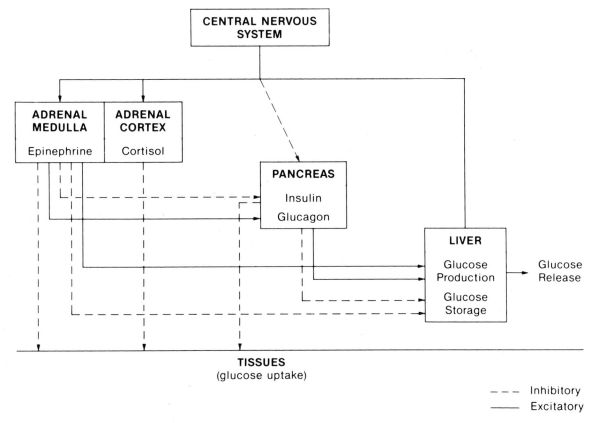

Figure 11-7. Flow chart.

sentations, and older presentations can easily be changed or updated. Easy storage and retrieval of slides is another advantage. Slides are portable and can be programmed with tapes to produce a slide-tape or audiovisual presentation.[11]

Filmstrips, like slides, are still images that can be adapted to audiotape, producing an audiovisual medium. The filmstrip is relatively outdated because of its fixed sequence of frames.

Audio Instruction

Records or audiotapes can be listened to individually or amplified for a group. Audio instruction rarely holds the attention of a group unless some type of visual aid is introduced. Tapes continue to be used in the classroom to record lectures for study purposes. The fragility of tapes and records

make this medium less desirable than the others. Compact discs, the most current advancement in sound and recording, produce outstanding audio quality.

Audiovisual Media

Motion pictures and the more recent videotape are particularly appropriate for displaying real-life action and complicated situations in sequence, such as cardiopulmonary resuscitation techniques. In addition to enhancing knowledge, they are one of the most effective media for working with affective forms of behavior (i.e., feelings or emotions). The learner can also view in a few moments what might have required a long time to produce, e.g., embryonic development during gestation, or see, with the naked eye, living images that normally need high-power magnification to be seen, e.g., cellular reproduction.[14] Because of the animation factor, audiovisual media can present sophisticated concepts such as health instruction to children in a manner they can relate to and understand (Fig. 11-8).

The dental health educator should always preview a film or tape before showing it to a group to (1) ensure its pertinence to the topic being addressed, (2) be able to prepare the group for what they are about to see and what important points should be looked for, (3) confirm its technical quality and time length, and (4) be able to field questions intelligently.[14]

Closed-circuit television enhances team teaching and laboratory instruction. A dental health educator in a television studio could present a demonstration or lecture to any number of schools in any geographic area. Prior to the lesson the dental health educator should communicate with classroom teachers so that teachers viewing the program with their students can explain things the students don't understand or take questions. Monitors in a laboratory enable students to see detailed procedures that would normally be difficult to see from a distance.

Computer Graphics

Computers are now being used to produce media such as camera-ready charts, graphs, illustrations, slides, transparencies, video graphics, and animation. The advantages of computer graphics include[18] speed of production, ease of revision, ability to explore alternate design layouts quickly, and reduced storage space.

Computer graphic systems have taken the advertising field by storm and are having a similar effect on instructional media development. In the time it would require a graphic designer to typeset and paste-up a word slide, for example, two slides could be generated using a computer.

Mass Media

The use of mass media to produce changes in behavior and to promote programs that will result in changes in health-related behaviors is gaining in importance. The mass media (newspapers, radio, and television) are effective in raising people's consciousness and interest levels in a program. Press releases, public service an-

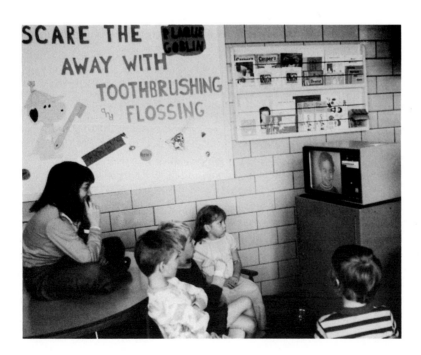

Figure 11-8. Videotape—an audiovisual instructional medium for augmenting the teaching of preventive dental health skills to children.

nouncements, and talk show appearances are effective promotional strategies for health education. Large numbers of people can be reached economically by media exposure. When used properly, the mass media can obtain spectacular results; when used improperly the outcome can be devastating.[11] It might be advisable for a dental health educator to prepare an approved statement for the press and do several rehearsed or simulated radio and television spots before actual taping occurs. Unfortunately, most dental health educators do not have any journalistic expertise and would benefit from the assistance of a qualified professional.

METHODS OF TEACHING

In the fifth century B.C., Lao Tzu counseled that "there can be teaching without words" which "few indeed can understand." Little has changed over the years, as the lecture method of teaching remains the most popular form of instruction among educators. Unfortunately, it appears to have minimal impact on the modification of behaviors.[24]

Method is defined by Webster as an orderly arrangement or an orderly procedure or process. Some view teaching as merely the dissemination of information using some type of method. This description lacks warmth and neglects to focus on the teacher-pupil (educator-patient) relationship that can be created when a mutual approach to a topic exists. Too often, says Paul Tillich, "we throw answers like stones to the heads of those who have not yet asked questions." The element of humanism is absent. Humanistic education helps individuals become more effective instruments in their community by encouraging introspection and interaction with others. A humanistic approach to education is an integral part of all methodologies that contribute to the health education effort.[24]

If the humanistic dimension is coupled with the cognitive elements of methodol-

ogy, health knowledge can flourish in a manner that enhances self-esteem, achievement, motivation, values, and human relations. Therefore, most dental health instruction objectives should be constructed to focus not only on knowledge acquisition and skill development, but on concept development, opinion expression and development, and values awareness.[10] Characteristics of humanistic instruction include:[24] (1) educator as facilitator, (2) consideration of the dignity and worth of students (patient), (3) respect for individuals with different lifestyles, (4) problem-solving and decision-making skills, (5) active learning through experiences, (6) intrapersonal skills for knowing oneself and handling inner feelings, and (7) interpersonal skills for relating effectively to others and being sensitive to their needs.

Criteria applied to teaching methodologies consist of a number of questions the educator should ask himself to discern if the particular method he has chosen will be effective:[14] (1) Will the method proposed promote the desired objectives? (2) Is the method adaptable to the various activities planned? (3) Does the method seem feasible when related to the instructional environment, equipment available, or time for presentation? (4) Will the method hold the interest of those being taught? (5) Do learners have enough background information to profit by the method chosen? (6) Are new ideas tried periodically to determine the ideal way to organize the learning experience so that good dental habits will result? and (7) Does the method used provide an opportunity for individual learning experiences to occur?

Lecture Method

The lecture as a method of teaching is a formal presentation of facts by a teacher. Its main function is to provide a foundation for initial learning and understanding about a particular topic. As the individual's knowledge base grows, new facets of the topic can be built on this foundation and other types of instruction should be used to assess the individual's transfer of learning. Unfortunately, most educators do not assess this integration process until test or demonstration time, when it might be too late. Likewise, participants in a dental health education program will be unable to perform proper oral hygiene procedures if, prior to that point, they have only been told how they are accomplished. Discussion, models, and guided demonstrations are needed to enhance the learning experience.

Lecturing is essentially an active process for the educator and a passive one for the learner. The absence of feedback makes this method an unidirectional one. With recitation in the form of discussion and questions rather than the simple reciting of information as traditional recitation usually implies, this method increases its effectiveness.

Guided Discovery Method

Whereas lecture-recitation is normally a direct way to "quiz" individuals about what they know, guided discovery employs a less direct questioning format to prod the learner into using logic or common sense to "discover" ideas and concepts rather than being told about them.

Guided discovery is an appropriate method for introducing new concepts once an initial foundation has been built. Discovery ultimately focuses on motivating students to reach the "correct" answer, but it is equally concerned with the manner in which the learner acquires the response. With lecture-recitation, the teacher accepts one set of responses; with guided discovery, several answers might be plausible and serve as the impetus for discussion. The same approach should be utilized when a dental health educator is attempting to stop a group of adolescents from using smokeless tobacco, for example. Rather than lecture to the group, the dental health educator should allow them to come up with the answers related to the dangers of its use; benefits, if they perceive the tobacco in that way, should also be addressed and disproven by logical thought.

Guided discovery is not merely a guessing game. Some degree of forethought must go into the guided discovery process. The educator must develop a list of facts, ideas, and concepts that he considers acceptable responses to the questions he uses to focus the lesson. Questions asked by the educator stimulate responses related to the content.[25]

Inquiry

True inquiry is a difficult method to execute. Experiencing the process of hypothesizing solutions to problems, testing the hypotheses, developing conclusions, and applying the conclusions to new problems is the goal of inquiry. Although guided discovery promotes the transfer of learning from one situation to another, responses must be acceptable. Inquiry, on the other hand, accepts all responses; there are no wrong answers. The major emphasis of inquiry entails the skillful use of process.

Simulations or role-play techniques can be designed to foster the inquiry process. Laboratories or field trips inadvertently involve inquiry, even if the educator has not planned it that way. When skillfully employed, the results of inquiry can be highly rewarding.

COMMUNITY SETTINGS FOR DENTAL HEALTH EDUCATION

Settings are locations where services are rendered or sought. Health services are provided in a large variety of settings. The settings where consumers receive care are primarily related to the type of service needed. Dental care has typically been provided in the private office setting, but the scope of dental service has broadened to include virtually all facets of life (Table 11-3).[7] These setting classifications serve as a guide for identifying career opportunities where community based dental health education programs can be established. The primary goal of alternative settings such as these is outreach; being able to provide dental services

Table 11-3. Classification of Settings for Provision of Dental Care

Health care settings	Education settings
"Solo" practice	Public and private primary and secondary
Group practice	schools
Independent contracting	Dental schools
Settings involving special populations	Dental hygiene programs
Day care centers	Schools of public health
Homebound programs	Other health programs
Nursing homes	Pharmacy
Long-term-care facilities	Nursing
General hospitals	Health education
Specialty hospitals for women or children	Government-funded settings
Rehabilitative centers	State health departments
Institutions for physically and mentally disabled	Local health departments
Institutions for the vision- and hearing-impaired	Federal level
	United States Public Health Service
	National Health Service Corps
Outreach centers and adaptive living facilities	Indian Health Service
Cancer centers	Head Start
Hospices	Neighborhood health centers
Business-oriented settings	Health systems agencies
Dental product companies	Professional standards review organizations
Industrial dental clinics	Health maintenance organizations
Dental instrument companies	Veterans hospitals
Computer companies	Armed forces
Book companies	Correctional facilities
Union dental clinics	
Department store dental clinics	
Corporation dental health promotion programs	

Adapted from Kostiw, U., Stephenson, M. M., and Zarkowski, P.: The Dental Health Consultant in Community Based Programs. Chicago, American Dental Hygienists' Association, 1982.

to a high percentage of the population. Those underserved population groups where need exceeds demand must be sought and treated. The options for dental professionals with strong health education skills in assessment, patient motivational techniques, and program development are limitless.

COMMENTS

Dental professionals involved in designing and implementing health education programs will experience challenging horizons ahead. To the dental health educator falls the task of health education and health promotion. Although these roles seem overwhelming, the needs and opportunities for dental care that exist in society make up the difference, balancing the scales, so to speak. As we approach the 21st century, now is the time for dental health educators to make a lasting contribution to the health and well-being of all Americans.

Remember, there are three kinds of people: those who make things happen, those who observe things happen, and those who wonder what happened. Dental health educators must strive to make things happen!

REFERENCES

1. Jong, A. W.: Community Dental Health. 2nd Ed. St. Louis, C. V. Mosby, 1988.
2. Boyle, P. G.: Planning Better Programs. New York, McGraw-Hill, 1981.

3. Knowles, M.: Modern Practice of Adult Education. Rev. ed. New York, Cambridge Books, 1980.

4. Lazes, P. M., Kaplan, L. H., and Gordon, K. A.: Handbook of Health Education. 2nd Ed. Rockville, MD, Aspen, 1987.

5. Dignan, M. B., and Carr, P. A.: Program Planning for Health Education and Health Promotion. Rev. ed. Philadelphia, Lea & Febiger, 1987.

6. Joki, R. A.: Health Education: Program development and implementation. Health Education, Oct./Nov.:31–33, 1988.

7. Kostiw, U., Stephenson, M. M., and Zarkowski, P.: The Dental Health Consultant in Community Based Programs. Chicago, American Dental Hygienists' Association, 1982.

8. Ahmann, J. S., and Glock, M. D.: Evaluating Student Progress: Principles of Test and Measurement. 6th Ed. Boston, Allyn and Bacon, 1981.

9. Striffler, D. F.: Planning a Survey to Secure a View of a State's Oral Health Problems. *In* Proceedings of the 4th Workshop on Dental Public Health: Objectives and Evaluation of a State's Dental Program. Edited by School of Public Health. Ann Arbor, University of Michigan, 1956.

10. Fodor, J. T., and Dalis, G. T.: Health Instruction: Theory and Application. 4th Ed. Philadelphia, Lea & Febiger, 1989.

11. Breckon, D. J., Harvey, J. R., and Lancaster, R. B.: Community Health Education. Rockville, MD, Aspen, 1985.

12. Gronland, N. E.: Stating Objectives for Classroom Instruction. 2nd Ed. New York, Macmillan, 1978.

13. Combs, A. W.: Myths in Education. Boston, Allyn and Bacon, 1979.

14. Stoll, F. A.: Dental Health Education. 5th Ed. Philadelphia, Lea & Febiger, 1977.

15. Simonson, M. R., and Volker, R. P.: Media Planning and Production. Columbus, Charles E. Merrill, 1984.

16. Brown, J. W., Lewis, R. B., and Harcleroad, F. F.: AV Instruction Technology, Media, and Methods. 5th Ed. New York, McGraw-Hill, 1977.

17. American Dental Hygienists' Association: ADHA Student Table Clinics. Brochure. Chicago, American Dental Hygienists' Association, 1977.

18. American Dental Association: The Creative Clinician: A Student's Guide to the Preparation of Table Clinics. York, PA, Alumni Association of Student Clinicians, 1983.

19. Kemp, J. E., and Smellie, D. C.: Planning, Producing, and Using Instructional Media. 6th ed. New York, Harper and Row, 1989.

20. Dreyer, R.: Center of attention. RDH, 7:44–45, 1987.

21. Department of Public Information: National children's dental health month 1987. J. Am. Dent. Assoc., 115:625–629, 1987.

22. American Dental Association: NCDHM In-Office Planning Guide. Chicago, Department of Public Information and Education.

23. Bethea, S. N.: Children's attitudes resulting from a dental health fair. J. Am. Dent. Hyg. Assoc., 61:556–561, 1987.

24. Willgoose, C. E.: Health Teaching in Secondary Schools. 3rd Ed. Philadelphia, W. B. Saunders, 1982.

25. Hyman, R. T.: Ways of Teaching. 2nd Ed. Philadelphia, J. B. Lippincott, 1974.

Chapter 12

LEGAL CONSIDERATIONS FOR THE DENTAL HEALTH EDUCATOR

Without law we cannot live; only with it can we insure the future which by right is ours. The best of man's hopes are enmeshed in its success; when it fails they must fail; the measure in which it can reconcile our passions, our wills, our conflicts, is the measure of our opportunity to find ourselves.

Learned Hand
1953
The Spirit of Liberty
edited by Irving Dilliard

Salus populi suprema lex.
The people's safety is the highest law.
Legal and political maxim

OVERVIEW

The 1990s are likely to witness advances unsurpassed by any other decade with regard to the health science fields. Never to be outdone, the litigation industry will scrutinize each advance to ensure that only the most qualified, most informed, and most proven methods serve the public.

The practice of dentistry is not immune to the malpractice risks that threaten all health care deliverers; therefore the safety net must be in place during every phase of the dental health process. Although most dental malpractice lawsuits are filed against dentists, it is important to view the dental office as a team. Whenever any member of the team is at risk from malpractice, the entire team is at risk as well.[1]

Consumer/patient protection concerns have spawned the new kid on the block—the risk-management team. An entity all its own, the team is composed of medicolegal professionals whose primary objective is to train health care practitioners to implement risk-management practices protecting not only themselves but the patient as well.

Licensing Requirements

Legislatures in every state have determined that public welfare requires those practicing in the dental profession to be licensed by a national board and state and/or regional board of examiners.[2]

Legislation to regulate the practice of dentistry is intended to afford protection to the patient against incompetent dentists (and hygienists and auxiliaries) and to promote the confidence of the public in the dental profession. Legislation is intended to assure that the practitioner will exercise a high degree of care and skill in the treatment of the patient and will adhere to a high standard of personal conduct.[3] Therefore, the dental professional must be properly licensed and registered, must comply with all laws regulating the practice of dentistry, and practice in a manner consistent with the code of ethics of the profession.[1]

Unlicensed Practice

The law provides various remedies against individuals who practice dentistry without a license. State dental boards, being statutory and constitutional entities, can seek injunctive relief to prohibit nonlicensed persons from performing dental services.[4] Practicing dentistry without a license constitutes a crime for which the unlicensed practitioner can be fined or imprisoned. Many of the cases involving practice by unlicensed persons have involved delegation of duties by a dentist to a nondentist such as a dental hygienist or denturist.[2]

Dentists, particularly orthodontists, must be careful about what acts they delegate to auxiliary workers. Because state laws differ, the licensee should examine the statutes in force in the state in which he is practicing to determine what acts may be lawfully delegated and what acts or services may be lawfully performed by a dental hygienist. In some instances, legislatures have set forth the acts that may be executed lawfully by a hygienist; other legislatures have set forth acts that a hygienist may not perform.[2]

ETHICAL CONSIDERATIONS

The surge of ethical consciousness, most acutely pronounced in the decline of many

a political career, pulsates through the professions. Certain practices performed by certain practitioners send a clear message to the society that becomes their victims—patient beware!

Health education plays a pivotal role between health care deliverers and the recipients of care. Thus, society creates a system of checks and balances defining the parameters of morals and ethics applied to the general public welfare and to those that concern fairness and equality for each individual.[5] The more educated, in theory, the greater protection afforded in almost all situations.

"Conflicts of interest, whistle-blowing on corruption, obligations to clients/patients versus duties to society, and the consequences of deception versus truthtelling"[6] comprise sources precipitating ethical questions. The escalation of health care costs and general inflation put pressure on health professionals to sacrifice quality for quantity, to minimize in order to maximize, and to take advantage of the all-trusting patient.

How then does the dental health educator maintain ethical practice amid the temptations to do otherwise? Through a moral decision-making process. "While morals often direct one's decisions and determine one's actions, they risk imposing one person's beliefs on another regardless of any consideration of ethical reasoning."[7] What "ought" to be done is not necessarily what is put into practice. Many factors must be weighed—essentially adding the pluses and minuses, or what legal scholars call a balancing test. For example, should more funds be directed to research to develop new and better treatments, or should funding be applied to a more expansive present-day health care delivery system?

Legislators and boards of directors make such decisions daily, and budgetary reasoning is often the crucial factor. On a societal level, it is a must. On a personal level it is only one of the myriad of ethical concerns between the professional and patient.

Perhaps no other profession deals with such difficult decisions, on a daily basis, as health care providers. Only when the practitioner is fully aware of his alternatives, including the risks, benefits, and probable outcomes of the available options can the "best" choice be made.[8]

Diagnosis and treatment might be the root of ethical and moral dilemmas, but dental professionals also face questions and concerns regarding (1) reporting communicable diseases to the health department;[9] (2) performing illegal services; (3) making false or fraudulent insurance claims; (4) reporting substandard care rendered by other dental health providers; (5) reporting instances of gross or continual maltreatment by others to a designated authority; (6) willingness to testify against another professional in a suit for negligence; and (7) departing from an accepted standard of care to save time or expense.[8]

So where do professionals turn for answers? Advice from an attorney might be the ultimate solution, but self-help is always the place to begin. Most professionals belong to or can consult local societies or can seek the advice of respected senior practitioners in their community. Every dental health professional's office should include in its library the *Principles of Ethics and Code of Professional Conduct* of the American Dental Association. This is an up-to-date text for instant referral.

Identifying and analyzing situations with no easy answers are daily challenges faced by health care providers. These situations often cause stress from indecision on what course to follow. If the professional will take the time to apply ethical considerations prescribed by the dental profession, look for guidance by moral consciousness, and use common sense, then the decision to act will be prudent. Benefits must always be weighed against risks with the realization that no decision will be universally accepted as right or wrong. Judgment, therefore, should be fair, impartial, and based on sound principles accessible to those who stay informed. Ethics, morals, and the law are never etched in stone. Societal advances and trends demand flexibility as each interacts with the decision-making process. Duty to the patient and society is paramount, and nothing less should ever be tolerated as the consciousness of all professions continues to rise.

PROFESSIONAL-PATIENT CONTRACT

In an article dealing with legal issues in the practice of dental hygiene,[1] a list of guidelines which serve as contractual responsibilities applicable to the entire dental office is provided. These obligations are:

1. Reasonable skill, care and judgment should be exercised, and a current level of knowledge is to be maintained.
2. Only standard drugs, materials, and techniques should be used; experimental procedures should never be used.
3. Only those procedures to which the patient agrees are to be performed.
4. The patient is to receive adequate instructions and be informed of the progress of treatment.
5. The professional is to keep accurate records of the treatment provided to the patient.
6. Emergency care should be available to the patient during a temporary absence of the professional.
7. The dental professional should provide appropriate referrals to specialists and request necessary consultations. The practitioner should not attempt a procedure for which he is not qualified or one that exceeds the scope of practice authorized by the professional's license.
8. Completion of the patient's treatment should be accomplished within a reasonable time.
9. The patient is never to be abandoned.
10. The professional should charge a reasonable fee for services.[1]

Patients also have responsibilities within the contractual relationship. Patients are expected to provide accurate information concerning their health history, keep dental professionals informed about changes in their health status, cooperate in their care, follow home care instructions, keep appointments, and pay a reasonable fee in a reasonable time period.[10]

A dental malpractice lawsuit can occur if someone fails to keep his part of a contract. Breaching (or breaking) a contract is, simply, failing to keep a promise.[11]

PATIENT RECORDS

The most important factor beyond the initial exam is the taking of a complete dental and medical history of the patient by the dental health educator. Oral care should never overlook the overall physical picture. In order for the dentist to properly diagnose and prescribe a particular treatment, he must be informed.

Good history-taking requires a detailed interview with the patient and follow-up on any area of concern or confusion. Data concerning the patient's overall health status are critical, especially when surgery is being considered or pharmaceuticals are to be prescribed. Simply failing to take and document a patient's blood pressure can form the basis of a malpractice action.

The dental record provides permanent documentation of patient care and must be maintained in a clear, concise, comprehensive, and accurate manner. This record should follow the patient throughout his treatment history. Entries made should be in ink and treated as though one were writing a check. Any changes should be carefully documented, and errors should be lined out with an explanation following the correction. The record must never appear to be altered or illegible, giving rise to a presumption that one has something to hide. Tampering with the patient's chart can never be condoned, but adding to it is acceptable and advisable if the entry is consistent and informative.[10] Memories fade, but a comprehensive patient record protects the health care deliverer should a lawsuit occur years after treatment.

All contacts with the patient must be recorded.[12] The following notations should be included in a patient record:

1. Broken appointments, cancellations, late arrivals, appointment changes (with the patient's reasons), and drop-in visits
2. Warnings, advice, or instructions to the patient
3. Tests ordered, prescriptions written, and recommendations made that the patient consult with either a medical or dental specialist
4. A brief summary of any letter sent to the patient
5. Any messages received from the patient, including phone calls, with date and reason for call, and response
6 Any refusal by the patient to accept recommended treatment, obey instructions, or take medications as directed
7. Any negative or positive comments made by the patient concerning his treatment, and, if appropriate, the dental health educator's response

As a general rule, too much is always better than too little. If a question arises regarding the appropriateness of an entry, the dental health educator should seek the advice of someone who should know or who has a primary responsibility for patient care.

Record-keeping has many uses, including providing meaningful medical information to other practitioners should the patient transfer to another practitioner or should the treating professional be unavailable.[13] Right to privacy applies to dental records as well as communications between professional and patient. Information obtained must not be disclosed to anyone outside the treatment relationship unless specifically authorized by the patient or, in the event of a legal action, by court order or subpoena. Confidentiality and common sense are the best guidelines to avoid liability for negligent conduct. To voluntarily disclose confidential information without the patient's consent constitutes invasion of the patient's right to privacy, justifying the bringing of a civil suit for damages. Failure to keep complete and adequate records amounts to unprofessional conduct on the part of the practitioner and justifies disciplinary action.[13]

PATIENTS' RIGHT OF PRIVACY

"Another person's secret is like another person's money: You are not as careful with it as you are with your own" (E. W. Howe).[14]

Public policy favors and protects the confidential and fiduciary (position of high trust) relationship existing between the professional and the patient. The patient's right of confidentiality and patient consent are inextricably tied together. This relationship is present so long as the patient can rest assured that he must give his consent before any of the information disclosed during the practitioner-patient relationship is released to a third party.[15]

Every health care provider has a duty to his patient not to disclose (except properly in the course of testimony in court or otherwise allowed or required by law) confidential information obtained in the course of providing treatment.[16] The public policy underlying this principle is intended to encourage patients to make full disclosure to the health care provider (including, but certainly not limited to, information concerning AIDS) in order to assure proper diagnosis and treatment. A dental health professional who divulges confidential information without the patient's consent has committed an actionable wrong.[17]

Patients and health professionals who are carriers of infectious diseases contribute to the risk of infectious disease transmission. How can each minimize the risk to others? One absolute method would be avoidance. A prospective patient with an infectious disease would not seek regular professional dental care, and an infectious dental practitioner would never engage in direct patient contact or at least refrain from conducting any invasive procedures. But is this the best solution to ensure infection control? Definitely not. What then can be done to prevent or minimize infectious disease transmission and the associated liability flowing therefrom?

The real threat of contracting AIDS, hepatitis B, or some other serious communicable disease results from lack of information and complacency. Every health professional must routinely use sterilization and barrier techniques to avoid transmittal and the legal implications certain to arise.

In the dental office, if an employee is infected within the scope of his employment, the dentist employer is liable under worker's compensation laws.[18]

Practitioner liability for patients who become infected is less clear because evidence of negligence is required. Recall that malpractice actions place the burden on the patient to prove the breach of a duty owed to them by the professional that resulted in the injury.[18] Damages or money awards to a patient who contracted, or is *likely* to test HIV-positive in the future, can be astronomical—and perhaps rightfully so if the transmittal could have or should have been prevented.

A fundamental issue of conflict matches the right to privacy against the duty to disclose. For instance, a patient who has contracted and been diagnosed with an infectious disease fails to report this when the medical history is taken. Is he liable if a dental hygienist, who is not otherwise in a high-risk group for the disease, contracts it? The above scenario makes a strong argument that infection-control procedures should be followed with all patients. The routine use of gloves, mask, protective eyewear, and sterilization has been recommended for some time by the Centers for Disease Control and recommended by the American Dental Association.[19]

There is no excuse (aside from medical reasons) for not being vaccinated for hepatitis B. The AIDS crisis remains unsolved, but to date there is no proven case of occupational transmission utilizing adequate precautions. The potential for this type of infectious transmittal is unclear, and until more is known, prevention must be a part of dental protocol.

Can a patient be refused treatment because he has AIDS or has tested positive for HIV? Can a dental professional continue in practice if he tests positive for HIV or contracts AIDS? These questions must be addressed and litigated through the judicial system. If the conclusion can be drawn that a person with AIDS is qualified as handicapped (under the Rehabilitation Act of

1973),[20] then certain rights and privileges are afforded them under the Act. The equal-protection provision of our Constitution also, when applied, grants specific benefits to handicapped individuals. Thus, all persons, regardless of the label attached describing their physical condition, should be afforded access to medical and dental care. To allow otherwise would be an obvious act of discrimination.[21]

Concluding that an AIDS patient, or other infectious disease carrier, must be treated, the assessment of the risk of transmission is also necessary. Unknowns continue in the research field, but what is presently known about transmittal can direct specific plans for protection when dealing with patients.

The medical, dental, and legal communities must develop strategies to afford health care to all who need it while minimizing associated risks of injuring the patient as well as the provider.[21]

INFORMED CONSENT

The doctrine of informed consent says that "before a physician (dentist or other health professional) may administer any treatment, the patient must be adequately informed about the proposed therapy and its effects and must freely consent to being treated."[22] Health care professionals have become frustrated and confused in the application of this doctrine because it has been legally created, defined, and applied in an adversarial system with which they are not accustomed.[23]

One frequently used model was formulated by Meisel, Roth, and Lidz.[24] This model says that when information is disclosed by a physician to a competent person, that person will understand the information and voluntarily make a decision to accept or refuse the recommended procedure. Five components are included in this model:

1. Voluntariness. Patients must not be coerced into making decisions and must be free from unfair persuasions and inducements. Health care providers are obligated to make patients aware that they have the right to make their own treatment decisions.

2. Information disclosure. The patient must be informed of the nature of the procedure, its risks and hazards, anticipated benefits, and alternatives.

3. Competence. It is assumed that all patients who are of legal age and manage their own affairs have the capacity to comprehend the disclosed information.

4. Understanding. It is assumed that once a competent patient is provided with information, he will understand it and be able to make a reasoned decision concerning treatment.

5. Decision. The patient has the right to decide to accept (i.e., consent) or not to accept (i.e., refuse) treatment.

It can be seen from this model that informed consent is a way in which society has regulated, through the law, the patient–health care provider relationship.[22] The doctrine has established limitations on practitioners' freedom in the interests of patients. A consequent tension has arisen between practitioners and the legal profession.[23]

This tension has resulted from the traditional view of health professionals as the dominant authoritarian figures in these relationships. This paternalism gave the physician both the right and the responsibility of making decisions in the best interests of the patient, with the simple requirement that patients consent to a procedure before it is done.[22]

According to the judge in the landmark Bessenger v Deloach case, "The rules governing the duty and liability of a dentist/hygienist to his patient correspond to the rules applicable to physicians and surgeons generally."[25] Similarly, the judge's ruling in the later Cobbs v Grant case included the observation that "an integral part of the dentist's overall obligation to the patient . . . is a duty of reasonable disclosure of the available choices with respect to proposed therapy and the dangers/risks inherently and potentially involved in each."[26] This comment indicates that the scope of the dental health educator's communications to the patient must be measured by the patient's "need to know" such information relevant to the decision-making process.

It is generally recognized that a patient's need to know defines the scope of the duty to reveal information regarding proposed treatment, alternative treatments, no treatment, and the associated risks of each. Only when the patient is fully informed can he exercise a reasonable choice.[27]

The concept of understanding goes hand-in-hand with informed consent. It is not enough for the professional to provide a laundry list of procedures and risks that the patient scans and signs routinely. Explanation, tailored to the level of sophistication and education of the patient, is a must. Many malpractice claims are brought alleging lack of informed consent resulting from misunderstanding.[28]

Physicians and dentists are not guarantors of the work they perform, nor are they required to advise the patient as to every conceivable possibility and eventuality that might stem from treatment. Medicine and dentistry are inexact fields of study. Consequently, following the most acceptable, proven, and appropriate methods of diagnosis and treatment is the standard to which a reasonably prudent practitioner must adhere in protecting himself and the patient.

The dental health team combines its members' areas of expertise, each assisting in total health care delivery. Thus when a patient claimed (in a malpractice action) that oral surgery was performed without informed consent because disclosure of the procedure and risks were made by the dentist's assistant rather than directly by the dentist, the court ruled that it was the totality of the information conveyed (of course determined by an objective standard) that was paramount and not who gave the information.[29]

munication among all members of the dental health team. Delegation of duties normally performed by a designated deliverer must be carefully scrutinized and supervised and must comport with the scope of the actual deliverer's authority and competence. A discussion of employee status versus independent contractor is beyond the scope of this text, but one fact is certain—if malpractice occurs, the attorney for the injured patient (plaintiff) will join everyone connected with the diagnosis and treatment in the lawsuit. This action leaves the defense attorneys the process of sorting out not only the negligent (liable) party, but who is ultimately responsible to pay damages.

CONCLUSION

In recent years the relationship between the medical and legal professions has become strained. The usual finger pointing occurs as to whose fault it might be, while the insurance industry stands on the sideline cheering for the team in the lead.

All professions, including dentistry, must practice risk management within their specialties, not only to avoid malpractice suits and other possible criminal litigation, but more important, to accomplish their ultimate goal—to safely and adequately provide a service or product to the consumer.

As technology takes mankind rocketing into the 21st century, common sense and decency need follow. For if economic, prejudicial, or mediocre standards outweigh the altruistic and safety-minded principles that guide our professions, then law will indeed have a greater and greater impact on them, and at a greater cost than society can afford.

MALPRACTICE AND LIABILITY

Liability of the dentist that is a direct result of the negligent act of a hygienist or auxiliary is a reality that requires complete com-

REFERENCES

1. Zarkowski, P.: Legal issues in the practice of dental hygiene. Semm. Dent. Hyg., 2:1–5, 1990.

2. Morris, W. O.: A decade of dental litigation—civil litigation. Part 1. J. Law Ethics Dent., *1*:65–81, 1988

3. Vining v Board of Governors of Alabama, 492 So2d 607 (Ala Civ App 1985).

4. Butler v Board of Governors of Registered Dentists of Oklahoma, 619 P2d 1262 (Okla 1980).

5. Breckon, D. J., Harney, J. R., and Lancaster, R. B.: Community Health Education. Rockville, MD, Aspen, 1985.

6. Callahan, D.: Applied ethics: A strategy for fostering professional responsibility. Carnegie Q, 28:2, 1980.

7. Lazes, P. M., Kaplan, L. H., and Gordon, K. A.: Handbook of Health Education. 2nd Ed. Rockville, MD, Aspen, 1987.

8. Pollack, B. R., and Marinelli, R. D.: Ethical, moral, and legal dilemmas in dentistry: The process of informed decision making. J. Law Ethics Dent. *1*:27–36, 1988.

9. New York State Public Health Law, § 2101, 2.12.

10. Pollack, B. R.: Risk Management Program. National Society of Dental Practitioners, 1986.

11. Black, H. C.: Black's Law Dictionary. 5th Ed. St. Paul, West Publishing, 1979.

12. Spital, S. E.: Reducing the risk of malpractice suits. Dent. Manage., *21*:50–55, 1981.

13. Schwarz v Board of Regents of the University of the State of New York, 453 NYS 2d 836 (1982).

14. Morris, W. O.: A decade of dental litigation—civil litigation. Part 2. J. Law Ethics Dent., *1*:126–142, 1988.

15. Petrillo v Syntex Laboratories, Inc., 148 Ill App 3d 581, 102 Ill Dec 172, 499 NE2d 952 (Ill App 1986).

16. Hope v Landau, 21 Mass App 248, 486 NE2d 89 (1985).

17. Tower v Hirschorn, 492 NE2d 728 (Mass 1986).

18. Sacred Heart Medical Center v Department of Labor, Etc., 92 Wash 2d 631 (1979).

19. Logan, M. K.: Legal implications of infectious disease in the dental office. J. Law Ethics Dent., *1*:92–98, 1988.

20. Rehabilitation Act of 1973, Pub L No 93-112, 87 Stat 355 (codified as amended at 29 USC § 701-796) (1985).

21. Keyes, G. G.: HIV-positive dental students and faculty: Their right to provide care in light of federal constitutional and antidiscrimination laws. J. Law Ethics Dent., *1*:199–210, 1988.

22. President's Commission for the Study of Ethical Problems in Medicine and Biomedical and Behavioral Research: Making Health Care Decisions, 1982.

23. Smith, T. J.: Informed consent doctorine in dental practice: A current case review. J. Law Ethics Dent., *1*:159–169, 1988.

24. Meisel, A., Roth, L., and Lidz, C.: Toward a model of the legal doctrine of informed consent. Am. J. Psychiatr., *134*:285–289, 1977.

25. Bessinger v Deloach, 230 S.C. 1–94 SE2d 3, 6 (1956).

26. Cobbs v Grant, 104 Cal Rptr 505, at 514, 502 P2d 1 (1972).

27. Miller v Kennedy, 11 Wash App 272, 282-286, 522 P2d 852, 860-862 (1974).

28. Willard v Hagemeister, 175 Cal Rptr 365, 121 Ca App 3d 406 (1981).

29. Bullman v Myers, 467 A2d 1353 (Pa Super 1983).

APPENDIXES

APPENDIX A   CHILD ABUSE AND NEGLECT RESOURCE LIST

American Humane Association Children's
  Division
9725 East Hampden Avenue
Denver, CO 80231

End Violence Against the Next Generation
977 Keeler Avenue
Berkeley, CA 94708-1498

Family Life Development Center
15 East 26th Street, 5th floor
Cornell University
New York, NY 10010-1565

Community School District
3961 Hillman Avenue
Bronx, NY 10466
Naomi Barber, Project Director

Institute for Family Research
  and Education
Syracuse University
Ed-U-Press
P.O. Box 583
Fayetteville, NY 13066

Minnesota Program for Victims of
  Sexual Assault
430 Metro Square Building
St. Paul, MN 55105

National Crime Prevention Council
Woodward Building
733 15th Street, NW
Washington, DC 20005

National Education Association
Professional Library
P.O. Box 509
West Haven, CT 06516

C. Henry Kempe National Center for
  Prevention and Treatment of Child
  Abuse and Neglect
1205 Oneida Street
Denver, CO 80220

Sex Information and Education Council of
  the United States
80 Fifth Avenue
New York, NY 10011

National School Board Association
1680 Duke Street
Alexandria, VA 22314

Adam Walsh Child Resource Center
1876 North University Drive
Suite 306
Fort Lauderdale, FL 33322

Child Find, Inc.
P.O. Box 277
New Paltz, NY 12561

National Center for Missing and Exploited
  Children
1835 K Street, NW
Suite 700
Washington, DC 20006

National Center on Child Abuse
and Neglect
332 South Michigan Avenue
Suite 1250
Chicago, IL 60604-4357

National Safety Council
44 North Michigan Avenue
Chicago, IL 60611

National Coalition for Children's Justice
2998 Shelburne Road
Shelburne, VT 05482

APPENDIX B   ADDITIONAL INFORMATION ON ANOREXIA NERVOSA AND BULIMIA

National Organizations

American Anorexia Nervosa Association
113 Cedar Lane
Teaneck, NJ 07666
(201) 836-1800
Publication: newsletter

National Association of Anorexia Nervosa
and Associated Disorders
Box 271
Highland Park, IL 60035
(312) 831-3438

National Anorexic Aid Society
P.O. Box 29461
Columbus, OH 43229
(614) 846-6810
Publication: newsletter

American Family Association
(Mental Health)
2250 M Street, NW
Washington, DC 20037
(202) 463-8510

BASH Treatment and Research Center for
Eating and Mood Disorders (Bulimia
Anorexia Self Help)
6150 Oakland Avenue
St. Louis, MO 63139
1-800-BASH-STL (24-hour line)
314-991-BASH (in Missouri)
1-800-762-3334 (Emergency line)

Overeaters Anonymous
World Service Office
2190 West 190th Street
Torrence, CA 90504
(213) 542-8363

Rader Institute Eating Disorder Program
Los Angeles, CA 90064
1-800-255-1818 (24-hour line)
(213) 478-8238 (in California)

Weight Watchers
Consumer Affairs Department
500 North Broadway
Jericho, NY 11753-2196

TOPS
P.O. Box 07360
4575 South Fifth Street
Milwaukee, WI 53207

American Association of Marriage and
Family Therapists
1717 K Street, NW
Washington, DC 20001

American Psychological Association
1200 17th Street, NW
Washington, DC 20001

Anorexia Nervosa and Related Eating
Disorders, Inc.
P.O. Box 5102
Eugene, OR 97405

Hopeline
K. Kim Lampson, M Ed
Providence Professional Building
550 16th Avenue, Suite 301
Seattle, WA 98122

State Contact

State Department of Health
State Mental Health Association
Private Hospital with an Eating Disorder
Unit

Other

Kruzas, A. T., Gill, K., and Backus K.
(Eds.): Medical Library, Medical and
Health Information Directory. Vols. 1, 2.

Gale Research Co., 835 Penobscott Building, Detroit, Michigan 48226-4094, 1985.
313-961-2242
1-800-347-4253
1-800-877-6253

APPENDIX C   SMOKING CESSATION RESOURCE LIST

Nonprofit Voluntary Health Agencies

American Lung Association
1740 Broadway
New York, NY 10019-4374
(212) 315-8700

American Cancer Society
1599 Clifton Road, North East
Atlanta, GA 30329

American Heart Association
7320 Greenville Avenue
Dallas, TX 75231
(214) 750-5300

Nonprofit Public Advocacy Organizations

New Jersey Group Against Smoking Pollution
105 Mountain Avenue
Summit, NJ 07901
(201) 273-9368

Americans for Nonsmokers' Rights
2054 University Avenue, Suite 500
Berkeley, CA 94704
(415) 841-3032

Action on Smoking and Health
2013 H Street, NW
Washington, DC 20006
(202) 659-4310

Environmental Improvement Associates
109 Chestnut Street
Salem, NJ 08079
(609) 935-4200

Government Agencies

Office on Smoking and Health
Park Building, Room 1-58
5600 Fishers Lane
Rockville, MD 20857
Public inquiries (301) 443-5287
Technical information (301) 443-1690

Indoor Air Office
U.S. Environmental Protection Agency
ANR 445
401 M Street, SW
Washington, DC 20460
(202) 475-7174

National Cancer Institute
Bethesda, MD 20205
Mark Manley, MD, MPH (301) 496-8520
Robert Mecklenburg, DDS, MPH (301) 330-9409
Publication: *How to Help Your Patients Stop Using Tobacco: A National Cancer Institute Manual for the Oral Health Team*

National Heart, Lung, and Blood Institute
Smoking Education Program
9000 Rockville Pike
Building 31, 4A-21
Bethesda, MD 20892
(301) 496-4236

Local Nonprofit Voluntary Health Agencies

APPENDIX D   AIDS-RELATED SERVICE ORGANIZATIONS

American Academy of Pediatrics
141 Northwest Point Boulevard
P.O. Box 927
Elk Grove Village, IL 60007

American College Health Association
15879 Crabbs Branch Way
Rockville, MD 20855
(301) 963-1100

American Foundation for AIDS Research
Executive Office
9601 Wilshire Boulevard, Mezzanine
Los Angeles, CA 90210
(213) 273-5547

American Public Health Association
1015 15th Street, NW
Washington, DC 20005
(202) 789-5600

American School Health Association
1521 South Water Street
P.O. Box 708
Kent, OH 44240-0708
(216) 678-1601

Centers for Disease Control
AIDS Headquarters
Building 16, Room G-29
Executive Park
1600 Clifton Road
Atlanta, GA 30333
(404) 639-0902
(404) 330-3020 (24-hour recorded message)

National Association of Independent
  Schools
18 Tremont Street
Boston, MA 02108
(617) 723-6900

National Education Association
1201 16th Street, NW
Washington, DC 20036
(202) 833-4000

National Gay and Lesbian Task Force
666 Broadway
Suite 410
New York, NY 10012
(212) 741-5800

National Institute of Allergy and
  Infectious Diseases
National Institutes of Health
Building 31
9000 Rockville Pike
Bethesda, MD 20892
(301) 496-2263

1-800-342-AIDS (U.S. Public Health
  Service AIDS Hotline)

United States Conference of Mayors
1620 Eye Street, NW
Washington, DC 20006
(202) 293-7330

APPENDIX E DENTAL ANXIETY CLINICS

Dental School Fear Clinic
UCLA Dental Fear and Anxiety Center
University of Southern California
Los Angeles, CA

Fear Clinic
University of Florida
Shands Teaching Hospital
Gainesville, FL

Behavioral Sciences Clinic
Dental School
Northwestern University
Chicago, IL

Dental Care Center
Our Lady of Mercy Hospital
Dyer, IN

Dental Fear Treatment Clinic
University of Kentucky
Lexington, KY

Dental Phobia Clinic
Mt. Sinai Medical Center
New York, NY

Dental Fear Clinic
Eastern Carolina Family Medicine Center
Greenville, NC

Phobia Clinic
University Hospitals of Cleveland
Cleveland, OH

Dental Fears Clinic
Evaluation and Treatment Center
University of Pittsburgh
Pittsburgh, PA

Pain Control Clinic
University of Texas
Dallas, TX

Dental Fears Research Clinic
University of Washington
Seattle, WA

APPENDIX F ALCOHOL RECOVERY RESOURCE LIST

Al-Anon Family Group Headquarters
One Park Avenue
New York, NY 10016

Alcoholics Anonymous World Services
P.O. Box 459, Grand Central Station
New York, NY 10163

National Association for Children of
Alcoholics
31706 Coast Highway (Suite 201)
South Laguna, CA 92677

National Association of Recovered
Alcoholics
P.O. Box 95
Staten Island, NY 10305

United States Department of Health and
Human Services
Public Health Service
Alcohol, Drug Abuse, and Mental Health
Administration
National Institute on Alcohol Abuse and
Alcoholism
NIAAA National Clearinghouse for
Alcohol Information
P.O. Box 2345
Rockville, MD 20852

APPENDIX G   RESOURCES FOR DEAF PERSONS

National

National Academy of Gallaudet College
National Center for Law and the Deaf
Gallaudet College
Florida Avenue at Seventh Street, NE
Washington, DC 20002

Registry of Interpreters for the Deaf
American Deafness and Rehabilitation
Association
International Association of Parents of the
Deaf
814 Thayer Avenue
Silver Spring, MD 20910

Deafness Research Foundation
55 East 34th Street
New York, NY 10016

National Black Deaf Advocates
4250 North Marine Drive, Room 832
Chicago, IL 60613

Alexander Graham Bell Association for the
Deaf
3417 Volta Place, NW
Washington, DC 20007
(202) 337-5220

Captioned Films for the Deaf
Distribution Center
5034 Wisconsin Avenue, NW
Washington, DC 20016
Information and catalog of films available
for the deaf

National Captioning Institute
5203 Leesburg Pike, Suite 1500
Falls Church, VA 22041
Information on captioned TV shows

National Theatre of the Deaf
305 Great Neck Road
Waterford, CT 06385
Touring schedule and information on a
one-person show

Local

Interpreter service
Message relay service
School/classes for deaf students
Association of/for deaf persons
Community agencies
Churches and temples

APPENDIX H   AGENCIES FOR THE BLIND

American Association of Workers for the
Blind
206 North Washington Street
Alexandria, VA 22314

American Council of the Blind
1211 Connecticut Avenue, NW
Washington, DC 20036

American Foundation for the Blind
15 West 16th Street
New York, NY 10010
Alphabet cards, films, publications and
aids

American Printing House for the Blind
1830 Frankfort Avenue
Louisville, KY 40206

Association for Education of the Visually
  Handicapped, Inc.
206 North Washington Street
Alexandria, VA 22314

Library of Congress, Division for the
  Blind
1291 Taylor Street, NW
Washington, DC 20542
(202) 882-5500

National Federation of the Blind
Suite 212, DuPont Circle Building
1346 Connecticut Avenue, NW
Washington, DC 20036
(202) 785-2974
Braille cards, literature, and information

APPENDIX I LEARNING DISABILITIES RESOURCE LIST

Books

Albert, Louise: *But I'm Ready to Go*

Barden, Annie: *What Child is He?*

Corcoran, Barbara: *Axe-time, Sword-time*

Hayes, Marvel Lo: *Tuned In—Turned On*

Pamphlets

"All About Me." Oppenheimer, J.:
  Learning Disabil. *1*:68–81, 1968

"Learning Disabilities." U.S. Department
  of Health and Human Services. U.S.
  Government Printing Office,
  Washington, DC 20402

"Special People. Basic Facts to Help
  Children Accept Their Handicapped
  Peers," New Jersey Association for
  Children with Learning Disabilities
  (1973). P.O. Box 249, Convent Station,
  NJ 07961

"What's Wrong with Joey?" Massachusetts
  Association for Children with Learning
  Disabilities. Box 908, 1296 Worchester
  Road, Framington, MA 01701

Agencies

Association of Learning Disabled Adults
P.O. Box 9722
Friendship Station
Washington, DC 20016

Council for Learning Disabilities
Council for Exceptional Children
1920 Association Drive
Reston, VA 22091
Publication: Learning Disability Quarterly

National Association for Children with
  Learning Disabilities
4156 Library Road
Pittsburgh, PA 15234
(412) 341-1515

Orton Dyslexia Society
8415 Bellona Lane
Baltimore, MD 21204
(301) 296-0232

APPENDIX J NATIONAL AGENCIES SERVING THE DISABLED

American Civil Liberties Union
132 West 43rd Street
New York, NY 10036

Coordinating Council for Handicapped
  Children
220 South Street, Room 412
Chicago, IL 60604

Council for Exceptional Children
1920 Association Drive
Reston, VA 22091

Developmental Disabilities Office
U.S. Department of Health and Human
  Services
200 Independence Avenue, SW
Room 338 E

Washington, DC 20201
Local offices: University Affiliated Centers
for Developmental Disabilities

Library of Congress
Division for the Blind and Physically
Handicapped
1291 Taylor Street, NW
Washington, DC 20542

National Easter Seal Society
2023 West Ogden Avenue
Chicago, IL 60612

National Information Center for
Handicapped Children and Youth
Box 1492
Washington, DC 20013

National Rehabilitation Association
633 South Washington Street
Alexandria, VA 22314

Office for Handicapped Individuals
U.S. Department of Health and Human
Services
200 Independence Avenue, SW
Washington, DC 20201

Office of Rehabilitation Services
U.S. Department of Education
400 Maryland Avenue, SW
Washington, DC 20202

President's Committee on Employment of
People with Disabilities
1111 20th Street, NW
Washington, DC 20005

President's Committee on Mental
Retardation
Wilber J. Cohen Federal Building, Room
4723
330 Independence Avenue, SW
Washington, DC 20201

Special Education Programs
U.S. Department of Education
400 Maryland Avenue, SW
Washington, DC 20202

Candlelighters
Childhood Cancer Foundation
2025 Eye Street, NW, Suite 1011
Washington, DC 20006

International Association of
Laryngectomees
c/o American Cancer Society
90 Park Avenue
New York, NY 10017

United Ostomy Association, Inc.
2001 West Beverly Boulevard
Los Angeles, CA 90057-2491

Make Today Count
P.O. Box 222
Osage Beach, MI 65065

Leukemia Society of America, Inc.
National Headquarters
733 Third Avenue
New York, NY 10017

Association of Brain Tumor Research
6232 North Pulaski Road, Suite 200
Chicago, IL 60646

Society for the Right to Die
250 West 57th Street
New York, NY 10107

National Hospice Organization
1901 North Fort Meyer Drive, Suite 402
Arlington, VA 22091

Cancer Care Inc. and the National Cancer
Foundation
One Park Avenue
New York, NY 10016

One/Fourth
The Alliance for Cancer Patients and
Their Families
1540 North State Parkway
Chicago, IL 60610

Office of Cancer Communications
National Cancer Institute
Building 31, Room 10A 24
Bethesda, MD 20892
1-800-4-CANCER

APPENDIX K ONCOLOGY SELF-HELP ORGANIZATIONS

American Cancer Society
Local chapters

APPENDIX L RESOURCE LIST ON AGING

American Association of Retired Persons
1909 K Street, NW

Washington, DC 20049
(202) 872-4700

American Geriatric Society
770 Lexington Avenue, Suite 400
New York, NY 10021
(212) 308-1414

National Institute on Aging
900 Rockville Pike, Building 31
Bethesda, MD 20892

National Council on Aging
600 Maryland Avenue, SW
West Wing 100
Washington, DC 20024
(202) 479-1200

American Society on Aging
833 Market Street, Suite 516
San Francisco, CA 94103
(415) 543-2617

Alzheimer's Disease and Related
  Disorders Associations, Inc., National
  Office
360 North Michigan Avenue
Chicago, IL 60606
1-800-621-0379

Arthritis Foundtaion
3400 Peachtree Road, NE
Room 1101
Atlanta, GA 30326

Self Help for Hard of Hearing People
  (Shhh)
7800 Wisconsin Avenue
Bethesda, MD 20814

National Caucus and Center for the Black
  Aged
1424 K Street, NW, Suite 500
Washington, DC 20005

National Indian Council on Aging
P.O. Box 2088
Albuquerque, NM 87103

National Pacific/Asian Resource Center on
  Aging
1341 G Street, NW, Suite 311
Washington, DC 20009

Associacion Nacional Pro Personas
  Mayores
1730 West Olympic Boulevard, Suite 401
Los Angeles, CA 90015

INDEX

Page numbers in *italics* indicate illustrations; numbers followed by "t" indicate tables.